Macrophages - Celebrating 140 Years of Discovery

Edited by Vijay Kumar

Published in London, United Kingdom

Macrophages - Celebrating 140 Years of Discovery
http://dx.doi.org/10.5772/intechopen.98074
Edited by Vijay Kumar

Contributors
Ragini Sinha, Marcelo J. Kuroda, Elizabeth S. Didier, Pijush K. Das, Arunima Biswas, Anindita Bhattacharya, Gianluca Cipriani, Suraj Pullapantula, Dženan Kovačić, Adna Softić, Jovana Jotanović, Adna Salihović, Stephan F. van Eeden, Don D. Sin, Marcela F. Lopes, Natalia S. Vellozo, Flavia L. Lima Ribeiro-Gomes, Lesley M. Forrester, Shyam Sushama Jose, Patrícia Sampaio Tavares Veras, Thiago Castro Gomes, Juliana Perrone Bezerra de Menezes, Milan Fiala, Mary Dover, Michael Kishek, Miranda Eddins, Naneeta Desar, Ranjan Bhadra, Avi Petroff, Jean-Louis Mege, Soraya Mezouar, Perla Abou Atmeh, Raghunathan Jagannathan, Balaji Thodur Madapusi, Cakku Jalliah Venkatakrishnan, Lakshmipriya Sridhar, Saranya Varadarajan, Swaminathan Rajendran, Dale Feldman, Parastoo Yousefi, Alireza Tabibzadeh, Wadih Arap, Tracey Smith, Anupama Hooda-Nehra, Pranela Rameshwar, Renata Pasqualini, Alejandra Ferrer, Fernanda Staquicini, Roland Osei Saahene, Samuel Victor Nuvor, Precious Barnes

First published in London, United Kingdom, 2022 by IntechOpen
IntechOpen is the global imprint of INTECHOPEN LIMITED, registered in England and Wales, registration number: 11086078, 5 Princes Gate Court, London, SW7 2QJ, United Kingdom

British Library Cataloguing-in-Publication Data
A catalogue record for this book is available from the British Library

Additional hard and PDF copies can be obtained from orders@intechopen.com

Macrophages - Celebrating 140 Years of Discovery
Edited by Vijay Kumar
p. cm.
Print ISBN 978-1-80355-624-6
Online ISBN 978-1-80355-625-3
eBook (PDF) ISBN 978-1-80355-626-0

For EU product safety concerns:
IN TECH d.o.o., Prolaz Marije Krucifikse Kozulić 3, 51000 Rijeka, Croatia,
info@intechopen.com or visit our website at intechopen.com.

Meet the editor

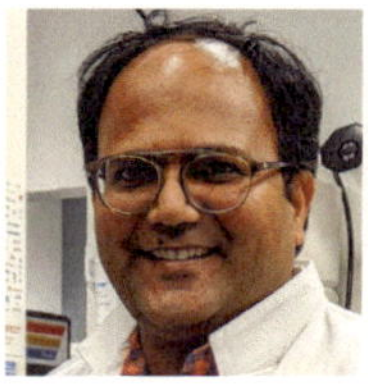

Dr. Vijay Kumar, Ph.D., has more than 17 years of research experience in bacterial infections, including sepsis and pneumonia, innate immunity, immunopharmacology, immunomodulation, and inflammation. He obtained his Ph.D. from the Department of Microbiology, Panjab University, India in 2009. Dr. Kumar is the recipient of the prestigious "Piero Periti review article award" for 2008, awarded by the *Journal of Chemotherapy* in the field of immunomodulation and antimicrobials for the article entitled "Innate immunity in sepsis pathogenesis and its modulation: new immunomodulatory targets revealed." He received junior research and senior research fellowships (2004–2009) from the Indian Council for Medical Research (ICMR), New Delhi, India. He has received seventeen international travel awards for attending various international conferences in infection and immunity. He has published seventy-five publications in peer-reviewed international journals as well as book chapters on macrophages and innate immunity. He is an associate editor for *Frontiers in Immunology* (Inflammation section), executive guest editor for the journal *Coronaviruses*, Biocell (special issue: Neuroimmune Interactions at the Crossroads of Health and Disease), and editorial board member of *Frontiers in Biosciences* and other journals. He is also an invited reviewer for several immunology journals like *Scientific Reports, British Journal of Pharmacology, Pharmacological Reports, Frontiers in Immunology, Frontiers in Medicine, Journal of Inflammation Research, Cellular and Cellular and Molecular Immunology, Immunology,* and *Innate Immunity.*

Contents

Preface **XI**

Section 1
Introduction **1**

Chapter 1 **3**
Introductory Chapter: Macrophages – More than Sentinel Innate Immune Cells
by Vijay Kumar

Section 2
Macrophages in Vertebrate Immunity **17**

Chapter 2 **19**
Macrophage: A Key Player of Teleost Immune System
by Ragini Sinha

Chapter 3 **39**
The Interactive Role of Macrophages in Innate Immunity
by Roland Osei Saahene, Precious Barnes and Samuel Victor Nuvor

Chapter 4 **55**
Lung Macrophages: Pivotal Immune Effector Cells Orchestrating Acute and Chronic Lung Diseases
by Stephan F. van Eeden and Don D. Sin

Chapter 5 **81**
Macrophages in the Smooth Muscle Layers of the Gastrointestinal Tract
by Gianluca Cipriani and Suraj Pullapantula

Chapter 6 **103**
The Tale of Mastering Macrophage Environment through the Control of Inflammasome-Mediated Macrophage Activation and cAMP Homeostasis by the Protozoan Parasite *Leishmania*
by Anindita Bhattacharjee, Arunima Biswas and Pijush K. Das

Chapter 7 123
Inflammation-Associated Wound Healing through a Monocytic Lens
by Avi Petroff

Chapter 8 135
The Role of Macrophages in Controlling the Adaptive Response to Injury: Regeneration Vs. Scarring
by Dale Feldman

Section 3
Macrophages in Parasitic Infections 155

Chapter 9 157
Elucidating the Complex Interrelationship on Early Interactions between *Leishmania* and Macrophages
by Patrícia Sampaio Tavares Veras, Thiago Castro-Gomes and Juliana Perrone Bezerra de Menezes

Chapter 10 179
Shifting Macrophage Phenotypes in Leishmaniasis
by Natália S. Vellozo, Flávia L. Ribeiro-Gomes and Marcela F. Lopes

Chapter 11 197
Macrophage as the Game Changer of the (Future) Therapeutic Paradigm
by Ranjan Bhadra

Section 4
Macrophages in Bacterial Infections 219

Chapter 12 221
The Ambiguous Role of Macrophages in Pulmonary Tuberculosis
by Dženan Kovačić, Adna Softić, Adna Salihović and Jovana Jotanović

Chapter 13 253
Role of CD14+ CD16+ Monocytes in the Pathogenesis of Periodontitis Associated Systemic Diseases
by Raghunathan Jagannathan, Balaji Thodur Madapusi, Cakku Jalliah Venkatakrishnan, Lakshmipriya Sridhar, Saranya Varadarajan and Swaminathan Rajendran

Section 5
Macrophages in Viral Infections 269

Chapter 14 271
Interaction of Ebola Virus with the Innate Immune System
by Parastoo Yousefi and Alireza Tabibzadeh

Chapter 15 **283**
Macrophage Polarization in Viral Infectious Diseases: Confrontation with the Reality
by Perla Abou Atmeh, Soraya Mezouar and Jean-Louis Mège

Chapter 16 **303**
Macrophages and HIV/AIDS Pathogenesis: Lessons from the Rhesus Macaque Model
by Elizabeth S. Didier and Marcelo J. Kuroda

Section 6
Macrophages in Neurological Diseases **319**

Chapter 17 **321**
The Role of M1- and M2-Type Macrophages in Neurological and Infectious Diseases
by Mary Dover, Michael Kishek, Miranda Eddins, Naneeta Desar and Milan Fiala

Section 7
Macrophages in Breast Cancer **333**

Chapter 18 **335**
Targeted Regulation and Cellular Imaging of Tumor-Associated Macrophages in Triple-Negative Breast Cancer: From New Mechanistic Insights to Candidate Translational Applications
by Anupama Hooda-Nehra, Tracey L. Smith, Alejandra I. Ferrer, Fernanda I. Staquicini, Wadih Arap, Renata Pasqualini and Pranela Rameshwar

Section 8
Stem Cells-Derived Macrophages **359**

Chapter 19 **361**
Pluripotent Stem Cell Derived Macrophages: Current Applications and Future Perspectives
by Shyam Sushama Jose and Lesley M. Forrester

Preface

Macrophages are potent innate immune cells. In 1882, Elia Metchnikoff first discovered them as phagocytes in starfish larvae and the water flea (*Daphnia*). This discovery revolutionized the field of immunology and gave birth to innate immunity. Before this discovery, researchers were mainly focused on adaptive immunity (B and T cells). Now, macrophages are considered the most plastic cells in the hematopoietic system. They are present in every organ and tissue, previously regarded as an immune privilege. For example, they are present in the testes, brain (microglia), and eye retina. The liver macrophages are called Kupffer cells. The advancement in the biology of macrophages has established their role in different areas of biology, including reproduction, embryonic development, regeneration, neurosciences, metabolism, immunity, infection, and inflammation.

Macrophage biology and its role in different biological processes are ever-changing due to advances in the field and new technologies. The book covers the role of macrophages in various areas of biology in health and disease.

The book opens with Section 1, "Introduction" which includes the introductory chapter describing essential aspects of macrophages in the male and female reproductive system, embryonic development, tissue or organ regeneration, neurological learning and behavioral mechanisms, and systemic metabolism. These functions of macrophages highlight their role beyond being innate immune cells.

Section 2, "Macrophages in Vertebrate Immunity", includes seven chapters. Each chapter in this section describes essential aspects of macrophages in vertebrate biology. For example, they play a crucial immune function in lower vertebrates, including teleost fish. Other chapters in the section describe the importance of macrophages (pulmonary) in acute and chronic lung inflammatory diseases, wound healing, and innate immunity, as well as their regulatory role in gastrointestinal muscle layers.

Section 3, "Macrophages in Parasitic Infections," describes the regulatory role of macrophages in parasitic infections. It focuses on macrophages and leishmaniasis (Kala-Azar), a protozoan parasitic infection most prevalent in developing countries, including India, Brazil, and South Africa.

Section 4, "Macrophages in Bacterial Infections," focuses on the role of macrophages in bacterial infections. This section includes two chapters. The first chapter describes the role of macrophages in bacterial periodontitis, and the second chapter describes their function in pulmonary tuberculosis. Both these diseases affect a large portion of the population worldwide. For example, periodontal diseases affect 20%–50% of the global population. Similarly, 1.5 million people worldwide died from tuberculosis in 2020. Tuberculosis is the 13th leading cause of death in the world.

Section 5, "Macrophages in Viral Infections," discusses the role of macrophages in viral diseases. It includes three chapters. The first chapter discusses macrophage polarization during viral diseases, and the second chapter discusses Ebola virus interaction with the innate immune system and the third chapter discusses Macrophages and HIV/AIDS Pathogenesis.

Section 6, "Macrophages in Neurological Diseases," includes one chapter that discusses the role of macrophages in different neurological disorders, including neurodegenerative diseases.

Section 7, "Macrophages in Breast Cancer," includes a chapter that discusses macrophages in triple-negative breast cancer, their imaging, and their translating applications.

Finally, Section 8, "Stem Cells-Derived Macrophages," includes one chapter that examines pluripotent stem cell-derived macrophages, their current applications, and future perspectives.

This book provides updated information for biomedical researchers working with macrophages in different conditions, including infections, regeneration, wound healing, neurosciences, cancer, and stem cell biology. It is a useful resource for researchers and scientists in the field.

Dr. Vijay Kumar, Ph.D.
Department of Interdisciplinary Oncology,
School of Medicine,
Stanley S. Scott Cancer Center,
Louisiana State University Health Science Center (LSUHSC),
New Orleans, LA, USA

Section 1

Introduction

Chapter 1

Introductory Chapter: Macrophages – More than Sentinel Innate Immune Cells

Vijay Kumar

1. Introduction

Elia or Ilya Metchnikoff first described macrophages as phagocytes (eating cells) in 1882 in starfish larvae inserted with the tangerine tree thorns and later (1883–1884) in *Daphnia magna* or common water flea infected with fungal/yeast spores due to its transparent outer carapace [1–4]. Metchnikoff considered macrophages/phagocytes as homeostatic agents of the body, which continuously vigil on foreign invaders and maintain the host's internal environment (homeostasis) and tissue/organ remodeling [5]. However, the term phagocytosis or phagocytes (Greek derivative for devouring cells) was not introduced by Elia Metchnikoff, instead given by Carl or Karl Claus (a German Zoology professor, who invited Elia Metchnikoff to publish his findings in his journal in 1883) [6, 7]. Elia Metchnikoff won the Noble prize (Physiology and Medicine) for this discovery with Paul Ehrlich in 1908. Thus, macrophages were first discovered as phagocytes or devouring cells that engulf any foreign material (size $\geq$0.5 μm) entering the host almost 140 years ago [8, 9]. These comprise first innate immune cells responding in response to the invasion of the host by foreign particles (pathogens, allergens, and xenobiotics). Hence, macrophages are considered one of the sentinel innate immune cells of the immune system. They play a crucial role in immune homeostasis maintenance, host defense, inflammation, and different inflammatory and infectious diseases through different mechanisms (phagocytosis, secretion of different inflammatory mediators, and interacting directly with different immune (innate and adaptive) and non-immune cells) [10–14]. Hence, macrophages are potent innate immune cells with diverse immunological functions. This chapter discusses emerging non-immunological functions of macrophages.

2. Macrophages in the human reproduction and reproductive cycle

Macrophages are present in the male (testes) and female reproductive organs/tract (ovaries, fallopian tubes, uterus, and vagina) and serve as crucial accessory cells for reproduction (**Figure 1**) [15–17]. In the embryonic life of a male fetus, the yolk-sac macrophages regulate testes morphogenesis and vascularization [18]. Further studies have shown that the macrophage-specific genes/transcription factors Mafb and Maf are crucial mediators of morphogenesis and vascularization of testes during the embryonic development [19, 20]. The process involves distortion of the myeloid cell

IntechOpen

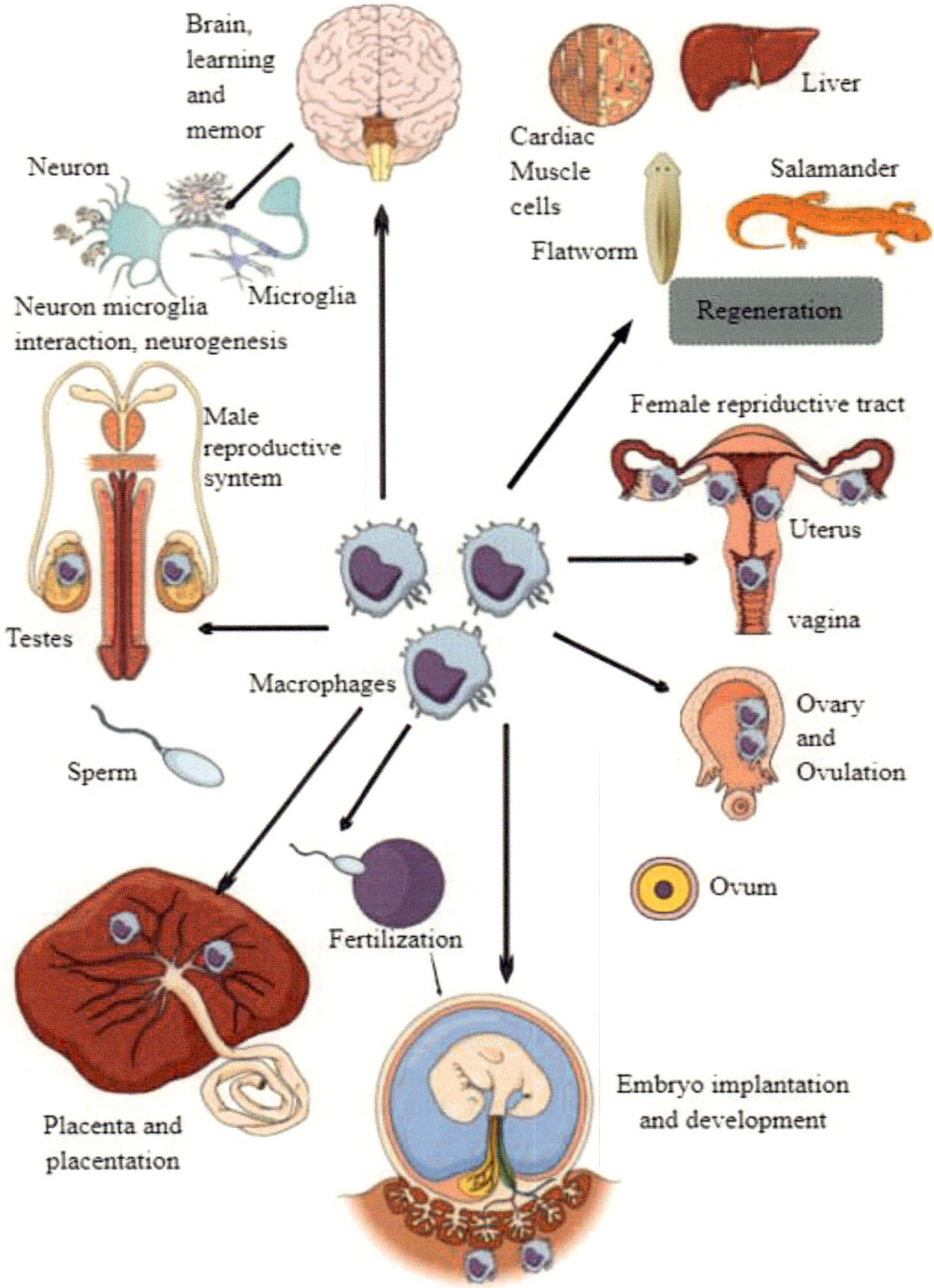

Figure 1.
Macrophages are crucial for different physiological process (sperm production, ovulation, fertilization, placentation, embryonic development, regeneration, neurogenesis, learning and memory) other than playing crucial role in immune function. Details are mentioned in the text.

ratios (profound increase in gonadal macrophages in the absence of Mafb) as Mafb regulates macrophages' differentiation. The Maf loss causes testicular hypervascularization, defective testis cord formation, deficiency of Leydig cells, and decreased germ cell number [19]. Mafb also regulates the cholesterol efflux in macrophages and can control the Leydig cell function by regulating the 2—hydroxycholesterol (25-HC) secretion [21]. However, Mafb or macrophages are not crucial for the maintenance of spermatogenesis in the adult mice [22, 23]. Notably, the resident macrophages of adult testes are the derivatives of embryonic precursors of macrophages (fetal macrophages) under normal conditions, and bone marrow-derived macrophages do not infiltrate testes [23]. On the other hand, in postnatal mice, testicular macrophages are crucial for steroidogenesis (sex hormone synthesis) by controlling Leydig cell proliferation and differentiation in the prepubertal stage [24–29]. For example, depletion of interstitial macrophages in testes inhibits Leydig cell development, and pro-inflammatory activation of macrophages also inhibits steroidogenesis by Leydig cells by producing a lipophilic factor that controls steroidogenesis or testosterone production.

The testicular macrophages secrete 25-HC, converted to testosterone by the neighboring Leydig cells [30]. However, the overproduction of 25-HC by testicular macrophages during infection or other inflammatory conditions impacting the testes inhibits the steroidogenic function of Leydig cells. The macrophage and Leydig cell interaction details are mentioned elsewhere [31]. The macrophage ubiquitin-specific protease 2 (USP2) contributes to the sperm motility, hyperactivation, capacitation, and fertilization capacity of the murine sperm, and myeloid-selective USP2 knockout (msUSP2KO) mice sperm has a decreased mitochondrial membrane potential for ovum fertilization [32]. The treatment of sperms derived from msUSP2KO mice with granulocyte macrophage-colony stimulating factor (GM-CSF) rescued their potential for fertilizing the ovum. Thus, testicular macrophages regulate steroidogenesis, spermatogenesis (maintenance of spermatogonial niche in adult testes), sperm motility, capacitation, and *in vitro* fertilization of mouse sperm that are crucial for sexual reproduction in mammals, including humans (**Figure 1**) [33–35]. Hence, testicular macrophages (peritubular macrophages) are close to peritubular myoid cells in seminiferous tubules where spermatogenesis takes place, and interstitial macrophages are located within the testicular interstitium in close contact with Leydig cells crucial for male reproductive function.

Macrophages are abundant in the mesenchymal and connective tissue stroma of the gravid and non-gravid uterus, comprising the necessary amount of villous or labyrinthine mesenchymal cells of human and mouse placenta (**Figure 1**) [36, 37]. The large (10–30 μm) human placental macrophages present in the fetal villi of the placenta (from the first trimester until birth) are called Hofbauer cells and maintain placental and fetal development and homeostasis (**Figure 1**) [38]. Thus, placental macrophages are composed of two different populations: (1) decidual macrophages and (2) Hofbauer cells [39]. Detailed ontogeny and function of placental macrophages have been discussed elsewhere [40, 41]. Recently identified, three different subsets of macrophages ($CCR2^{-}CD11c^{low}$, $CCR2^{-}CD11c^{hi}$, and $CCR2^{+}CD11c^{hi}$) express CD45 and CD14 differently in the human uterus during early pregnancy maintain maternal-fetal homeostasis [42, 43]. In the absence of pregnancy, these uterine or endometrial macrophages play a crucial role in menstruation and the maintenance of tissue integrity to prepare the uterus for reproductive events, including fertilization and implantation (**Figure 1**) [44]. However, the macrophage number varies (1–15%) in the endometrium depending on the stage of the menstrual cycle [45]. The number of macrophages also increases in the uterus and cervix preceding the parturition, indicating their involvement in childbirth through releasing several biological mediators [46]. A recent human study has indicated that women with recurrent pregnancy loss have alternatively activated $CD45^{+}CD14^{+}ICAM3^{-}$ macrophages expressing low levels of CD209 and CD206 expression and have high expression of TNF-α in their proinflammatory $CD45^{+}CD14^{+}CD80^{+}HLA\text{-}DR^{+}$ macrophages in their uterus at the maternal-fetal interface [47]. Hence, any imbalance in the uterine/decidual macrophages in human females and in experimental mammals prevents pregnancy/blastocyst implantation and induces recurrent pregnancy loss [48, 49].

In addition to the uterus and placenta, macrophages are also present in the ovary and regulate the ovarian cycle (ovulation, corpus luteum formation, and luteolysis) through different processes, including the phagocytosis of the apoptotic cells and the release of different mediators (**Figure 1**) [50, 51]. The details are beyond the scope of this introductory chapter and have been discussed elsewhere [50, 51]. The macrophage-derived multinucleated giant cells increase in the ovaries of aged mice indicating ovarian aging and a decline in its reproductive potential or ovum production and release [52]. Of note, in aged male mice, the testicular macrophages show lipofuscin granule accumulation and altered morphology that are absent in testicular macrophages of young adult mice [53]. The lipofuscin granule accumulation in the testicular macrophages of aged mice occurs due to altered metabolism but not due to its phagocytosis.

Further studies are required to indicate the role of testicular macrophages in the event of andropause. However, the expression of transient receptor potential vanilloid 2 (TRPV2, a cation channel) increased in CD206+MHC II+ testicular macrophages of aged mice due to inflammaging in the testes microenvironment may play a crucial role in andropause [54]. The TRPV2 expression affects the phagocytic potential of macrophages by controlling cytosolic Ca2+ levels and their motility [55–57]. In addition, aging impacts Leydig cell functions, including steroidogenesis (testosterone synthesis), and testicular interstitial macrophages are crucial in affecting these cells [58]. Hence, macrophages are crucial for sexual reproduction and developmental process.

3. Macrophages in organ and tissue regeneration

Abraham Trembley, a naturalist in the eighteen century, gave the idea of regeneration and wanted to know about the process responsible for regressing the heads of hydra and earthworms [59]. Hence, the regeneration process involves regressing the lost tissue or organ in animals when they lose it. However, some animals (planarians (a class of flatworms considered masters of regeneration and can rebuild any body part once it is lost or cut) and cnidarians) are considered immortal under the edge of a knife [60–62]. Amphibians, including salamanders and axolotls, also regenerate their body parts [63]. In reptiles, regeneration is proper for lizards, geckos, and iguanas as they regenerate their lost tails, but it is not valid for snakes and crocodiles [64]. Birds can regenerate their lost mechanoreceptive sensory (auditory) hair cells in the inner ear responsible for hearing that is absent in mammals [65, 66]. Hence, the loss of auditory hair cells in humans leads to permanent deafness. In humans, liver and cardiac muscle cells have the power of regeneration only. Hence, the loss of auditory hair cells in humans leads to permanent deafness. In humans, liver and cardiac muscle cells only have the power of regeneration. The biology of regeneration is beyond the scope of this chapter.

Macrophages also play a crucial role in the process of tissue or organ regeneration (**Figure 1**). For example, macrophages have been shown to play a crucial role in the regeneration process in Salamanders (**Figure 1**) [67]. In these organisms, their recruitment at the site of limb amputation peaks around 6 days after the amputation in response to the profound release of macrophage chemoattractants [68]. Even heart regeneration in salamanders requires macrophage infiltration, which is essential for fibroblast activation and the extracellular landscape without affecting cardiomyocyte proliferation [69]. Macrophage depletion prevents heart regeneration and induces fibroblast activation, and alters collagenase deposition and arrangement process that may lead to fibrosis, a condition that may lead to organ malfunction and mortality [69, 70]. The details of macrophage function in tissue and organ (skin, heart, and liver) regeneration in mammals, including humans, have been described elsewhere [71–75].

4. Microglia or brain macrophages in neurogenesis, learning, and memory

Microglia are resident brain macrophages of the central nervous system (CNS), which solely originate from the embryonic yolk sac erythromyeloid precursors under normal conditions, which also give rise to macrophages in other tissues and organs [76, 77]. Of note, adult hematopoietic progenitors do not significantly contribute to the maintenance of microglia in the adult brain. In addition to their primary function as local innate immune cells of the brain and the maintenance of brain homeostasis, microglia also play a crucial role in neurogenesis, learning, and memory [78–80]. Recent studies have suggested the role of microglia in brain development or neurogenesis (**Figure 1**), and their dysregulation induces different neurodevelopmental diseases and other neurological diseases later in life [81–83]. The activation of the phosphatidylinositol 3-kinase (PI3K)/protein kinase B or AKT (PI3K-AKT) signaling pathway in microglia is crucial for inducing neurogenic protein expression in primary cortical cells [84]. For example, microglia in the CNS control synaptic pruning, which is crucial to promote synapse formation and the regulation of neuronal and synaptic plasticity *via* different signals involving complement proteins and CX3CR1 signaling [85, 86]. The microglia-based regulation of synaptic pruning, plasticity, and neuronal activity is beyond the current chapter's scope and has been discussed in detail elsewhere [87].

Deleting the circadian clock gene Bmal1, specifically in mice's microglia (the circadian clock regulates their function), increases their learning potential and memory in mice fed a high-fat diet [88]. On the other hand, the microglia-specific brain-derived neurotrophic factor (BDNF) depletion promotes working memory and stimulates neural precursor proliferation following traumatic brain injury (TBI) [89]. However, under normal conditions, BDNF depletion, specifically from microglia, impairs memory and reduces motor-learning-dependent synapse formation [90]. Thus, microglia's memory and synaptic plasticity function vary with the brain's homeostatic alteration. Further studies have shown that the repopulation of microglia in the rat brain after their depletion significantly improves their learning and memory performance [91]. Of note, microglia depletion does not impact short-term memory in rats acutely.

The microglia also regulate learning and memory through IL-33 (expressed in adult hippocampal neurons and also secreted by astrocytes) as they express IL-33 receptor (IL-33R) along with controlling spine plasticity, synapse homeostasis during CNS development, newborn neuron integration, and remote fear memories [92, 93]. The IL-33 binding to the microglial IL-33R induces uptake of extracellular matrix (ECM), and its loss causes over-accumulation of ECM in contact with synapses that affect synaptic plasticity and memory. Microglia inhibition in rodents with neurodegenerative diseases, including Alzheimer's disease (AD) and other neuroinflammatory conditions with minocycline (a centrally penetrant tetracycline antibiotic), affects long-term potentiation (LTP), synaptic plasticity, neurogenesis, and hippocampal-dependent spatial memory [94–97]. However, the treatment with minocycline impairs human spatial and temporal memory by disrupting striatal processing [98]. Hence, modulating the microglial function in humans is not a straightforward approach and is a two-edge sword to restoring memory and learning associated with different neurodegenerative diseases. The details of microglia in neurogenesis, learning, and memory are mentioned elsewhere [87, 99–101].

5. Macrophages regulating systemic metabolism

Metabolism plays a crucial role in the organism's well-being and homeostasis. The disruption in the metabolic pathways through different factors (including intake of high-calorie or high-fat diet, lack of exercise, insulin tolerance, and different genetic factors) in individuals predispose them to type 1 or type 2 diabetes mellitus (T1DM or T2DM), obesity, hypertension, and atherosclerosis. However, the potential pro-inflammatory action of macrophages in the pathogenesis of metabolic syndrome (obesity, insulin resistance, T2DM, atherosclerosis) has been well studied and established due to their direct involvement in the pathogenesis of inflammation and inflammatory diseases [102–105]. This section is not intended to describe the immunological function of macrophages in metabolism but to discuss their non-immune role in regulating systemic metabolism.

The anti-inflammatory drugs show a modest effect on metabolism, as shown by many clinical trials that indicate the limited impact of inflammation on the metabolism [106, 107]. However, the depletion of liver macrophages (LMs) or Kupffer cells in obese mice affects their metabolism and improves fatty liver, indicating their role in insulin sensitivity [108–110]. Notably, the pro-inflammatory phenotype of LMs does not play a significant role in obesity and insulin resistance in flies, mice, and humans [111]. Instead, LMs produce non-inflammatory insulin-like growth factor-binding protein 7 (IGFBP7) that directly controls liver metabolism. The IGFBP7 released from LMs binds to the insulin receptor, which induces lipogenesis and gluconeogenesis by activating extracellular-signal-related kinase (ERK) signaling [111]. Hence, LMs contribute to systemic metabolism and associated diseases independent of their immune functions. Thus, the discovery of other non-immune factors in other macrophages, including adipose-tissue macrophages (ATMs) in obese people controlling systemic metabolism, may serve as a better therapeutic approach where their inflammatory role is secondary in the pathogenesis. Further studies are required in this direction.

6. Conclusion

Macrophages are first discovered as phagocytic innate immune cells. After 140 years of their discovery, they are ruling the world of immunology as a potent innate immune cell in almost every organ. They are present in even organs considered previously devoid of immune cells (brain, testes, and retina). Along with potent innate immune cells, which protect the host from foreign invasion, they also control the adaptive immune response by serving as potent antigen-presenting cells (APC). In addition, they also serve as potent immune cells, which control different non-immune functions (reproduction and embryonic development, regeneration, neurogenesis, and neurological functions, including learning and memory and systemic metabolism) that I have described in this chapter. Thus, macrophages are not only the body's guards against pathogens but also maintain homeostasis through different mechanisms *via* controlling different biological functions varying from reproduction to regeneration and from metabolism to learning and memory. Thus, after 140 years of their discovery, macrophages sit over the top in immunology and biology.

Author details

Vijay Kumar[1,2]

1 Department of Pharmaceutical Sciences, College of Pharmacy, University of Tennessee Health Science Center (UTHSC), Memphis, TN, USA

2 Department of Interdisciplinary Oncology, Stanley S. Scott Cancer Center, School of Medicine, Louisiana State University Health Science Center (LSUHSC), New Orleans, LA, USA

*Address all correspondence to: vkuma2@lsuhsc.edu; vij_tox@yahoo.com

References

[1] Hirsch JG. Phagocytosis. Annual Review of Microbiology. 1965;**19**:339-350

[2] Gordon S. Elie Metchnikoff: Father of natural immunity. European Journal of Immunology. 2008;**38**:3257-3264

[3] Metchnikoff E. The Overtime of Life: Optimistic Studies. London, United Kingdom: Edition William Heinemann; 1907

[4] Brown GD. How fungi have shaped our understanding of mammalian immunology. Cell Host & Microbe. 2010;**7**:9-11

[5] Teti G, Biondo C, Beninati C. The phagocyte, Metchnikoff, and the foundation of immunology. Microbiology Spectrum. 2016;**4**

[6] Cavaillon JM. The historical milestones in the understanding of leukocyte biology initiated by Elie Metchnikoff. Journal of Leukocyte Biology. 2011;**90**:413-424

[7] Tauber AI. Metchnikoff and the phagocytosis theory. Nature Reviews Molecular Cell Biology. 2003;**4**:897-901

[8] Flannagan RS, Jaumouille V, Grinstein S. The cell biology of phagocytosis. Annual Review of Pathology. 2012;**7**:61-98

[9] Kumar V. Phagocytosis: Phenotypically simple yet a mechanistically complex process. International Reviews of Immunology. 2020;**39**:118-150

[10] Bhat A, Wooten RM, Jayasuriya AC. Secretion of growth factors from macrophages when cultured with microparticles. Journal of Biomedical Materials Research. Part A. 2013;**101**: 3170-3180

[11] Shimokado K, Raines EW, Madtes DK, Barrett TB, Benditt EP, Ross R. A significant part of macrophage-derived growth factor consists of at least two forms of PDGF. Cell. 1985;**43**:277-286

[12] Nathan CF. Secretory products of macrophages. The Journal of Clinical Investigation. 1987;**79**:319-326

[13] Franken L, Schiwon M, Kurts C. Macrophages: Sentinels and regulators of the immune system. Cellular Microbiology. 2016;**18**:475-487

[14] Kumar V. Chapter 1: Macrophages: The potent immunoregulatory innate immune cells. In: Khalid Hussain B, editor. Macrophage Activation. London, UK, Rijeka: IntechOpen; 2019

[15] Cohen PE, Nishimura K, Zhu L, Pollard JW. Macrophages: Important accessory cells for reproductive function. Journal of Leukocyte Biology. 1999;**66**:765-772

[16] Nguyen PV, Kafka JK, Ferreira VH, Roth K, Kaushic C. Innate and adaptive immune responses in male and female reproductive tracts in homeostasis and following HIV infection. Cellular & Molecular Immunology. 2014;**11**:410-427

[17] Monin L, Whettlock EM, Male V. Immune responses in the human female reproductive tract. Immunology. 2020;**160**:106-115

[18] DeFalco T, Bhattacharya I, Williams AV, Sams DM, Capel B. Yolk-sac-derived macrophages regulate fetal testis vascularization

and morphogenesis. Proceedings of the National Academy of Sciences of the United States of America. 2014;**111**:E2384-E2393

[19] Li SY, Gu X, Heinrich A, Hurley EG, Capel B, DeFalco T. Loss of Mafb and Maf distorts myeloid cell ratios and disrupts fetal mouse testis vascularization and organogenesis. Biology of Reproduction. 2021;**105**:958-975

[20] Hamada M, Tsunakawa Y, Jeon H, Yadav MK, Takahashi S. Role of MafB in macrophages. Experimental Animals. 2020;**69**:1-10

[21] Kim H. The transcription factor MafB promotes anti-inflammatory M2 polarization and cholesterol efflux in macrophages. Scientific Reports. 2017;7:7591

[22] Shawki HH, Oishi H, Usui T, Kitadate Y, Basha WA, Abdellatif AM, et al. MAFB is dispensable for the fetal testis morphogenesis and the maintenance of spermatogenesis in adult mice. PLoS One. 2018;**13**:e0190800

[23] Lokka E, Lintukorpi L, Cisneros-Montalvo S, Mäkelä J-A, Tyystjärvi S, Ojasalo V, et al. Generation, localization and functions of macrophages during the development of testis. Nature Communications. 2020;**11**:4375

[24] Bhushan S, Meinhardt A. The macrophages in testis function. Journal of Reproductive Immunology. 2017;**119**:107-112

[25] Hales DB. Testicular macrophage modulation of Leydig cell steroidogenesis. Journal of Reproductive Immunology. 2002;**57**:3-18

[26] Mossadegh-Keller N, Sieweke MH. Testicular macrophages: Guardians of fertility. Cellular Immunology. 2018;**330**:120-125

[27] Gaytan F, Bellido C, Aguilar E, van Rooijen N. Requirement for testicular macrophages in Leydig cell proliferation and differentiation during prepubertal development in rats. Journal of Reproduction and Fertility. 1994;**102**:393-399

[28] Nes WD, Lukyanenko YO, Jia ZH, Quideau S, Howald WN, Pratum TK, et al. Identification of the lipophilic factor produced by macrophages that stimulates steroidogenesis. Endocrinology. 2000;**141**:953-958

[29] Hutson JC, Garner CW, Doris PA. Purification and characterization of a lipophilic factor from testicular macrophages that stimulates testosterone production by Leydig cells. Journal of Andrology. 1996;**17**:502-508

[30] Lukyanenko YO, Chen JJ, Hutson JC. Production of 25-hydroxycholesterol by testicular macrophages and its effects on Leydig cells. Biology of Reproduction. 2001;**64**:790-796

[31] Hutson JC. Physiologic interactions between macrophages and Leydig cells. Experimental Biology and Medicine. 2006;**231**:1-7

[32] Hashimoto M, Kimura S, Kanno C, Yanagawa Y, Watanabe T, Okabe J, et al. Macrophage ubiquitin-specific protease 2 contributes to motility, hyperactivation, capacitation, and in vitro fertilization activity of mouse sperm. Cellular and Molecular Life Sciences: CMLS. 2021;**78**:2929-2948

[33] DeFalco T, Potter SJ, Williams AV, Waller B, Kan MJ, Capel B. Macrophages contribute to the spermatogonial niche in the adult testis. Cell Reports. 2015;**12**:1107-1119

[34] Meistrich ML, Shetty G. The new director of "the spermatogonial niche": Introducing the peritubular macrophage. Cell Reports. 2015;**12**:1069-1070

[35] de Oliveira SA, Cerri PS, Sasso-Cerri E. Impaired macrophages and failure of steroidogenesis and spermatogenesis in rat testes with cytokines deficiency induced by diacerein. Histochemistry and Cell Biology. 2021;**156**:561-581

[36] Hunt JS, Pollard JW. Macrophages in the uterus and placenta. In: Russell SW, Gordon S, editors. Macrophage Biology and Activation. Berlin, Heidelberg: Springer Berlin Heidelberg; 1992. pp. 39-63

[37] Chambers M, Rees A, Cronin JG, Nair M, Jones N, Thornton CA. Macrophage plasticity in reproduction and environmental influences on their function. Frontiers in Immunology. 2021;**11**

[38] Zulu MZ, Martinez FO, Gordon S, Gray CM. The elusive role of placental macrophages: The Hofbauer cell. Journal of Innate Immunity. 2019;**11**:447-456

[39] Mezouar S, Katsogiannou M, Ben Amara A, Bretelle F, Mege J-L. Placental macrophages: Origin, heterogeneity, function and role in pregnancy-associated infections. Placenta. 2021;**103**:94-103

[40] Thomas JR, Naidu P, Appios A, McGovern N. The ontogeny and function of placental macrophages. Frontiers in Immunology. 2021;**12**:771054

[41] Reyes L, Golos TG. Hofbauer cells: Their role in healthy and complicated pregnancy. Frontiers in Immunology. 2018;**9**

[42] Jiang X, Du M-R, Li M, Wang H. Three macrophage subsets are identified in the uterus during early human pregnancy. Cellular & Molecular Immunology. 2018;**15**:1027-1037

[43] Jiang X, Wang H. Macrophage subsets at the maternal-fetal interface. Cellular & Molecular Immunology. 2020;**17**:889-891

[44] Thiruchelvam U, Dransfield I, Saunders PTK, Critchley HOD. The importance of the macrophage within the human endometrium. Journal of Leukocyte Biology. 2013;**93**:217-225

[45] Salamonsen LA, Zhang J, Brasted M. Leukocyte networks and human endometrial remodelling. Journal of Reproductive Immunology. 2002;**57**:95-108

[46] Mackler AM, Iezza G, Akin MR, McMillan P, Yellon SM. Macrophage trafficking in the uterus and cervix precedes parturition in the mouse. Biology of Reproduction. 1999;**61**:879-883

[47] Gomez-Lopez N, Garcia-Flores V, Chin PY, Groome HM, Bijland MT, Diener KR, et al. Macrophages exert homeostatic actions in pregnancy to protect against preterm birth and fetal inflammatory injury. JCI Insight. 2021;**6**:e146089

[48] Robertson SA, Jasper MJ, Bromfield JJ, Care AS, Nakamura H, Ingman WV. The role of macrophages in implantation and early pregnancy success. Biology of Reproduction. 2008;**78**:274-275

[49] Sun F, Wang S, Du M. Functional regulation of decidual macrophages during pregnancy. Journal of Reproductive Immunology. 2021;**143**:103264

[50] Wu R, Van der Hoek KH, Ryan NK, Norman RJ, Robker RL. Macrophage

contributions to ovarian function. Human Reproduction Update. 2004;**10**:119-133

[51] Pepe G, Locati M, Della Torre S, Mornata F, Cignarella A, Maggi A, et al. The estrogen–macrophage interplay in the homeostasis of the female reproductive tract. Human Reproduction Update. 2018;**24**:652-672

[52] Foley KG, Pritchard MT, Duncan FE. Macrophage-derived multinucleated giant cells: Hallmarks of the aging ovary. Reproduction. 2021;**161**:V5-V9

[53] Giannessi F, Giambelluca MA, Scavuzzo MC, Ruffoli R. Ultrastructure of testicular macrophages in aging mice. Journal of Morphology. 2005;**263**:39-46

[54] Eubler K, Rantakari P, Gerke H, Herrmann C, Missel A, Schmid N, et al. Exploring the ion channel TRPV2 and testicular macrophages in mouse testis. International Journal of Molecular Sciences. 2021;**22**

[55] Link TM, Park U, Vonakis BM, Raben DM, Soloski MJ, Caterina MJ. TRPV2 has a pivotal role in macrophage particle binding and phagocytosis. Nature Immunology. 2010;**11**:232-239

[56] Koyasu S. Vanilloid flavor for a good appetite? Nature Immunology. 2010;**11**:187-189

[57] Lévêque M, Penna A, Le Trionnaire S, Belleguic C, Desrues B, Brinchault G, et al. Phagocytosis depends on TRPV2-mediated calcium influx and requires TRPV2 in lipids rafts: Alteration in macrophages from patients with cystic fibrosis. Scientific Reports. 2018;**8**:4310

[58] Wang Y, Chen F, Ye L, Zirkin B, Chen H. Steroidogenesis in Leydig cells: Effects of aging and environmental factors. Reproduction. 2017;**154**:R111-R122

[59] MacCord K, Maienschein J. Understanding regeneration at different scales. eLife. 2019;**8**:e46569

[60] Dalyell JG. Observations on some Interesting Phenomena in Animal Physiology, Exhibited by Several Species of Planariae. Edinburgh: Dyer Press; 2007

[61] Holstein TW, Hobmayer E, Technau U. Cnidarians: An evolutionarily conserved model system for regeneration? Developmental Dynamics. 2003;**226**:257-267

[62] Reddien PW. The cellular and molecular basis for planarian regeneration. Cell. 2018;**175**: 327-345

[63] Joven A, Elewa A, Simon A. Model systems for regeneration: Salamanders. Development (Cambridge, England). 2019;**146**:dev167700

[64] Alibardi L. Regeneration in reptiles and its position among vertebrates. In: Alibardi L, editor. Morphological and Cellular Aspects of Tail and Limb Regeneration in Lizards: A Model System with Implications for Tissue Regeneration in Mammals. Berlin, Heidelberg: Springer Berlin Heidelberg; 2010. pp. 1-49

[65] Stone JS, Rubel EW. Cellular studies of auditory hair cell regeneration in birds. Proceedings of the National Academy of Sciences. 2000;**97**:11714-11721

[66] Menendez L, Trecek T, Gopalakrishnan S, Tao L, Markowitz AL, Yu HV, et al. Generation of inner ear hair cells by direct lineage conversion of primary somatic cells. eLife. 2020;**9**:e55249

[67] Bolaños-Castro LA, Walters HE, García Vázquez RO, Yun MH. Immunity in salamander regeneration: Where are we standing and where are we headed? Developmental Dynamics. 2021;**250**:753-767

[68] Godwin JW, Pinto AR, Rosenthal NA. Macrophages are required for adult salamander limb regeneration. Proceedings of the National Academy of Sciences. 2013;**110**:9415-9420

[69] Godwin JW, Debuque R, Salimova E, Rosenthal NA. Heart regeneration in the salamander relies on macrophage-mediated control of fibroblast activation and the extracellular landscape. npj Regenerative Medicine. 2017;**2**:22

[70] Distler JHW, Györfi A-H, Ramanujam M, Whitfield ML, Königshoff M, Lafyatis R. Shared and distinct mechanisms of fibrosis. Nature Reviews Rheumatology. 2019;**15**:705-730

[71] Kumar V. Macrophages: The potent immunoregulatory innate immune cells. In: Macrophage Activation - Biology and Disease. 2019

[72] Wynn TA, Vannella KM. Macrophages in tissue repair, regeneration, and fibrosis. Immunity. 2016;**44**:450-462

[73] Leor J, Palevski D, Amit U, Konfino T. Macrophages and regeneration: Lessons from the heart. Seminars in Cell & Developmental Biology. 2016;**58**:26-33

[74] Ding J, Lei L, Liu S, Zhang Y, Yu Z, Su Y, et al. Macrophages are necessary for skin regeneration during tissue expansion. Journal of Translational Medicine. 2019;**17**:36

[75] Gao Y, Qian N, Xu J, Wang Y. The roles of macrophages in heart regeneration and repair after injury. Frontiers in Cardiovascular Medicine. 2021;**8**

[76] Ginhoux F, Guilliams M. Tissue-resident macrophage ontogeny and homeostasis. Immunity. 2016;**44**:439-449

[77] Ginhoux F, Greter M, Leboeuf M, Nandi S, See P, Gokhan S, et al. Fate mapping analysis reveals that adult microglia derive from primitive macrophages. Science. 2010;**330**:841-845

[78] Li Q, Barres BA. Microglia and macrophages in brain homeostasis and disease. Nature Reviews Immunology. 2018;**18**:225-242

[79] Prinz M, Priller J. Microglia and brain macrophages in the molecular age: From origin to neuropsychiatric disease. Nature Reviews Neuroscience. 2014;**15**:300-312

[80] Salter MW, Stevens B. Microglia emerge as central players in brain disease. Nature Medicine. 2017;**23**:1018-1027

[81] Reemst K, Noctor SC, Lucassen PJ, Hol EM. The indispensable roles of microglia and astrocytes during brain development. Frontiers in Human Neuroscience. 2016;**10**:566

[82] Derecki NC, Katzmarski N, Kipnis J, Meyer-Luehmann M. Microglia as a critical player in both developmental and late-life CNS pathologies. Acta Neuropathologica. 2014;**128**:333-345

[83] Sato K. Effects of microglia on neurogenesis. Glia. 2015;**63**:1394-1405

[84] Lorenzen K, Mathy NW, Whiteford ER, Eischeid A, Chen J, Behrens M, et al. Microglia induce neurogenic protein expression in primary cortical cells by stimulating PI3K/AKT intracellular signaling in vitro. Molecular Biology Reports. 2021;**48**:563-584

[85] Miyamoto A, Wake H, Ishikawa AW, Eto K, Shibata K, Murakoshi H, et al. Microglia contact induces synapse formation in developing somatosensory cortex. Nature Communications. 2016;**7**:12540

[86] Lehrman EK, Wilton DK, Litvina EY, Welsh CA, Chang ST, Frouin A, et al. CD47 protects synapses from excess microglia-mediated pruning during development. Neuron. 2018;**100**: 120-134.e6

[87] Cornell J, Salinas S, Huang HY, Zhou M. Microglia regulation of synaptic plasticity and learning and memory. Neural Regeneration Research. 2022;**17**:705-716

[88] Wang XL, Kooijman S, Gao Y, Tzeplaeff L, Cosquer B, Milanova I, et al. Microglia-specific knock-down of Bmal1 improves memory and protects mice from high fat diet-induced obesity. Molecular Psychiatry. 2021;**26**:6336-6349

[89] Harley SBR, Willis EF, Shaikh SN, Blackmore DG, Sah P, Ruitenberg MJ, et al. Selective ablation of BDNF from microglia reveals novel roles in self-renewal and hippocampal neurogenesis. The Journal of Neuroscience: The Official Journal of the Society for Neuroscience. 2021;**41**:4172-4186

[90] Parkhurst CN, Yang G, Ninan I, Savas JN, Yates JR, Lafaille JJ, et al. Microglia promote learning-dependent synapse formation through brain-derived neurotrophic factor. Cell. 2013;**155**:1596-1609

[91] De Luca SN, Soch A, Sominsky L, Nguyen T-X, Bosakhar A, Spencer SJ. Glial remodeling enhances short-term memory performance in Wistar rats. Journal of Neuroinflammation. 2020;**17**:52

[92] Nguyen PT, Dorman LC, Pan S, Vainchtein ID, Han RT, Nakao-Inoue H, et al. Microglial remodeling of the extracellular matrix promotes synapse plasticity. Cell. 2020;**182**:388-403.e15

[93] Vainchtein ID, Chin G, Cho FS, Kelley KW, Miller JG, Chien EC, et al. Astrocyte-derived interleukin-33 promotes microglial synapse engulfment and neural circuit development. Science. 2018;**359**:1269-1273

[94] Kohman RA, Bhattacharya TK, Kilby C, Bucko P, Rhodes JS. Effects of minocycline on spatial learning, hippocampal neurogenesis and microglia in aged and adult mice. Behavioural Brain Research. 2013;**242**:17-24

[95] Jiang Y, Liu Y, Zhu C, Ma X, Ma L, Zhou L, et al. Minocycline enhances hippocampal memory, neuroplasticity and synapse-associated proteins in aged C57 BL/6 mice. Neurobiology of Learning and Memory. 2015;**121**:20-29

[96] Hou Y, Xie G, Liu X, Li G, Jia C, Xu J, et al. Minocycline protects against lipopolysaccharide-induced cognitive impairment in mice. Psychopharmacology. 2016;**233**:905-916

[97] Lu Y, Giri PK, Lei S, Zheng J, Li W, Wang N, et al. Pretreatment with minocycline restores neurogenesis in the subventricular zone and subgranular zone of the hippocampus after ketamine exposure in neonatal rats. Neuroscience. 2017;**352**:144-154

[98] Berens SC, Bird CM, Harrison NA. Minocycline differentially modulates human spatial memory systems. Neuropsychopharmacology. 2020;**45**:2162-2169

[99] Rodríguez-Iglesias N, Sierra A, Valero J. Rewiring of memory circuits: Connecting adult newborn neurons with

the help of microglia. Frontiers in Cell and Developmental Biology. 2019;7

[100] Gupta N, Dheen S. A paradigm shift: Emerging roles of microglia, a non-neuronal cell, in learning and memory. Neural Regeneration Research. 2021;**16**:1992-1993

[101] Morris GP, Clark IA, Zinn R, Vissel B. Microglia: A new frontier for synaptic plasticity, learning and memory, and neurodegenerative disease research. Neurobiology of Learning and Memory. 2013;**105**:40-53

[102] Chawla A, Nguyen KD, Goh YPS. Macrophage-mediated inflammation in metabolic disease. Nature Reviews. Immunology. 2011;**11**:738-749

[103] McNelis JC, Olefsky JM. Macrophages, immunity, and metabolic disease. Immunity. 2014;**41**:36-48

[104] Bhargava P, Lee CH. Role and function of macrophages in the metabolic syndrome. Biochemical Journal. 2012;**442**:253-262

[105] Qin Y, Jia L, Liu H, Ma W, Ren X, Li H, et al. Macrophage deletion of Noc4l triggers endosomal TLR4/TRIF signal and leads to insulin resistance. Nature Communications. 2021;**12**:6121

[106] Everett BM, Donath MY, Pradhan AD, Thuren T, Pais P, Nicolau JC, et al. Anti-inflammatory therapy with Canakinumab for the prevention and management of diabetes. Journal of the American College of Cardiology. 2018;**71**:2392-2401

[107] Esser N, Paquot N, Scheen AJ. Anti-inflammatory agents to treat or prevent type 2 diabetes, metabolic syndrome and cardiovascular disease. Expert Opinion on Investigational Drugs. 2015;**24**:283-307

[108] Chen L, Ye H, Zhao X, Miao Q, Li Y, Hu R. Selective depletion of hepatic Kupffer cells significantly alleviated hepatosteatosis and intrahepatic inflammation induced by high fat diet. Hepato-Gastroenterology. 2012;**59**:1208-1212

[109] Papackova Z, Palenickova E, Dankova H, Zdychova J, Skop V, Kazdova L, et al. Kupffer cells ameliorate hepatic insulin resistance induced by high-fat diet rich in monounsaturated fatty acids: The evidence for the involvement of alternatively activated macrophages. Nutrition & Metabolism. 2012;**9**:22

[110] Zeng TS, Liu FM, Zhou J, Pan SX, Xia WF, Chen LL. Depletion of Kupffer cells attenuates systemic insulin resistance, inflammation and improves liver autophagy in high-fat diet fed mice. Endocrine Journal. 2015;**62**:615-626

[111] Morgantini C, Jager J, Li X, Levi L, Azzimato V, Sulen A, et al. Liver macrophages regulate systemic metabolism through non-inflammatory factors. Nature Metabolism. 2019;**1**: 445-459

Section 2

Macrophages in Vertebrate Immunity

Chapter 2

Macrophage: A Key Player of Teleost Immune System

Ragini Sinha

Abstract

Fish, the free-living organisms, residing in aquatic environment, are earliest vertebrates with fully developed innate and adaptive immunity. Immune organs homologous to those of mammalian immune system are found in fish. Macrophages are best known for their role in immunity, basic function of which being cytokine production and phagocytosis. Due to environmental adaptation and whole genome duplication, macrophages in teleost are differently modulated (pro-inflammatory, M1-type, and anti-inflammatory/regulatory, M2-type) and perform a variety of different functions as compared with those of mammals. Phagocytosis is a major mechanism for removing pathogens and/or foreign particles in immune system and therefore is a critical component of the innate and adaptive immune system. One of the most competent phagocytes in teleost is found to be macrophages/monocytes. Increasing experimental evidence demonstrates that teleost phagocytic cells can recognize and destroy antigens to elicit adaptive immune responses that involve multiple cytokines. A detail understanding of teleost macrophages and phagocytosis would not only help in understanding the immune mechanism but will also help in disease prevention in teleost.

Keywords: inflammatory response, cytokine production, macrophages, phagocytosis, teleost

1. Introduction

Fish, the first vertebrate group, appeared in evolution after adaptive radiation during the Devonian period, presenting the most successful and diverse group of vertebrates. Importantly, immune organs homologous to those of the mammalian system are found in fish. This population possesses complicated innate immune networks and are the earliest vertebrates that have fully developed both arms of the immune system, i.e., innate and adaptive immunity [1]. Macrophage lineage cells are integral to fish immune responses like any other vertebrate, and hence, recent fish immunology research focuses on fish macrophage biology. Macrophages are one of the most important immune cells that bridge the innate and adaptive immunity. It plays a crucial role in tight regulation of immune response by secreting different immune mediators [2, 3]. Macrophages are present in most animal tissues and play crucial roles in host protection and homeostasis. They are known by different names such as amebocytes, hemocytes, coelomocytes, granulocytes, monocytes, and macrophages, but have similar morphology and comparable functions [4–6]. Due to whole genome duplication and environmental adaptation, teleost monocyte/macrophages possess a variety of different functions and modulation compared with those of mammals. The basic functions of macrophages are production of cytokines and phagocytosis in vertebrates. Monocytes give rise to macrophages during inflammatory conditions in both mammals and fish [7]. Macrophages play multiple roles in immune system. Macrophages are potent innate immune cells, which exert a crucial antimicrobial defense through phagocytosis and release of different antimicrobial mediators, including reactive oxygen and nitrogen species (ROS and RNS). Additionally, they also serve as professional antigen presenting cells (APCs) to activate the adaptive immune system (T and B cells) [8]. Macrophages pose the phagocytic activity, which is the initial step in the immune response in fish and is the major line of defense for all foreign material, including pathogenic agents [9]. Measurement of macrophage activation serves as a bio-indicator and reveals the impact of environmental stress as well as chemical contamination of the aquatic bodies.

2. Development of macrophages

Teleost blood cell development occurs within primitive waves of hematopoiesis [7]. In mammals, macrophages are predominantly derived from the hematopoietic precursors born in the yolk sac (YS) and the aorta-gonad-mesonephros (AGM) where embryonic and adult hematopoiesis occurs [10–14]. Likewise, macrophages originate from the rostral blood island (RBI) and ventral wall of dorsal aorta (VDA), the fish hematopoietic tissue equivalent to the mammalian YS and AGM for myelopoiesis, respectively [15–19]. During primitive hematopoiesis, embryonic mesoderm becomes committed to produce monopotent hematopoietic precursors in the rostral blood island that give rise to macrophages [20–22]. Following monopoiesis, first multilineage progenitor cells arise, known as erythromyloid progenitors (EMPs), which can develop into both erythroid and myeloid cells. Later, a population of hematopoietic stem cells (HSCs) arises in the AGM. The existence of renal marrow-derived HSCs has been documented in both zebrafish and ginbuna carp [23, 24]. The progenitor cells that are found in the kidney have been shown to be able to differentiate into erythrocytes, lymphocytes, thrombocytes, granulocytes, and monocytes. Monocytes mainly exist in the bone marrow, blood, and spleen. They can differentiate into inflammatory macrophages and dendritic cells during inflammation [25, 26]. Macrophages reside in a variety of tissues including lymphoid and non-lymphoid ones. Until recently, tissue macrophages were believed to arise from circulation monocyte precursors in response to different stimuli [27]. Recent evidence by fate-mapping blood cell lineages suggests that contribution of monocytes is limited in maintaining the population of tissue macrophages. Instead, tissue macrophages are "seeded" during primary haematopoiesis and self-maintain the resident population like that of the mammals [28–30]. There is a specific group of cytokines that act as hematopoietic group of cytokine, which can regulate the development of multiple cell lineages and can act individually or concurrently to stimulate a specific response. Hematopoietic cytokines are produced by a variety of cell types, which can act in paracrine, endocrine, juxtracrine, or autocrine manner on the target cells for their renewal and development [31, 32]. Cytokine sensitivity is determined by a complex regulatory network, a hematopoietic cytokine may induce different developmental changes in different circumstances. Specific cell lineage can be responsive to certain cytokines.

3. Role of transcription factor in macrophage development

The regulation of hematopoiesis is carried out in and orchestrated manner involving cell-cell and cell-extracellular matrix. Transcription factors play a critical role in determining the fate of development of macrophages. Transcription factors are DNA-binding proteins that recognize specific domains. Improper expression of transcription factors and activity results in serious consequences within the hematopoietic system including inhibition of proliferation [33, 34]. Synergistic interactions between transcription factors are generally required for the activation of specific genes. Apart from that, negative interaction between transcription factors is also necessary for the control of hematopoiesis [31].

3.1 Role of colony-stimulating factor-1

Macrophage colony-stimulating factor-1 (CSF-1) is an important growth and differentiation factor of both fish and mammalian macrophages [35]. The survival, proliferation, differentiation, and functionality of most of the macrophage lineage cells are governed by CSF-1 through binding to its cognate receptor (CSF-1R). CSF-1R is expressed exclusively on committed myeloid precursors and derivative macrophage populations [36–42]. CSF-1 has recently been identified in several fish species including trout [43], zebrafish [43], and goldfish [43, 44]. Recombinant trout CSF-1 was found to promote the proliferation of trout head kidney leucocytes [43]. Reports suggest that the recombinant goldfish CSF-1 (rg-CSF-1) induced chemotactic response and enhanced antimicrobial functions of macrophages. It plays a central role in regulation of goldfish pro-inflammatory macrophage responses [35]. Many teleost fish species have two distinct CSF-1 genes (CSF-1.1 and CSF-1.2) [43], which happen to work by upregulating pro-inflammatory components [45, 46]. A variety of cytokines can induce the production of CSF-1 by monocytes and macrophages, such as GM-CSF [47], TNF-α [48], IL-1 [49, 50], and INF-γ [51, 52]. The capacity of monocyte/macrophages to produce CSF-1 suggests that these cells can auto-regulate their own proliferation and functions [31]. CSF-1 also stimulates the production of several cytokines including G-CSF, GM-CSF, IL-1, IL-6, IL-8, and TNF-α and interferons [38, 53]. Cyprinid fish produce a soluble CSF-1 receptor (sCSF-1R) that downregulates their pro-inflammatory responses by reducing available soluble CSF-1. The sCSF-1R is produced by mature macrophages and not by monocytes and efficiently removes a variety of inflammatory events including macrophage chemotaxis, phagocytosis, and production of ROS intermediates and recruitment of leukocytes [54]. Circulating CSF-1 can effectively be cleared by the process of CSF-1 receptor-mediated internalization followed by intracellular destruction of the growth factor. Liver and splenic macrophages have been demonstrated to be capable of absorbing approximately 94% of the circulating CSF-1 [55, 56]. Adding CSF-1 to primary cultures has proven to increase the longevity of the cultures and can drive the culture from a heterogeneous population of progenitor monocyte and macrophage cells, toward a homogeneous population of macrophages [57].

4. Activation of macrophages

Macrophage activation occurs under various intracellular as well as environmental influences. Based on the activation cue and the following effector functions, macrophages have been broadly classified in two types: classically activated macrophages (M1) induced in a T helper 1 (T_H1) cytokine environment and alternatively activated macrophages (M2) induced in a T helper 2 (T_H2) cytokine environments [58]. In a different terminology, M1 macrophages have been termed to be "inflammatory," whereas M2 macrophages have been termed to be "healing" in nature. There have been studies indicating four different phenotypes of macrophages, which are innate activated, classically activated, and alternatively activated and regulatory macrophages. Classically activated macrophages present higher respiratory burst activity and iNOS expression as compared with innate activated macrophages [59]. Macrophages that are activated by microbial stimulus and innate danger signals without any influence of adaptive immune cells lead to the formation of the M1 population [5, 59]. M2 macrophages that form in the presence of T_H2 cytokines can again be classified into three groups: activated by IL-4/IL-13 or M2a macrophages [60], stimulated by Toll-like receptor (TLR) ligands in combination with second signal or M2b, developed in response to IL-10 or M2c [60].

4.1 M1 macrophage activation

Innate activation of M1 macrophages is induced by microbial stimulus, which can be detected by various receptors on the macrophage surface [61]. These microbial stimuli can activate macrophages through a large array of pattern recognition receptors (PRRs) [62]. Fish species poses a wide variety of PRRs both putative mammalian orthologues and fish-specific family members [63] and can be activated in the absence of exogenous cytokines. M1 macrophages are induced by pathogen associated molecular patterns (PAMPs) such as lipopolysaccharides (LPSs), a major component of outer membrane of Gram-negative bacteria [5, 6]. A number of publications show that in vitro stimulation of fish macrophages with LPS leads to increased respiratory burst activity and increased secretion of pro-inflammatory cytokines [64]. Classically activated macrophages require a microbial stimulus plus the presence of the cytokine INFγ (**Figure 1**) [65]. INFγ has been sequenced in fugu [66], rainbow trout [67], zebrafish [68], Atlantic salmon [69], catfish [70], common carp [71], goldfish [72], Atlantic cod [73], and flounder [74]. Certain fish species possess two distinct types of INFs. Both the isoforms, initially named INFγ1 and INFγ2, contain typical INFγ motifs and are now referred to as INFγ- related (INFγrel) and INFγ, respectively [75]. In carp and in grass carp, both isoforms are regulated by different stimuli [71, 76], *in vivo* bacterial infection in zebrafish embryo indicated that INFγ and INFγrel act partly redundantly, they have largely overlapping functions [77]. Goldfish INFγrel induced significantly higher phagocytosis and nitrite production in monocytes and macrophages, respectively, when compared with INFγ [72]. Research studies suggest that most probably INFγrel proteins are antiviral proteins without direct effects on M1/M2 polarization in fish [78]. It is particularly notable that certain teleosts possess two INFγ-receptor-binding chains (IFNGR1-1 and IFNGR1-2) in comparison to other vertebrates that have a single INFγ receptor 1 (INFGR1) [72, 79, 80]. These suggest that fish have adopted very unique strategies surrounding their M1 activation cytokine system. INFγ as a combination stimulus with LPS induces inflammatory M1 population. These macrophages show higher respiratory burst activity and nitric oxide synthase expression [62].

Classically activated macrophages are induced by a combination of INFγ and TNFα [81, 82]. Like its mammalian counterpart, teleost TNFα is one of the markers of M1 macrophages [83, 84]. Multiple isoforms of TNFα have been found in a

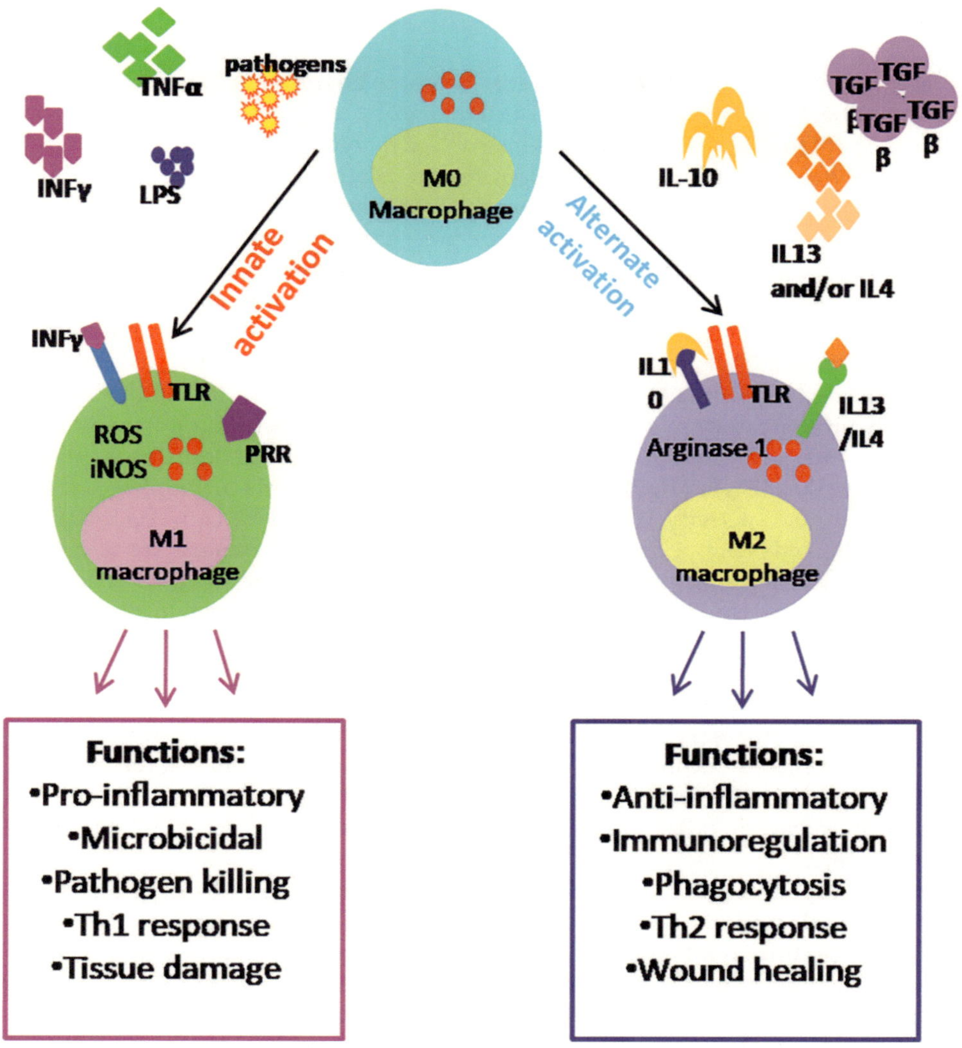

Figure 1.
M1 and M2 macrophage activation.

variety of fishes. These isoforms have been shown to enhance inflammatory gene expressions, macrophage chemotaxis, and phagocytosis [85–96]. Functional evaluation of fish TNFα has discovered some contradictory results. In some fish species, recombinant TNFα (rTNFα) was found to hardly activate macrophages [97–99], whereas the trout and goldfish TNFα1 and 2 are shown to be active in macrophages [87, 100]. Two different TNF receptors have been found in goldfish, namely TNF-R1 and TNF-R2, which bind the goldfish TNFα1 and TNFα2 in a homodimeric conformation unlike the trimeric conformations of mammalian TNF ligands and receptors [101]. The bacterial LPS readily induces the TNFα gene expression, which in turn plays a major role in polarizing the macrophages [99, 102]. From different studies it is clearly understood that fish possess a well-defined M1 polarization upon microbial stimuli.

4.2 M2 macrophage activation

M2 macrophages also known as alternatively activated macrophages can be generally characterized as having "anti-inflammatory" or "pro-healing" phenotypes (**Figure 1**) when developed in the presence of T_H2 cytokines IL-4 and/or IL-13 [103]. To date, at least two genes have been identified in fish that share homology with both the mammalian IL-4 and IL-13 cytokines (IL-4/13A and IL-4/13B) [104] even though variable number of copies of these genes are present in different fish due to genome duplication events [105]. Of the two may be IL-4/13A shows complete synteny with other genes in T_H2 cytokine complex [106]. There is a common homodimeric receptor subunit called IL-4Rα for both cytokines (IL-4 and IL-13) found in mammalian vertebrates [107], paralogues of which, IL-13Rα1 and IL-13Rα2, have also been identified in teleosts [108, 109]. Teleost recombinant IL-4/13A and IL-4/13B have anti-inflammatory roles including upregulation of immunosuppressive genes (TGF-β, IL-10, SAP1, and SOC3) and downregulation of pro-inflammatory cytokine gene expressions (TNFα, IL-1β, and INFγ) [110–112]. These M2 macrophages show increased arginase activity. In M1 macrophage, the iNOS enzyme converts L-arginine to L-cutrulin and NO. By contrast, in M2 macrophages, the enzyme arginase, a manganese metallo-enzyme, converts L-arginine to L-ornithine and urea [113, 114]. Mammals possess two arginase isoforms including arginase-1 located in cytosol and arginase-2 located in mitochondria [115]. Teleosts possess both the forms arginase-1 and arginase-2, which are found to be mitochondrial forms unlike that of their vertebrate counterparts. In carp, arginase-1 gene expression was found mainly in the mid kidney, whereas arginase-2 expression was found in all organs with the liver having the maximum expression [116]. Under stimulation of exogenous cAMP, carp head kidney-derived macrophages show upregulation of arginase-2 but not arginase-1 expression, suggesting that arginase-2 might be an excellent marker of M2 macrophages in fish.

M2 macrophages that are deactivated by glucocorticoids or by cytokines such as TGF-β or IL-10 are also referred to as regulatory macrophages. Glucocorticoids diffuse across plasma membrane and alter the expression of immune-related genes [60]. It has been shown to be a strong inhibitor of NO production in goldfish macrophages [117] and increases fish susceptibility to diseases due to its immunosuppressive nature [118–120]. Grass carp recombinant IL-10 and recombinant TGF-β1 have found to attenuate LPS-stimulated inflammatory gene expressions in monocyte/macrophages [121]. The goldfish TGFβ downregulates the nitric oxide response of TNFα-activated macrophages [122]. Mammalian IL-10 functions through IL-10R1 and IL-10R2 leading to activation of STAT3 [123]. Similar to mammalian IL-10, carp IL-10 acts through a signaling pathway involving phosphorylation of STAT3 and leading to upregulation of SOCS-3 expression [124]. An IL-10R1 has been found in zebrafish, goldfish, and grass carp [125, 126], whereas IL-10R2 has been found in rainbow trout [127]. These cytokines demonstrate an evolutionary conserved role in fish immunology.

5. Function of macrophages

Macrophages and monocytes serve as professional phagocytes in fish [128]. Phagocytosis is a specific type of endocytic process by which cell engulfs solid particulate targets. These solid particles (including microbial pathogens) are internalized to form phagolysosome followed by antigen degradation [129–132]. Phagocytosis plays an essential role of linking the innate and adaptive immune response in vertebrates. It is well established that fish have both the innate and adaptive immune system in which macrophages happen to play a crucial role. The phagocytic mechanism depends on recognition of the foreign particle by cell surface receptors and killing by oxygen radicals [133, 134]. Phagocytosis plays a crucial role in the macrophage inflammatory immune response through hydrophobic interaction between the phagocytic membrane and the target particles. The multiple receptors present on the phagocyte can recognize their targets coated with opsonin molecules and form the phagosome by engulfing them [135]. Lysosome then fuses with the phagosome to form the phagolysosome, the vesicles in which the internalized microbes would be killed and degraded. Potent antimicrobial compounds including degradative enzymes (proteases, nucleases, phosphatases, lipases) and antimicrobial peptides (basic proteins and neutrophilic peptides) are generated by active phagocytes, which help in destruction of the phagocytosed pathogens [136–141]. Both M1 and M2-type macrophages form phagolysosomes. Reports suggest that M1 macrophages form a phagosome with relatively neutral pH as compared with M2 macrophages that form phagosomes with acidic pH [142]. Macrophages are known to be "professional" phagocytes along with polymorphonuclear cells (PMNs), monocytes, and dendritic cells in vertebrates. Apart from this, some "amateur" phagocytic cells (epithelial cells, fibroblasts, and B lymphocytes) show a lower degree phagocytic activity [129, 143]. Research suggests that succinate is critical in controlling phagocytosis in macrophages. Exogenous methyl-succinate was found to enhance phagocytosis, pro-inflammatory cytokine production, and expression of phagocytic genes [46].

The destruction of the internalized microorganism occurs by robust production of ROS (reactive oxygen species) by active macrophages. The multi-component enzyme NADPH assembles on the phagosome membrane during macrophage respiratory burst, which transfers electrons from NADPH to molecular oxygen-producing superoxide anion [144]. The functional sites of fish and mammalian NADPH oxidase are highly conserved. All of the components of NADPH oxidase have been found in teleosts, and fish ROS generation has been well documented following PAMP stimulation [145–148] and antimicrobial responses [149, 150].

Classically activated M1 macrophages abundantly express high levels of inducible nitric oxide synthase enzyme iNOS, which catalyze the conversion of L-arginine to L-citruline, resulting in the production of nitric oxide (NO) [151]. iNOS serves as a marker of M1 macrophage and is upregulated in response to INFγ, TNFα, and microbial compounds [82]. The fish iNOS has been characterized with marked similarity to the mammalian enzyme counterpart. The fish iNOS gene expression is induced by antimicrobial and inflammatory stimuli including cleaved transferring products [152, 153]. iNOS plays an important role in protection of fish from a variety of pathogens.

Another hallmark of M1 macrophages is upregulation of the expression of indoleamine2,3-dioxygenase (IDO) enzyme that depletes local tryptophan levels [154]. Tryptophan degradation produces certain metabolites that may inhibit T cell proliferation. Teleost IDO is less effective in tryptophan degradation as compared with their mammalian counterparts [155].

6. Conclusion

Teleosts are found throughout the world and are highly susceptible to variations caused by natural as well as man-made external changes, which affect their immune system. Macrophages are one of the basic immune cells found in teleosts like their mammalian counterparts, which play a crucial role in bridging the innate and adaptive immunity in fish. Macrophages of teleost fish exhibit many functions from that of homeostasis to host immune defense. They possess the phagocytic activity, which is initial step of defense in fish immunity. Measurement of macrophage activation serves as a bioindicator of fish health. Teleosts have shown to have different macrophage polarizations (M1 and M2) pathways under different stimuli, which provides a great support in understanding the evolutionary development of fish immune system. Despite having multiple isoforms of key macrophage cytokines in fish, functional studies of these have been limited. Whole-genome duplication events are responsible for the availability of multiple isoforms of immune mediators in different fish [156]. A greater understanding of teleost macrophages and their function with growing genetic resources would help widely in deciphering the minutes of fish immune system and its evolutionary linkage with that of their mammalian counterparts.

Acknowledgements

RS is thankful to the Council of Scientific and Industrial Research (CSIR), Human Resource Development Group, Govt. of India for her NET-SRF fellowship (Grant No. 09/202(0078)/2018-EMR-I). The author is thankful to Prof. Dipak Kumar Mandal for his guidance and support and to Monisha Das and Nibedita Sharma for their constant encouragement.

Conflict of interest

The author declares no conflict of interest.

Note/thanks/other declarations

The author thanks the Head of the Department of Zoology, for providing the assistance in the research work.

Author details

Ragini Sinha
Department of Zoology, Visva-Bharati University, Santiniketan, West Bengal, India

*Address all correspondence to: raginniissinha5@gmail.com

References

[1] Zhu L, Nie L, Zhu G, Xiang L, Shao J. Advances in research of fish immune-relevant genes: A comparative overview of innate and adaptive immunity in teleosts. Developmental and Comparative Immunology. 2013;**39**:39-62. DOI: 10.1016/j.dci.2012.04.001

[2] Rajaram MV, Ni B, Dodd CE, Schlesinger LS. Macrophage immunoregulatory pathways in tuberculosis. Seminars in Immunology. 2014;**26**:471-485. DOI: 10.1016/j.smim.2014.09.010

[3] Oishi Y, Manabe I. Macrophages in inflammation, repair and regeneration. International Immunology. 2018;**30**:511-528. DOI: 10.1093/intimm/dxy054

[4] Bilej M, De Baetselier P, Beschin A. Antimicrobial defense of the earthworm. Folia Microbiologica. 2000;**45**(4):283-300. DOI: 10.1007/BF02817549

[5] Wiegertjes GF, Wentzel AS, Spaink HP, Elks PM, Fink IR. Polarization of immune responses in fish: The 'macrophages first' point of view. Molecular Immunology. 2016;**69**(3):146-156. DOI: 10.1016/j.molimm.2015.09.026

[6] Lu XJ, Chen J. Specific function and modulation of teleost monocytes/macrophages: Polarization and phagocytosis. Zoological Research. 2019;**40**(3):146-150

[7] Hodgkinson JW, Grayfer L, Belosevic M. Biology of bony fish macrophages. Biology. 2015;**4**(4):881-906. DOI: 10.3390/biology4040881

[8] Joerink M, Ribeiro CMS, Stet RJM, Hermsen T, Savelkoul HFJ, Wiegertjes GF. Head kidney-derived macrophages of common carp (*Cyprinus carpio* L.) show plasticity and functional polarization upon differential stimulation. The Journal of Immunology. 2006;**177**(1):61-69. DOI: 10.4049/jimmunol.177.1.61

[9] Bennani N, Alliana AS, Lafaurie M. Evaluation of phagocytic activity in a teleost fish, *Dicentrachus labrax*. Fish and Shellfish Immunology. 1995;**5**:237-246. DOI: 10.1016/S1050-4648(05)80017-8

[10] Boisset JC, van Cappellen W, Andrieu-Soler C, Galjart N, Dzierzak E, Robin C. In vivo imaging of haematopoietic cells emerging from the mouse aortic endothelium. Nature. 2010;**464**(7285):116-120. DOI: 10.1038/nature08764

[11] de Bruijn MF, Speck NA, Peeters MC, Dzierzak E. Definitive hematopoietic stem cells first develop within the major arterial regions of the mouse embryo. The EMBO Journal. 2000;**19**(11):2465-2474. DOI: 10.1093/emboj/19.11.2465

[12] Medvinsky A, Dzierzak E. Definitive hematopoiesis is autonomously initiated by the AGM region. Cell. 1996;**86**(6):897-906. DOI: 10.1016/s0092-8674(00)80165-8

[13] Bertrand JY, Jalil A, Klaine M, Jung S, Cumano A, Godin I. Three pathways to mature macrophages in the early mouse yolk sac. Blood. 2005;**106**(9):3004-3011. DOI: 10.1182/blood-2005-02-0461

[14] Palis J, Chan RJ, Koniski A, Patel R, Starr M, Yoder MC. Spatial and temporal emergence of high proliferative potential hematopoietic precursors during murine embryogenesis. Proceedings of the National Academy of Sciences of the United States of America.

2001;**98**(8):4528-4533. DOI: 10.1073/pnas.071002398

[15] Herbomel P, Thisse B, Thisse C. Ontogeny and behaviour of early macrophages in the zebrafish embryo. Development. 1999;**126**(17):3735-3745

[16] Herbomel P, Thisse B, Thisse C. Zebrafish early macrophages colonize cephalic mesenchyme and developing brain, retina, and epidermis through a M-CSF receptor-dependent invasive process. Developmental Biology. 2001;**238**(2):274-288. DOI: 10.1006/dbio.2001.0393

[17] Jin H, Sood R, Xu J, et al. Definitive hematopoietic stem/progenitor cells manifest distinct differentiation output in the zebrafish VDA and PBI. Development. 2009;**136**(4):647-654. DOI: 10.1242/dev.029637

[18] Xu J, Du L, Wen Z. Myelopoiesis during zebrafish early development. The Journal of Genetics and Genomics. 2012;**39**(9):435-442. DOI: 10.1016/j.jgg.2012.06.005

[19] Yu T, Guo W, Tian Y, Xu J, Chen J, Li L, et al. Distinct regulatory networks control the development of macrophages of different origins in zebrafish. Blood. 2017;**129**(4):509-519. DOI: 10.1182/blood-2016-07-727651

[20] Bertrand JY, Kim AD, Violette EP, Stachura DL, Cisson JL, Traver D. Definitive hematopoiesis initiates through a committed erythromyeloid progenitor in the zebrafish embryo. Development. 2007;**134**:4147-4156. DOI: 10.1242/dev.012385

[21] Lieschke GJ, Oates AC, Paw BH, Thompson MA, Hall NE, Ward AC, et al. Zebrafish SPI-1 (PU.1) marks a site of myeloid development independent of primitive erythropoiesis: Implications for axial patterning. Development Biology. 2002;**246**:274-295. DOI: 10.1006/dbio.2002.0657

[22] Willett CE, Cortes A, Zuasti A, Zapata AG. Early hematopoiesis and developing lymphoid organs in the zebrafish. Developmental Dynamics. 1999;**214**:323-336

[23] Kobayashi I, Kuniyoshi S, Saito K, Moritomo T, Takahashi T, Nakanishi T. Long-term hematopoietic reconstitution by transplantation of kidney hematopoietic stem cells in lethally irradiated clonal ginbuna crucian carp (*Carassius auratus* langsdorfii). Developmental and Comparative Immunology. 2008;**32**:957-965. DOI: 10.1016/j.dci.2008.01.006

[24] Traver D, Winzeler A, Stern HM, Mayhall EA, Langenau DM, Kutok JL, et al. Effects of lethal irradiation in zebrafish and rescue by hematopoietic cell transplantation. Blood. 2004;**104**:1298-1305. DOI: 10.1182/blood-2004-01-0100

[25] Ray R, Rai V. Lysophosphatidic acid converts monocytes into macrophages in both mice and humans. Blood. 2017;**129**(9):1177-1183. DOI: 10.1182/blood-2016-10-743757

[26] Shi C, Pamer EG. Monocyte recruitment during infection and inflammation. Nature Reviews Immunology. 2011;**11**(11):762-774. DOI: 10.1038/nri3070

[27] Van Furth R, Cohn ZA, Hirsch JG, Humphrey JH, Spector WG, Langevoort HL. Mononuclear phagocytic system: New classification of macrophages, monocytes and of their cell line. Bulletin of World Health Organization. 1972;**47**:651-658

[28] Ginhoux F, Jung S. Monocytes and macrophages: Developmental pathways and tissue homeostasis. Nature Reviews Immunology. 2014;**14**:392-404. DOI: 10.1038/nri3671

[29] Hashimoto D, Chow A, Noizat C, Teo P, Beasley MB, Leboeuf M, et al. Tissue-resident macrophages self-maintain locally throughout adult life with minimal contribution from circulating monocytes. Immunity. 2013;**38**:792-804. DOI: 10.1016/j.immuni.2013.04.004

[30] Yona S, Kim KW, Wolf Y, Mildner A, Varol D, Breker M, et al. Fate mapping reveals origins and dynamics of monocytes and tissue macrophages under homeostasis. Immunity. 2013;**38**:79-91. DOI: 10.1016/j.immuni.2012.12.001

[31] Hanington PC, Tam J, Katzenback BA, Hitchen SJ, Barreda DR, Belosevic M. Development of macrophages of cyprinid fish. Development and Comparative Immunology. 2009;**33**(4):411-429. DOI: 10.1016/j.dci.2008.11.004

[32] Ihle JN. Pathways in cytokine regulation of hematopoiesis. Annals of the New York Academy of Sciences. 2001;**938**:129-130. DOI: 10.1111/j.1749-6632.2001.tbo3581.x

[33] Gewirtz AM, Calabretta B. A c-myb antisense oligodeoxynucleotide inhibits normal human hematopoiesis in vitro. Science. 1988;**242**(4883):1303-1306. DOI: 10.1126/science.2461588

[34] Anfossi G, Gewirtz AM, Calabretta B. An oligomer complementary to c-myb-encoded mRNA inhibits proliferation of human myeloid leukemia cell lines. Proceedings of the National Academy of Sciences of the United States of America. 1989;**86**(9):3379-3383. DOI: 10.1073/pnas.86.9.3379

[35] Grayfer L, Hanington PC, Belosevic M. Macrophage colony-stimulating factor (CSF-1) induces pro-inflammatory gene expression and enhances antimicrobial responses of goldfish (*Carassius auratus* L.) macrophages. Fish and Shellfish Immunology. 2009;**26**(3):406-413. DOI: 10.1016/j.fsi.2008.12.001

[36] Garceau V, Smith J, Paton IR, Davey M, Fares MA, Sester DP, et al. Pivotal advance: Avian colony-stimulating factor 1 (CSF-1), interleukin-34 (IL-34), and CSF-1 receptor genes and gene products. The Journal of Leukocyte Biology. 2010;**87**:753-764. DOI: 10.1189/jlb.0909624

[37] Hanington PC, Wang T, Secombes CJ, Belosevic M. Growth factors of lower vertebrates: Characterization of goldfish (*Carassius auratus* L.) macrophage colony-stimulating factor-1. Journal of Biological Chemistry. 2007;**282**:31865-31872. DOI: 10.1074/jbc.M706278200

[38] Pixley FJ, Stanley ER. CSF-1 regulation of the wandering macrophage: Complexity in action. Trends in Cell Biology. 2004;**14**:628-638. DOI: 10.1016/j.tcb.2004.09.016

[39] Petit J, Embregts CWE, Forlenza M, Wiegertjes GF. Evidence of trained immunity in a fish: Conserved features in carp macrophages. The Journal of Immunology. 2019;**203**(1):216-224. DOI: 10.4049/jimmunol.1900137

[40] Dai XM, Ryan GR, Hapel AJ, Dominguez MG, Russell RG, Kapp S, et al. Targeted disruption of the mouse colony-stimulating factor 1 receptor gene results in osteopetrosis, mononuclear phagocyte deficiency, increased primitive progenitor cell frequencies, and reproductive defects. Blood. 2002;**99**: 111-120. DOI: 10.1182/blood.V99.1.111

[41] Guilbert LJ, Stanley ER. Specific interaction of murine colony-stimulating factor with mononuclear phagocytic cells. Journal of Cell Biology. 1980;**85**:153-159. DOI: 10.1083/jcb.85.1.153

[42] Lichanska AM, Browne CM, Henkel GW, Murphy KM, Ostrowski MC, McKercher SR, et al. Differentiation of the mononuclear phagocyte system during mouse embryogenesis: The role of transcription factor PU.1. Blood. 1999;**94**:127-138. DOI: 10.1182/blood.V94.1.127.413k07_127_138

[43] Wang T, Hanington PC, Belosevic M, Secombes CJ. Two macrophage colony-stimulating factor genes exist in fish that differ in gene organization and are differentially expressed. The Journal of Immunology. 2008;**181**(5):3310-3322. DOI: 10.4049/jimmunol.181.5.3310

[44] Neumann NF, Barreda DR, Belosevic M. Generation and functional analysis of distinct macrophage sub-populations from goldfish (*Carassius auratus* L.) kidney leukocyte cultures. Fish and Shellfish Immunology. 2000;**10**:1-20. DOI: 10.1006/fsim.1999.0221

[45] Grayfer L, Kerimoglu B, Yaparla A, Hodgkinson JW, Xie J, Belosevic M. Mechanisms of fish macrophage antimicrobial immunity. Frontiers in Immunology. 2018;**9**:1105. DOI: 10.3389/fimmu.2018.01105

[46] Yang DX, Yang H, Cao YC, Jiang M, Zheng J, Peng B. Succinate promotes phagocytosis of monocytes/macrophages in teleost fish. Frontiers in Molecular Biosciences. 2021;**8**:644957. DOI: 10.3389/fmolb.2021.644957

[47] Horiguchi J, Warren MK, Kufe D. Expression of the macrophage-specific colony-stimulating factor in human monocytes treated with granulocyte macrophage colony-stimulating factor. Blood. 1987;**69**:1259-1261

[48] Oster W, Lindemann A, Horn S, Mertelsmann R, Herrmann F. Tumor necrosis factor (TNF)-alpha but not TNF-beta induces secretion of colony stimulating factor for macrophages (CSF-1) by human monocytes. Blood. 1987;**70**:1700-1703

[49] Harrington M, Konicek BW, Xia XL, Song A. Transcriptional regulation of the mouse CSF-1 gene. Molecular Reproduction and Development. 1997;**46**:39-44 [discussion 5]. DOI: 10.1002/(SICI)1098-2795(199701)46:1<39::AID-MRD7>3.0.CO;2-S

[50] Gruber MF, Williams CC, Gerrard TL. Macrophage-colony-stimulating factor expression by anti-CD45 stimulated human monocytes is transcriptionally up-regulated by IL-1 beta and inhibited by IL-4 and IL-10. The Journal of Immunology. 1994;**152**:1354-1361

[51] Horiguchi J, Warren MK, Ralph P, Kufe D. Expression of the macrophage specific colony-stimulating factor (CSF-1) during human monocytic differentiation. Biochemical and Biophysics Research Communication. 1986;**141**:924-930. DOI: 10.1016/s0006-291x(86)80131-0

[52] Oster W, Lindemann A, Mertelsmann R, Herrmann F. Regulation of gene expression of M-, G-, GM-, and multi-CSF in normal and malignant hematopoietic cells. Blood Cells. 1988;**14**:443-462

[53] Chitu V, Stanley ER. Colony-stimulating factor-1 in immunity and inflammation. Current Opinion in Immunology. 2006;**18**:39-48. DOI: 10.1016/j.coi.2005.11.006

[54] Rieger AM, Hanington PC, Belosevic M, Barreda DR. Control of CSF-1 induced inflammation in teleost fish by a soluble form of the CSF-1 receptor. Fish and Shellfish Immunology. 2014;**41**:45-51. DOI: 10.1016/j.fsi.2014.03.035

[55] Bartocci A, Mastrogiannis DS, Migliorati G, Stockert RJ, Wolkoff AW, Stanley ER. Macrophages specifically regulate the concentration of their own growth factor in the circulation. Proceedings of the National Academy of Sciences. 1987;**84**:6179-6183

[56] Tushinski RJ, Oliver IT, Guilbert LJ, Tynan PW, Warner JR, Stanley ER. Survival of mononuclear phagocytes depends on a lineage-specific growth factor that the differentiated cells selectively destroy. Cell. 1982;**28**:71-81. DOI: 10.1016/0092-8674(82)90376-2

[57] Hanington PC, Hitchen SJ, Beamish LA, Belosevic M. Macrophage colony stimulating factor (CSF-1) is a central growth factor of goldfish macrophages. Fish and Shellfish Immunology. 2009;**26**(3):406-413. DOI: 10.1016/j.fsi.2008.12.001

[58] Forlenza M, Fink IR, Raes G, Wiegertjes GF. Heterogeneity of macrophage activation in fish. Developmental and Comparative Immunology. 2011;**35**:1246-1255. DOI: 10.1016/j.dci.2011.03.008

[59] Gordon S. Alternative activation of macrophages. Nature Reviews Immunology. 2003;**3**:23-35. DOI: 10.1038/nri978

[60] Mantovani A, Sica A, Sozzani S, Allavena P, Vecchi A, Locati M. The chemokine system in diverse forms of macrophage activation and polarization. Trends in Immunology. 2004;**25**(12):677-686. DOI: 10.1016/j.it.2004.09.015

[61] Janeway CA Jr, Medzhitov R. Innate immune recognition. Annual Review of Immunology. 2002;**20**:197-216. DOI: 10.1146/annurev.immunol.20.083001.084359

[62] Taylor PR, Martinez-Pomares L, Stacey M, Lin HH, Brown GD, Gordon S. Macrophage receptors and immune recognition. Annual Reviews of Immunology. 2004;**23**:901-944. DOI: 10.1146/annurev.immunol.23.021704.115816

[63] van der Vaart M, Spaink HP, Meijer AH. Pathogen recognition and activation of the innate immune response in zebrafish. Advances in Hematology. 2012;**2012**:159807. DOI: 10.1155/2012/159807

[64] Rieger AM, Barreda DR. Antimicrobial mechanisms of fish leukocytes. Developmental and Comparative Immunology. 2011;**35**:1238-1245. DOI: 10.1016/j.dci.2011.03.009

[65] Dalton DK, Pitts-Meek S, Keshav S, Figari IS, Bradley A, Stewart TA. Multiple defects of immune cell function in mice with disrupted interferon gamma genes. Science. 1993;**259**(5102):1739-1742. DOI: 10.1126/science.8456300

[66] Zou J, Yoshiura Y, Dijkstra JM, Sakai M, Ototake M, Secombes C. Identification of an interferon gamma homologue in Fugu, *Takifugu rubripes*. Fish and Shellfish Immunology. 2004;**17**:403-409. DOI: 10.1016/j.fsi.2004.04.015

[67] Zou J, Carrington A, Collet B, Dijkstra JM, Yoshiura Y, Bols N, et al. Identification and bioactivities of IFN-γ in rainbow trout *Oncorhynchus mykiss*: The first Th1- type cytokine characterized functionally in fish. The Journal of Immunology. 2005;**175**:2484-2494. DOI: 10.4049/jimmunol.175.4.2484

[68] Igawa D, Sakai M, Savan R. An unexpected discovery of two interferon gamma-like genes along with interleukin (IL)-22 and -26 from teleost: IL-22 and -26 genes have been described for the first time outside mammals. Molecular Immunology. 2006;**43**:999-1009. DOI: 10.1016/j.molimm.2005.05.009

[69] Robertsen B. The interferon system of teleost fish. Fish and Shellfish Immunology. 2006;**20**:172-191. DOI: 10.1016/j.fsi.2005.01.010

[70] Milev-Milovanovic I, Long S, Wilson M, Bengten E, Miller NW, Chinchar VG. Identification and expression analysis of interferon gamma genes in channel catfish. Immunogenetics. 2006;**58**:70-80. DOI: 10.1007/s00251-006-0081-x

[71] Stolte EH, Savelkoul HFJ, Wiegertjes G, Flik G, van Kemenade BM. Differential expression of two interferon-γ genes in common carp (*Cyprinus carpio* L.). Developmental and Comparative Immunology. 2008;**32**:1467-1481. DOI: 10.1016/j.dci.2008.06.012

[72] Grayfer L, Garcia EG, Belosevic M. Comparison of macrophage antimicrobial responses induced by type II interferons of the goldfish (*Carassius auratus* L.). Journal of Biological Chemistry. 2010;**285**:23537-23547

[73] Furnes C, Seppola M, Robertsen B. Molecular characterisation and expression analysis of interferon gamma in Atlantic cod (*Gadus morhua*). Fish and Shellfish Immunology. 2009;**26**:285-292. DOI: 10.1016/j.fsi.2008.12.002

[74] Jung CY, Hikima J, Ohtani M, Jang HB, del Castillo CS, Nho SW, et al. Recombinant interferon-γ activates immune responses against *Edwardsiella tarda* infection in the olive flounder, *Paralichthys olivaceus*. Fish and Shellfish Immunology. 2012;**33**:197-203. DOI: 10.1016/j.fsi.2012.04.015

[75] Savan R, Ravichandran S, Collins JR, Sakai M, Young HA. Structural conservation of interferon gamma among vertebrates. Cytokine & Growth Factor Reviews. 2009;**20**(2):115-124. DOI: 10.1016/j.cytogfr.2009.02.006

[76] Chen WQ, Xu QQ, Chang MX, Zou J, Secombes CJ, Peng KM, et al. Molecular characterization and expression analysis of the IFN-gamma related gene (IFN-gammarel) in grass carp *Ctenopharyngodon idella*. Veterinary Immunology and Immunopathology. 2010;**134**(3-4):199-207. DOI: 10.1016/j.vetimm.2009.09.007

[77] Sieger D, Stein C, Neifer D, van der Sar AM, Leptin M. The role of gamma interferon in innate immunity in the zebrafish embryo. Disease Model and Mechanism. 2009;**2**(11-12):571-581. DOI: 10.1242/dmm.003509

[78] Shibasaki Y, Yabu T, Araki K, Mano N, Shiba H, Moritomo T, et al. Peculiar monomeric interferon gammas, IFN _rel 1 and IFN _rel 2, inginbuna crucian carp. FEBS Journal. 2014;**281**:1046-1056. DOI: 10.1111/febs.12666

[79] Aggad D, Stein C, Sieger D, Mazel M, Boudinot P, Herbomel P, et al. In vivo analysis of IFN-γ1 and IFN-γ2 signaling in zebrafish. The Journal of Immunology. 2010;**185**:6774-6782. DOI: 10.4049/jimmunol.1000549

[80] Yabu T, Toda H, Shibasaki Y, Araki K, Yamashita M, Anzai H, et al. Antiviral protection mechanisms mediated by ginbuna crucian carp interferon gamma isoforms 1 and 2 through two distinct interferon γ-receptors. Journal of Biochemistry. 2011;**150**:635-648. DOI: 10.1093/jb/mvr108

[81] Mosser DM. The many faces of macrophage activation. The Journal of Leukocyte Biology. 2003;**73**(2):209-212. DOI: 10.1189/jlb.0602325

[82] Mosser DM, Edwards JP. Exploring the full spectrum of macrophage activation. Nature Reviews Immunology. 2008;**8**(12):958-969. DOI: 10.1038/nri2448

[83] Nguyen-Chi M, Laplace-Builhe B, Travnickova J, Luz-Crawford P, Tejedor G, Phan QT, et al. Identification of polarized macrophage subsets in zebrafish. Elife. 2015;**4**:e07288. DOI: 10.7554/eLife.07288

[84] Ronza P, Losada AP, Villamarin A, Bermudez R, Quiroga MI. Immunolocalization of tumor necrosis factor alpha in turbot (*Scophthalmus maximus*, L.) tissues. Fish and Shellfish Immunology. 2015;**45**:470-476. DOI: 10.1016/j. fsi. 2015.04.032

[85] García-Castillo J, Pelegrín P, Mulero V, Meseguer J. Molecular cloning and expression analysis of tumor necrosis factor α from a marine fish reveal its constitutive expression and ubiquitous nature. Immunogenetics. 2002;**54**:200-207. DOI: 10.1007/s00251-002-0451-y

[86] Hirono I, Nam BH, Kurobe T, Aoki T. Molecular cloning, characterization, and expression of TNF cDNA and gene from Japanese flounder *Paralychthys olivaceus*. The Journal of Immunology. 2000;**165**:4423-4427. DOI: 10.4049/jimmunol.165.8.4423

[87] Grayfer L, Walsh JG, Belosevic M. Characterization and functional analysis of goldfish (*Carassius auratus* L.) tumor necrosis factor-alpha. Developmental and Comparative Immunology. 2008;**32**:532-543. DOI: 10.1016/j.dci.2007.09.009

[88] Kadowaki T, Harada H, Sawada Y, Kohchi C, Soma GI, Takahashi Y, et al. Two types of tumor necrosis factor-α in bluefin tuna (*Thunnus orientalis*) genes: Molecular cloning and expression profile in response to several immunological stimulants. Fish and Shellfish Immunology. 2009;**27**:585-594. DOI: 10.1016/j.fsi.2008.12.006

[89] Laing KJ, Wang T, Zou J, Holland J, Hong S, Bols N, et al. Cloning and expression analysis of rainbow trout *Oncorhynchus mykiss* tumour necrosis factor-α. European Journal of Biochemistry. 2001;**268**:1315-1322. DOI: 10.1046/j.1432-1327.2001.01996.x

[90] Lam FWS, Wu SY, Lin SJ, Lin CC, Chen YM, Wang HC, et al. The expression of two novel orange-spotted grouper (*Epinephelus coioides*) TNF genes in peripheral blood leukocytes, various organs, and fish larvae. Fish and Shellfish Immunology. 2011;**30**:618-629. DOI: 10.1016/j.fsi.2010.12.011

[91] Nascimento DS, Pereira PJB, Reis MIR, do Vale A, Zou J, Silva MT, et al. Molecular cloning and expression analysis of sea bass (*Dicentrarchus labrax* L.) tumor necrosis factor-α (TNF-α). Fish and Shellfish Immunology. 2007;**23**:701-710. DOI: 10.1016/j.fsi.2010.12.011

[92] Ordás MC, Costa MM, Roca FJ, López-Castejón G, Mulero V, Meseguer J, et al. Turbot TNFα gene: Molecular characterization and biological activity of the recombinant protein. Molecular Immunology. 2007;**44**:389-400. DOI: 10.1016/j.molimm.2006.02.028

[93] Saeij JP, Stet RJ, Groeneveld A, van Kemenade LB, van Muiswinkel WB, Wiegertjes GF. Molecular and functional characterization of a fish inducible-type nitric oxide synthase. Immunogenetics.

2000;**51**:339-346. DOI: 10.1007/s002510050628

[94] Savan R, Kono T, Igawa D, Sakai M. A novel tumor necrosis factor (TNF) gene present in tandem with the TNF-α gene on the same chromosome in teleosts. Immunogenetics. 2005;**57**:140-150. DOI: 10.1007/s00251-005-0768-4

[95] Zhang A, Chen D, Wei H, Du L, Zhao T, Wang X, et al. Functional characterization of TNF-α in grass carp head kidney leukocytes: Induction and involvement in the regulation of NF-κB signaling. Fish and Shellfish Immunology. 2012;**33**:1123-1132. DOI: 10.1016/j.fsi.2012.08.029

[96] Hong S, Li R, Xu Q, Secombes CJ, Wang T. Two types of TNF-α exist in teleost fish: Phylogeny, expression, and bioactivity analysis of type-II TNF-α3 in rainbow trout *Oncorhynchus mykiss*. The Journal of Immunology. 2013;**191**:5959-5972. DOI: 10.4049/jimmunol.1301584

[97] Wang T, Secombes CJ. The cytokine networks of adaptive immunity in fish. Fish and Shellfish Immunology. 2013;**35**(6):1703-1718. DOI: 10.1016/j.fsi.2013.08.030

[98] Roca FJ, Mulero I, López-Muñoz A, Sepulcre MP, Renshaw SA, Meseguer J, et al. Evolution of the inflammatory response in vertebrates: Fish TNF-alpha is a powerful activator of endothelial cells but hardly activates phagocytes. The Journal of Immunology. 2008;**181**:5071e81. DOI: 10.4049/jimmunol.181.7.5071

[99] Forlenza M, Magez S, Scharsack JP, Westphal A, Savelkoul HF, Wiegertjes GF. Receptor-mediated and lectin-like activities of carp (*Cyprinus carpio*) TNFalpha. The Journal of Immunology. 2009;**183**:5319e32. DOI: 10.4049/jimmunol.0901780

[100] Zou J, Peddie S, Scapigliati G, Zhang Y, Bols NC, Ellis AE, et al. Functional characterisation of the recombinant tumor necrosis factors in rainbow trout, *Oncorhynchus mykiss*. Developmental and Comparative Immunology. 2003;**27**:813e22. DOI: 10.1016/s0145-305x(03)00077-6

[101] Grayfer L, Belosevic M. Molecular characterization of tumor necrosis factor receptors 1 and 2 of the goldfish (*Carassius aurutus* L.). Molecular Immunology. 2009;**46**:2190-21999. DOI: 10.1016/j.molimm.2009.04.016

[102] Roca FJ, Mulero I, Lopez-Munoz A, Sepulcre MP, Renshaw SA, Meseguer J, et al. Evolution of the inflammatory response in vertebrates: Fish TNF-alpha is a powerful activator of endothelial cells but hardly activates phagocytes. The Journal of Immunology. 2008;**181**(7):5071-5081. DOI: 10.4049/jimmunol.181.7.5071

[103] Gordon S, Martinez FO. Alternative activation of macrophages: Mechanism and functions. Immunity. 2010;**32**(5):593-604. DOI: 10.1016/j.immuni.2010.05.007

[104] Ohtani M, Hayashi N, Hashimoto K, Nakanishi T, Dijkstra JM. Comprehensive clarification of two paralogous interleukin 4/13 loci in teleost fish. Immunogenetics. 2008;**60**:383-397. DOI: 10.1007/s00251-008-0299-x

[105] Wang T, Secombes CJ. The evolution of IL-4 and IL-13 and their receptor subunits. Cytokine. 2015;**75**:8-13. DOI: 10.1016/j.cyto.2015.04.012

[106] Yamaguchi T, Takizawa F, Fischer U, Dijkstra JM. Along the axis between Type 1 and Type 2 immunity: Principles conserved in evolution from fish to mammals. Biology (Basel).

2015;**4**(4):814-859. DOI: 10.3390/biology4040814

[107] Mueller TD, Zhang JL, Sebald W, Duschl A. Structure, binding, and antagonists in the IL-4/IL-13 receptor system. Biochimica et Biophysica Acta. 2002;**1592**(3):237-250. DOI: 10.1016/s0167-4889(02)00318-x

[108] Wang T, Huang W, Costa MM, Martin SAM, Secombes CJ. Two copies of the genes encoding the subunits of putative interleukin (IL)-4/IL-13 receptors, IL-4Rα, IL-13Rα1 and IL-13Rα2, have been identified in rainbow trout (*Oncorhynchus mykiss*) and have complex patterns of expression and modulation. Immunogenetics. 2011;**63**:235-253. DOI: 10.1007/s00251-010-0508-2

[109] Zhu L, Pan P, Fang W, Shao J, Xiang L. Essential role of IL-4 and IL-4Rα interaction in adaptive immunity of zebrafish: Insight into the origin of Th2-like regulatory mechanism in ancient vertebrates. The Journal of Immunology. 2012;**188**:5571-5584. DOI: 10.4049/jimmunol.1102259

[110] Wang T, Johansson P, Abos B, Holt A, Tafalla C, Jiang Y, et al. First in-depth analysis of the novel Th2-type cytokines in salmonid fish reveals distinct pat-terns of expression and modulation but overlapping bioactivities. Oncotarget. 2016;**7**:10917-10946

[111] Yang ZJ, Li CH, Chen J, Zhang H, Li MY, Chen J. Molecular characterization of an interleukin-4/13B homolog in grass carp (*Ctenopharyngodon idella*) and its role in fish against Aeromonas hydrophila infection. Fish and Shellfish Immunology. 2016;**57**:136-147. DOI: 10.1016/j.fsi.2016.08.022

[112] Stocchi V, Wang T, Randelli E, Mazzini M, Gerdol M, Pallavicini A, et al. Evolution of Th2 responses: Characterization of IL-4/13 in sea bass (*Dicentrarchus labrax* L.) and studies of expression and biological activity. Scientific Reports. 2017;**7**:2240

[113] Green SJ, Crawford RM, Hockmeyer JT, Meltzer MS, Nacy CA. Leishmania major amastigotes initiate the L-arginine-dependent killing mechanism in IFN-gamma-stimulated macrophages by induction of tumor necrosis factor-alpha. The Journal of Immunology. 1990;**145**:4290-4297

[114] Barksdale AR, Bernard AC, Maley ME, Gellin GL, Kearney PA, Boulanger BR, et al. Regulation of arginase expression by T-helper II cytokines and iso-proterenol. Surgery. 2004;**135**:527-535. DOI: 10.1016/j.surg.2003.10.007

[115] Jenkinson CP, Grody WW, Cederbaum SD. Comparative properties of arginases. Comparative Biochemistry and Physiology Part B: Biochemistry and Molecular Biology. 1996;**114**:107-132. DOI: 10.1016/0305-0491(95)02138-8

[116] Joerink M, Savelkoul HFJ, Wiegertjes GF. Evolutionary conservation of alternative activation of macrophages: Structural and functional characterization of arginase 1 and 2 in carp (*Cyprinus carpio* L.). Molecular Immunology. 2006;**43**:1116-1128. DOI: 10.1016/j.molimm.2005.07.022

[117] Wang R, Belosevic M. The in vitro effects of estradiol and cortisol on the function of a long-term goldfish macrophage cell line. Developmental and Comparative Immunology. 1995;**19**:327-336. DOI: 10.1016/0145-305x(95)00018-o

[118] Maule AG, Tripp RA, Kaattari SL, Schreck CB. Stress alters immune function and disease resistance in chinook salmon (*Oncorhynchus*

tshawytscha). The Journal of Endocrinology. 1989;**120**:135-142. DOI: 10.1677/joe.0.1200135

[119] Pickering AD, Pottinger TG. Cortisol can increase the susceptibility of brown trout, *Salmo trutta* L., to disease without reducing the white blood cell count. The Journal of Fish Biology. 1985;**27**:611-619. DOI: 10.1111/j.1095-8649.1985.tb03206.x

[120] Maciuszek M, Rydz L, Świtakowska I, Verburg-van Kemenade BML, Chadzińska M. Effects of stress and cortisol on the polarization of carp macrophages. Fish and Shellfish Immunology. 2019;**94**:27-37. DOI: 10.1016/j.fsi.2019.08.064

[121] Wei H, Yin L, Feng S, Wang X, Yang K, Zhang A, et al. Dual-parallelinhibition of IL-10 and TGF-beta1 controls LPS-induced inflammatory responsevia NF-kappaB signaling in grass carp monocytes/macrophages. Fish and Shellfish Immunology. 2015;**44**:445-452. DOI: 10.1016/j.fsi.2015.03.023

[122] Haddad G, Hanington PC, Wilson EC, Grayfer L, Belosevic M. Molecular and functional characterization of goldfish (*Carassius auratus* L.) transforming growth factor beta. Developmental and Comparative Immunology. 2008;**32**:654e63. DOI: 10.1016/j.dci.2007.10.003

[123] Ferrante CJ, Leibovich SJ. Regulation of macrophage polarization and wound healing. Advances in Wound Care. 2012;**1**:10-16

[124] Piazzon MC, Savelkoul HS, Pietretti D, Wiegertjes GF, Forlenza M. CarpIl10 has anti-inflammatory activities on phagocytes, promotes proliferation ofmemory T cells, and regulates B cell differentiation and antibody secretion. The Journal of Immunology. 2015;**194**:187-199. DOI: 10.4049/jimmunol.1402093

[125] Grayfer L, Belosevic M. Identification and molecular characterization of the interleukin-10 receptor 1 of the zebrafish (*Danio rerio*) and the goldfish (*Carassius auratus* L.). Developmental and Comparative Immunology. 2012;**36**:408-417. DOI: 10.1016/j.dci.2011.08.006

[126] Wei H, Wang S, Qin L, Wang X, Zhou H. Molecular characterization, 3D modeling of grass carp interleukin-10 receptor 1 (IL10R1). Engineering. 2013;**5**:214-219. DOI: 10.4236/eng.2013.510B045

[127] Monte MM, Wang T, Collet B, Zou J, Secombes CJ. Molecular characterisation of fourclass 2 cytokine receptor family members in rainbow trout, *Oncorhynchus mykiss*. Developmental and Comparative Immunology. 2015;**48**:43-54

[128] Esteban MÁ, Cuesta A, Chaves-Pozo E, Meseguer J. Phagocytosis in Teleosts. Implications of the new cells involved. Biology (Basel). 2015;**4**(4):907-922

[129] Wu L, Qin Z, Liu H, Lin L, Ye J, Li J. Recent advances on phagocytic B cells in Teleost fish. Frontiers in Immunology. 2020;**11**:824. DOI: 10.3389/fimmu.2020.00824

[130] Stuart LM, Ezekowitz RA. Phagocytosis: Elegant complexity. Immunity. 2005;**22**:539-550. DOI: 10.1016/j.immuni.2005.05.002

[131] Tauber AI. Metchnikoff and the phagocytosis theory. Nature Reviews Molecular Cell Biology. 2003;**4**:897-901. DOI: 10.1038/nrm1244

[132] Watts C, Amigorena S. Phagocytosis and antigen presentation. Seminars in

Immunology. 2001;**13**:373-379. DOI: 10.1006/smim.2001.0334

[133] Allen PG, Dawidowicz EA. Phagocytosis in Acanthamoeba: I. A mannose receptor is responsible for the binding and phagocytosis of yeast. The Journal of Cellular Physiology. 1990;**145**:508-513. DOI: 10.1002/jcp.1041450317

[134] Davies B, Chattings LS, Edwards SW. Superoxide generation during phagocytosis by *Acanthamoeba castellanii*: Similarities to the respiratory burst of immune phagocytes. The Journal of General Microbiology. 1991;**137**:705-710. DOI: 10.1099/00221287-137-3-705

[135] Moretti J, Blander JM. Insights into phagocytosis-coupled activation of pattern recognition receptors and inflammasomes. Current Opinion in Immunology. 2014;**26**:100-110. DOI: 10.1016/j.coi.2013.11.003

[136] Alberdi F Jr, Alderton MR, Coloe PJ, Smith SC. Characterization of immu-norelated peptides to porcidin P1. Immunology and Cell Biology. 1995;**73**:505-510. DOI: 10.1038/icb.1995.80

[137] Alberdi F Jr, Alderton MR, Korolik V, Coloe PJ, Smith SC. Antibacterial proteins from porcine polymorphonuclear neutrophils. Immunology and Cell Biology. 1995;**73**:38-43. DOI: 10.1038/icb.1995.6

[138] Kaplan DH, Greenlund AC, Tanner JW, Shaw AS, Schreiber RD. Identification of an interferon-gamma receptor alpha chain sequence required for JAK-1 binding. The Journal of Biological Chemistry. 1996;**271**:9-12. DOI: 10.1074/jbc.271.1.9

[139] Ganz T, Lehrer RI. Antimicrobial peptides of leukocytes. Current Opinion in Hematology. 1997;**4**:53-58. DOI: 10.1097/00062752-199704010-00009

[140] Borelli V, Banfi E, Perrotta MG, Zabucchi G. Myeloperoxidase exerts micro-bicidal activity against Mycobacterium tuberculosis. Infection and Immunity. 1999;**67**:4149-4152

[141] Sorensen OE, Follin P, Johnsen AH, Calafat J, Tjabringa GS, Hiemstra PS, et al. Human cathelicidin, hCAP-18, is processed to the antimicrobial peptide LL-37 by extracellular cleavage with proteinase 3. Blood. 2001;**97**:3951-3959. DOI: 10.1182/blood.V97.12.3951

[142] Canton J, Khezri R, Glogauer M, Grinstein S. Contrasting phagosome pH regulation and maturation in human M1 and M2 macrophages. Molecular Biology of the Cell. 2014;**25**:3330-3341. DOI: 10.1091/mbc.E14-05-0967

[143] Rabinovitch M. Professional and non-professional phagocytes: An introduction. Trends in Cell Biology. 1995;**5**:85-87

[144] Briggs RT, Drath DB, Karnovsky ML, Karnovsky MJ. Localization of NADH oxidase on the surface of human polymorphonuclear leukocytes by a new cytochemical method. Journal of Cell Biology. 1975;**67**:566-586. DOI: 10.1083/jcb.67.3.566

[145] Jorgensen JB, Robertsen B. Yeast beta-glucan stimulates respiratory burst activity of Atlantic salmon (*Salmo salar* L.) macrophages. Developmental and Comparative Immunology. 1995;**19**:43-57. DOI: 10.1016/0145-305X(94)00045-H

[146] Stafford JL, Galvez F, Goss GG, Belosevic M. Induction of nitric oxide and respiratory burst response in activated goldfish macrophages

requires potassium channel activity. Developmental and Comparative Immunology. 2002;**26**:445-459. DOI: 10.1016/S0145-305X(01)00087-8

[147] Sepulcre MP, Lopez-Castejon G, Meseguer J, Mulero V. The activation of gilthead seabream professional phagocytes by different PAMPs underlines the behavioural diversity of the main innate immune cells of bony fish. Molecular Immunology. 2007;**44**:2009-2016. DOI: 10.1016/j.molimm.2006.09.022

[148] Boltana S, Donate C, Goetz FW, Mackenzie S, Balasch JC. Characterization and expression of NADPH oxidase in LPS-, poly(I:C)- and zymosan-stimu-lated trout (*Oncorhynchus mykiss* W.) macrophages. Fish and Shellfish Immunology. 2009;**26**:651-661. DOI: 10.1016/j.fsi.2008.11.011

[149] Sharp GJE, Secombes CJ. The role of reactive oxygen species in the killing of the bacterial fish pathogen Aeromonas salmonicida by rainbow trout macrophages. Fish and Shellfish Immunology. 1993;**3**:119-129. DOI: 10.1006/fsim.1993.1013

[150] Ardó L, Jeney Z, Adams A, Jeney G. Immune responses of resistant and sensitive common carp families following experimental challenge with Aeromonas hydrophila. Fish and Shellfish Immunology. 2010;**29**:111-116. DOI: 10.1016/j.fsi.2010.02.029

[151] John M, Qiao-Wen X, Nathan C. Nitric oxide and macrophage function. The Annual Review of Immunology. 1997;**15**:323-350. DOI: 10.1146/annurev.immunol.15.1.323

[152] Stafford JL, Neumann NF, Belosevic M. Products of proteolytic cleavage of transferrin induce nitric oxide response of goldfish macrophages. Developmental and Comparative Immunology. 2001;**25**:101-115. DOI: 10.1016/S0145-305X(00)00048-3

[153] Stafford JL, Wilson EC, Belosevic M. Recombinant transferrin induces nitric oxide response in goldfish and murine macrophages. Fish and Shellfish Immunology. 2004;**17**:171-185. DOI: 10.1016/j.fsi.2004.03.001

[154] Taylor MW, Feng GS. Relationship between interferon-gamma, indoleamine 2,3-dioxygenase, and tryptophan catabolism. The FASEB Journal. 1991;**5**:2516-2522. DOI: 10.1096/fasebj.5.11.1907934

[155] Yuasa HJ, Takubo M, Takahashi A, Hasegawa T, Noma H, Suzuki T. Evolution of vertebrate indoleamine 2,3-dioxygenases. The Journal of Molecular Evolution. 2007;**65**:705-714. DOI: 10.1007/s00239-007-9049-1

[156] MacKintosh C, Ferrier DEK. Recent advances in understanding the roles of whole genome duplications in evolution. F1000 Research. 2017;**6**:1623

Chapter 3

The Interactive Role of Macrophages in Innate Immunity

Roland Osei Saahene, Precious Barnes and Samuel Victor Nuvor

Abstract

Macrophages are critical effector cells of the innate immune system that play central roles in the initiation and resolution of inflammation. They mediate resistance in response to pathogens and "danger" signals mainly through phagocytosis. Macrophages and other cells co-operate and complement one another in host defense. As innate immune cells, they also contribute to the initiation of adaptive immune responses. Therefore, appropriate activation of macrophages would aid effective immune response in curbing many infections. This chapter explores how the interaction and roles of macrophages influence outcomes during infections. It is expected that understanding these fundamental mechanisms may help stimulate research to exploit macrophages for therapeutic benefits.

Keywords: macrophage, phagocytosis, infection, innate immunity

1. Introduction

Macrophages are effector cells of the innate immune system that play central roles in the initiation and resolution of inflammation. They secrete a wide range of cytokines, chemokines, and antimicrobial mediators in response to pathogens and "danger" signals largely through phagocytosis [1]. Additionally, macrophages eliminate diseased and damaged cells and present antigens to activate the acquired immune system. Macrophages differentiate from hematopoietic stem cell-derived monocytes and embryonic progenitor cells. However, tissue macrophages mainly arise from the embryonic yolk sac and occur at sites of primary pathogen exposure [2–5]. Macrophages exist in the tissues of vertebrates, and phenotypes respond differently to different stimuli to direct the immune response. They are critical for the commencement of inflammatory responses. Pattern recognition receptors (PRRs) on the surface of macrophages recognize pathogen-associated molecular patterns (PAMPs), danger-associated molecular patterns (DAMPs) and as a result, activate intracellular signaling cascades for host defense. Pattern recognition receptors such as mannose receptor, dectin-1, scavenger receptors, dendritic cell-specific intercellular adhesion molecule-3-grabbing nonintegrin, toll-like receptors in macrophages recognize pathogens and initiate phagocytosis [6]. Plasticity and functional polarization are characteristics of macrophages. Macrophages exist in two different functional phenotypes: classically activated or M1 macrophages and alternatively activated or M2 macrophages. The M1 are activated by PAMPs and DAMPs as well as Type 1 T helper (Th1) cytokines, such as interferon-gamma (IFN-γ) and tumor necrosis factor-alpha (TNF-α). They function as microbicidal and tumoricidal agents by producing proinflammatory cytokines such as interleukin-1β (IL-1β), IL-6, IL-12, IL-23, and TNF-α, and also activate cytotoxic T cells [7]. M2 are induced by IL-4 and/or IL-13 and plays a crucial role in phagocytosis, tissue remodeling, and wound repair and produces anti-inflammatory cytokines such as IL-10 and transforming growth factor-beta (TGF-β) and usually attract regulatory T cells [8, 9]. M1 potentially induces Type 1 T helper (Th1) and Th17 cells, while M2 induces Type 2 T helper (Th2) cells [10]. The interplay between macrophages and T cells is regarded as a critical link between the innate and adaptive immune systems and is essential for host defense. This chapter explores how the interaction and roles of macrophages influence outcomes during infections.

2. Macrophage-neutrophil co-operation

Macrophage and neutrophils originate from stem cells that differentiate through common myeloid progeny and play essential roles to protect the host. They employ a wide variety of antimicrobial mechanisms, such as the production of reactive oxygen species, reactive nitrogen species, and granules in their defense through phagocytosis. Macrophage-neutrophil interaction plays a critical role in both the initiation and resolution stages of inflammation. During the resolution of inflammation, macrophages produce IL-10 and downregulate IL-12, to promote tissue repair when apoptotic neutrophils are phagocytosed [11]. Macrophages secrete chemokines such as C-X-C motif chemokine ligand 8 (CXCL8) to attract neutrophils upon recognition of bacterial extracellular pathogens [12]. They secret granulocyte colony-stimulating factor (G-CSF), IL-1β, TNF-α, and granulocyte-macrophage colony-stimulating factor (GM-CSF) which prolongs survival of recruited neutrophils to the site of infection [13–16]. Moreover, as principal scavengers of aging and apoptotic neutrophils, they acquire potent neutrophil antimicrobial molecules to enhance their antimicrobial capacity [17]. Neutrophils transfer intracellular microbes to macrophages to be cleared when they are phagocytosed. Neutrophils also interact with macrophages by secreting antimicrobial agents to aid in the clearance of bacterial intracellular pathogens in mycobacteriosis [18–22], in oral [23] listeriosis, in salmonellosis [24], and in legionellosis [25]. Notably, the antimicrobial capacity of macrophages in macrophage-neutrophil interaction depends on the pathogen encountered during the immune response. These include the use of neutrophil acquired lactoferrin, myeloperoxidase, against *Candida albicans* [26, 27], or *Histoplasma capsulatum* [28] and human neutrophil peptide-1 against *Trypanosoma cruzi* [29]. Therefore, macrophage-neutrophil co-operation boosts the antimicrobial capacity of macrophages to restore inflammation and homeostasis in innate immunity.

3. Macrophage-dendritic cell interaction

Macrophages and dendritic cells may impact the Thl/Th2 response and respond to T and B cells, through cellular co-operation and cytokine secretion. These include the use of interferon γ, IL4, IL 13, and antibodies which modulate their phagocytic and microbicidal activities. A recent study indicated that macrophages could transfer phagocytosed antigens to dendritic cells for effective antigen presentation to enhance T cell activation [30].

4. Macrophage-basophil co-operation

Until recently, the function of basophils was not investigated as they were considered as small relatives of mast cells. Basophil-derived IL-4 causes monocyte differentiation into M2 macrophage which suppresses allergic inflammation or provides immunity against helminths [31]. Lung-basophil alveolar macrophage niche is essential in the differentiation, compartmentalization, and phagocytic effects of alveolar macrophage [32].

5. Macrophage and T cell interaction

Macrophages are professional antigen-presenting cells that initiate host protection by phagocytosing pathogens circulating in the host for destruction during inflammation. They recognize a broad array of PAMPs or DAMPs using PRRs. After phagocytosis, they present pieces of foreign antigens within a major histocompatibility complex (MHC I or II) bound to its membrane surface to activate T cells. T cell activation requires three main signals which include T cell receptor (TCR)-MHC peptide, costimulatory and polarizing cytokines. T cells recognize MHC–peptide complex through TCR complexed with a cluster of differentiation 3 (CD3) for onward transmission into the cell. TCR-MHC II-peptide interaction triggers several signaling cascades within T cells. The activation of Lck and zeta-chain associated protein 70 (ZAP-70) in turn activate downstream phospholipase C-γ. This gives rise to diacylglycerol and inositol trisphosphate to switch on the cell's transcription machinery [33]. The activation of phosphorylated tyrosine-based immunoreceptor motifs of TCR/CD3 complex activates various pathways such as Ras/ extracellular-signal-regulated kinase, mitogen-activated protein kinase cascade, the protein kinase C/nuclear factor-kappa B, and Ca/calcineurin/nuclear factor [34].

Macrophages express costimulatory and/or coinhibitory molecules to induce activation or inhibition of T cells. The modulation of costimulatory and coinhibitory molecules is vital to highlight the significance of macrophage functional role in T cell activation and suppression. The ultimate subset differentiation, survival, and role of T cell are determined by the costimulatory and coinhibitory ligand-receptor signal interaction between the macrophage and T cell. Different costimulatory molecules have been characterized, including coreceptor CD28, commonly expressed by naïve and primed T cells. CD28 interact with B7–1 (CD80) and B7–2 (CD86) on macrophages. The activation of T cells requires TCR-MHC–peptide complex and CD28-B7 costimulation. This interaction is essential as it promotes T cell proliferation, survival, and cytokine production. Moreover, it induces an increase in response to the production of B-cell lymphoma 2 (Bcl-2) and B-cell lymphoma-extra large (Bcl-xL) anti-apoptotic proteins [35]. However, failure of CD28-B7 interactions results in anergy and apoptosis of T cells.

On the contrary, several key coinhibitory molecules including cytotoxic T-lymphocyte antigen 4 (CTLA4; CD152), programmed cell death-1 (PD-1), and killer inhibitory receptors interact with ligands on macrophages to suppress T cell activation [36, 37]. CTLA-4 binds with a much higher affinity to the B7 proteins on antigen-presenting cells (APCs) than CD28. However, CTLA-4 expressed ensuing T cell activation is predominantly high compared to that of naive T cells. During the initial priming event, T cells experience cell-cycle arrest if CTLA-4 binds to the B7 proteins and prevent CD28 engagement. T cell-expressed PD-1 binds with PD-L1 on

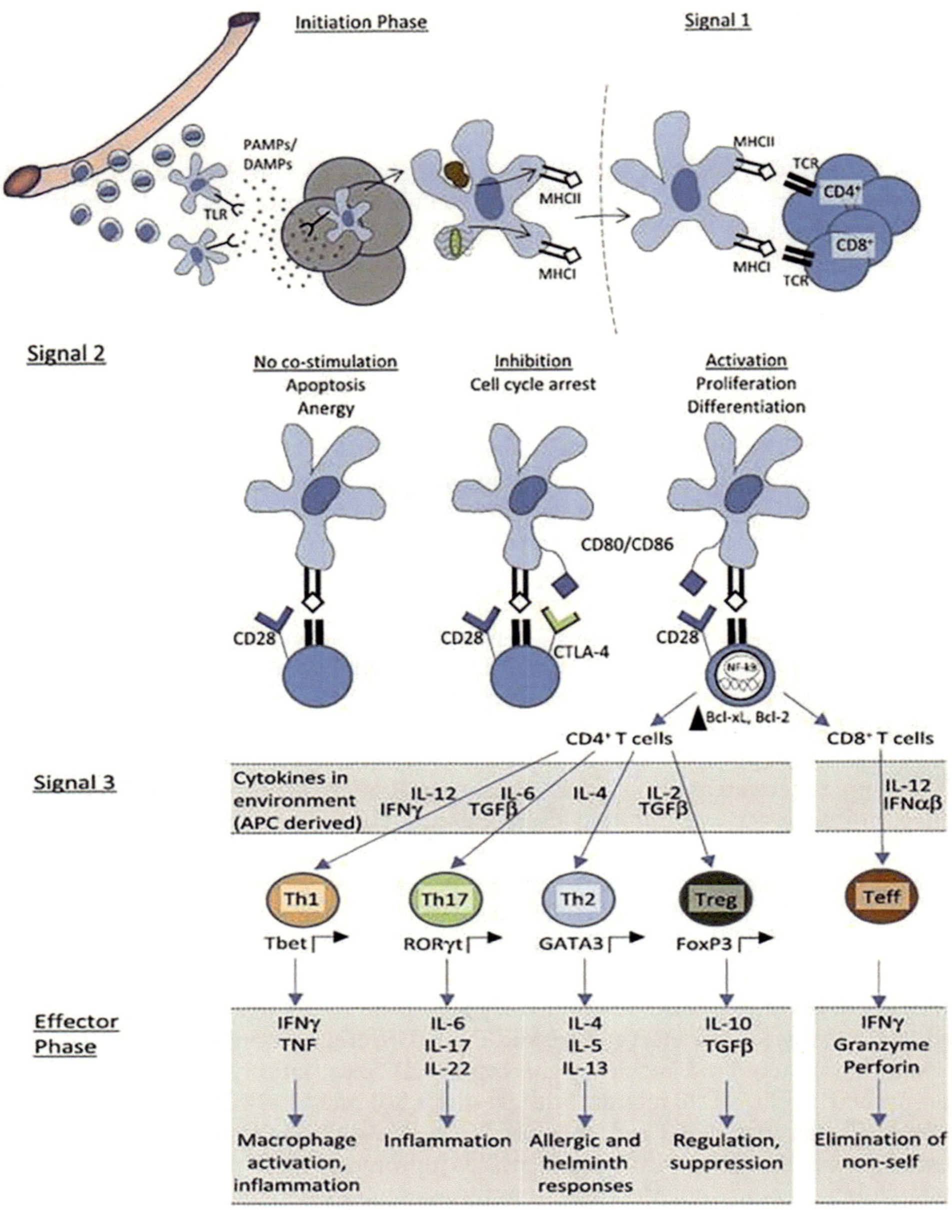

Figure 1.
Macrophages activate T cells through a series of critically important stepwise signals. *After phagocytosis, macrophages (APCs) present peptide antigen within major histocompatibility complex (MHC)-II for T cell recognition. Effector T cells develop following appropriate costimulation and release of polarizing cytokines in the environment which also activates macrophages [40].*

macrophages and serves as a negative regulator during T cell activation. This engagement can affect the positive signals between CD28 and CD80/CD86 and inhibit T cell activation [38].

Finally, simultaneous engagement of TCR-MHC–peptide complex and costimulatory molecules requires cytokines produced by macrophages, other cells as well as

T cells to effect cell activation. The activation of naïve CD4+ T cells by cytokines produces different subsets and dictates their functional outcome [39]. Th1 cells are produced by activation of CD4+ T cells with IL-12 and IFN-γ from APC (macrophages). Th1 cells secrete IFN-γ and TNF that activate macrophages to destroy pathogens and CD8+ T cells to combat infected cells. CD8+ T cells require cytokine signaling through IL-12 and type 1 IFN-α/β to maximize immune response. Effector CD8+ T cells kill infected cells through apoptosis by releasing perforin to act on membranes of the target cell and granzyme to enter and induce apoptosis (**Figure 1**) [41, 42].

6. Macrophages as a phagocytic cell

Macrophages defend the body against pathogens and play a key role in homeostasis through the removal of internal waste products and tissue repair. Phagocytosis, ingestion of large particles (>0.5 μm) into macrophages initiates the process of digestion and clearance. During phagocytosis, macrophages migrate in a chemotactic fashion toward the particles to be phagocytosed. Adhesion and particle uptake begin with the interaction of specific PRR with PAMPs or DAMPs of the particles or infected cells [6, 43]. Several PRRs have been identified to initiate phagocytosis upon recognition of PAMPs or DAMPs. These include scavenger receptor A (SR-A), c-type lectin receptors (dectin-1), and opsonin receptors (Fc receptor mainly immunoglobulin G (IgG) antibodies conserved domain, complement receptor 1 (CR1) and CR3) that binds to bacterial and fungal cell wall molecules [6, 43, 44]. The adhesion leads to polymerization of actin at the ingestion site, and the uptake through an actin-based technique [45, 46]. After absorption, F-actin is shed from the phagosome, and the newly formed phagosome matures through a series of fusion and fission events. The microbes and apoptotic cells are then destroyed by an oxygen-dependent or oxygen-independent killing mechanism.

The phagosomal NADPH-oxidase generates reactive oxygen species (ROS) and phospholipase A2 generates fatty acids for sterilization [47, 48]. Subsequently, myeloperoxidase (MPO), several hydrolases, and lysosomes fuse with the phagosome and deliver molecules that kill and degrade microbes. During this event, phagosomal pH is lowered by proton ATPase to activate an oxygen-dependent mechanism through halogenation or an oxygen-independent mechanism with lysosomal enzymes and basic sterilization proteins [49, 50]. Macrophages produce Fe2+ ions that bind with adenosine to substitute MPO.

7. The macrophage and complement system interaction

Macrophages and complement systems closely interact during which complement migrate in a chemotactic fashion and cover pathogens with C3b for efficient elimination through phagocytosis [51]. In human macrophages, a variety of complement components, including C1, C1q, C1s, C2, and C4 proteins, are expressed in the classical pathway; C3, factor B (FB) and factor D (FD) in the alternative pathway and C5 at the terminal pathway. Additionally, regulators such as factor H, factor P, factor I, and C1 inhibitor are secreted [52–55]. C2, C3, and FB are expressed, but C3 is upregulated if macrophages are stimulated with oxidized low-density lipoprotein, acetylated low-density lipoprotein, IgA or IgG immune complexes [56]. Complement regulators, such as CD46, CD55, and CD59, have been demonstrated to be expressed by cultured macrophages isolated from peripheral blood monocytes [57, 58]. Several complement receptors including the anaphylatoxin receptors C3aR, C5aR1, and C5aR2 [59–61] and the CR1, CR3, and CR4 have been found to be expressed on the surface of macrophages [62]. Complement immunoglobulin receptor (CRIg) an opsonin receptor is known to be expressed on several tissue-resident macrophages, such as Kupffer cells [63, 64].

8. Macrophage and infection

8.1 Bacterial infection

M1 macrophages have strong microbicidal and tumoricidal agents that promote resistance against bacterial toxins and destroy infected cells [65–67]. Pathogen-associated molecular patterns recognition by PRRs stimulates macrophages to secrete M1-like cytokines, including IFN-γ, TNF-α, IL-1, IL-6, and IL-12 [68]. These induce M1 polarization to promote prolonged production of ROS to kill invading microbes [7]. However, some intracellular bacteria promote the production of IL-4, IL-13, IL-10, and TGF-β to induce M2 phenotype polarization to reduce Th1 inflammatory response [69]. Mycobacterium tuberculosis (MTB) induces M2 phenotype by stimulating the production of IL-10 to inhibit the maturation of phagosomes and promote their survival [70, 71]. Alveolar macrophages have distinctive M2 phenotypic characteristics that promote the secretion of IL-10 and TGF-β with low oxidants and small antigen presentation capacity [72]. M1 promotes the potential bactericidal properties of macrophages during MTB infection and M2 the vice versa [73, 74]. Granulomatous macrophages within the lungs of MTB patients polarize to co-express proinflammatory and anti-inflammatory markers, signifying polarization is not binary and can occur continuously [75]. *Helicobacter(H) pylori*, induce M1 phenotype in patients with atrophic gastritis [76]. However, a mixture of M1/M2 phenotypes has been observed in the biopsy of the gastric mucosa in patients infected with *H. pylori* [77]. *Salmonella typhi*-infected patients have also demonstrated M1-like/M2-like phenotypic transition [78].

8.2 Viral infection

Viruses attack macrophages and polarize their activation during viral infections. Polarization is essential in reducing damage to tissues. M1 phenotype polarization is key in anti-viral immunity [79]. In acute and chronic human immunodeficiency (HIV) infection, M1 macrophages are crucial in early and late anti-viral immune responses. Additionally, macrophages infected with HIV are associated with the clearance of CD8+ T cells [79–82]. Hepatitis B virus (HBV) and hepatitis C virus (HCV) disease induce M2 phenotype [83, 84]. However, HCV suppressed monocyte polarization to M1-like or M2-like phenotype via TLR2. This leads to an impaired transducer and activator of the STAT pathway [85] or promotes a mixture of M1-like/M2-like cytokines [86]. Abnormal function of M1-like and M2-like phenotypes results in HCV infections. During human cytomegalovirus infection, infected monocytes are induced to promote M1-like/M2-like polarization in favor of M1 phenotype to upregulate IL-1, IL-6, and TNF-α secretion [87]. However, viral elimination is restricted in the late phase of the infection because of upregulated IL-10 secretion that promotes M2 phenotype activation [88]. M1 and M2 macrophages play crucial roles in both early and late viral infection. Therefore, therapies that can inhibit M1/M2 polarization will promote better clinical outcomes.

8.3 Parasitic infection

Macrophages undergo a shift toward M1 or M2 with respect to the causative agent. M1 phenotype promotes parasite clearance and resistance to leishmaniasis while M2 phenotype mediates the growth and survival of the parasite in the host [56, 58]. Th2-derived IL-4 and IL-13 mediate worm killing in granulomas and induce clearance by the contraction of smooth muscle [89–91]. M2 macrophages in hookworm disease suppress glucose absorption and function in various immune responses [69, 92]. M2-polarized macrophage in helminthic infection plays an important role in worm elimination but predisposes infected organs to cancer [89–91]. Protozoans, such as *Plasmodium, Toxoplasma, Leishmania,* and *Trypanosoma*, induce M1 macrophage phenotype that destroys the parasite to control the infection. M1 to M2 switch occurs partially to inhibit inflammatory-associated tissue damages but promotes chronic infection [9, 71, 89–91, 93–95].

8.4 Fungal infection

Disease-causing microbes induce a favorable environment inside their host to support proliferation, invasion, and survival of the microbes [96]. Activation of macrophage polarization is a mechanism used by the fungus to aid invasion and colonization of the host [96]. The macrophage polarization state of fungal pathogens within the lungs control disease progression or resolution [72]. M2-polarized macrophages possess a potent fungicidal effect against *Pneumocystis pneumonia*. M2 polarization inhibition can suppress the growth of *Aspergillus* and several fungal pulmonary diseases that result in allergic airway infection [96]. *Aspergillus fumigatus, Cryptococcus neoformans*, and *Histoplasma capsulatum* infections are favored by M1 polarized phenotypes [96]. *Candida albicans* induce an M1-like to M2-like phenotype to evade the host immune response [97].

9. Conclusions

Macrophages, other cells, and complement systems have overlapping and complementary potentials that are employed in a concerted first-line defense to fight infections. Macrophage-neutrophil co-operation aid each other to fight intracellular and extracellular pathogens, respectively. Macrophages play central roles in T cell activation by initiating a cascade of step-wise signals without which T cell apoptosis or anergy occurs. Macrophage activation is not fixed as they integrate many signals, such as those from microbes, dead cells, damaged and dying cells, and the normal tissue micro-environment to dictate phenotypes and direct the immune response. Different macrophage phenotypes have both protective and pathogenic decisive roles in a large array of infections. Therefore, appropriate activation of macrophages would aid effective immune response in curbing many infections developing to diseases.

Conflict of interest

The authors declare no conflict of interest.

Author details

Roland Osei Saahene[1], Precious Barnes[2] and Samuel Victor Nuvor[1]*

1 Department of Microbiology and Immunology, School of Medical Sciences, College of Health and Allied Sciences, University of Cape Coast, Cape Coast, Ghana

2 Department of Physician Assistant Studies, School of Allied Health Sciences, College of Health and Allied Sciences, University of Cape Coast, Cape Coast, Ghana

*Address all correspondence to: s.v.nuvor@uccsms.edu.gh

References

[1] Hume DA. The mononuclear phagocyte system. Current Opinion in Immunology. 2006;**18**:49-53

[2] Yona S, Kim K-W, Wolf Y, Mildner A, Varol D, Breker M, et al. Fate mapping reveals origins and dynamics of monocytes and tissue macrophages under homeostasis. Immunity. 2013;**38**:79-91

[3] Epelman S, Lavine KJ, Beaudin AE, Sojka DK, Carrero JA, Calderon B, et al. Embryonic and adult-derived resident cardiac macrophages are maintained through distinct mechanisms at steady state and during inflammation. Immunity. 2014;**40**:91-104

[4] Hashimoto D, Chow A, Noizat C, Teo P, Beasley MB, Leboeuf M, et al. Tissue-resident macrophages self-maintain locally throughout adult life with minimal contribution from circulating monocytes. Immunity. 2013;**38**:792-804

[5] Ginhoux F, Guilliams M. Tissue-resident macrophage ontogeny and homeostasis. Immunity. 2016;**44**: 439-449

[6] Fu YL, Harrison RE. Microbial phagocytic receptors and their potential involvement in cytokine induction in macrophages. Frontiers in Immunology. 2021;**12**:662063

[7] Shapouri-Moghaddam A, Mohammadian S, Vazini H, Taghadosi M, Esmaeili SA, Mardani F, et al. Macrophage plasticity, polarization, and function in health and disease. Journal of Cellular Physiology. 2018;**233**:6425-6440

[8] Balkwill F. Cancer and the chemokine network. Nature Reviews Cancer. 2004;**4**:540-550

[9] Mantovani A, Sica A, Sozzani S, Allavena P, Vecchi A, Locati M. The chemokine system in diverse forms of macrophage activation and polarization. Trends in Immunology. 2004;**25**:677-686

[10] Arnold CE, Gordon P, Barker RN, Wilson HM. The activation status of human macrophages presenting antigen determines the efficiency of Th17 responses. Immunobiology. 2015;**220**:10-19

[11] Persson YAZ, Blomgran-Julinder R, Rahman S, Zheng L, Stendahl O. Mycobacterium tuberculosis-induced apoptotic neutrophils trigger a pro-inflammatory response in macrophages through release of heat shock protein 72, acting in synergy with the bacteria. Microbes and Infection. 2008;**10**:233-240

[12] Veckman V, Miettinen M, Matikainen S, Lande R, Giacomini E, Coccia EM, et al. Lactobacilli and streptococci induce inflammatory chemokine production in human macrophages that stimulates Th1 cell chemotaxis. Journal of Leukocyte Biology. 2003;**74**:395-402

[13] Simon HU. Neutrophil apoptosis pathways and their modifications in inflammation. Immunological Reviews. 2003;**193**:101-110

[14] Colotta F, Re F, Polentarutti N, Sozzani S, Mantovani A. Modulation of granulocyte survival and programmed cell death by cytokines and bacterial products. Blood. 1992;**80**:2012-2020

[15] Dibbert B, Weber M, Nikolaizik WH, Vogt P, Schöni MH, Blaser K, et al. Cytokine-mediated Bax deficiency and consequent delayed neutrophil apoptosis: A general mechanism to accumulate

effector cells in inflammation. Proceedings of the National Academy of Sciences. 1999;**96**:13330-13335

[16] Ward C, Dransfield I, Chilvers ER, Haslett C, Rossi AG. Pharmacological manipulation of granulocyte apoptosis: Potential therapeutic targets. Trends in Pharmacological Sciences. 1999;**20**:503-509

[17] Savill JS, Wyllie AH, Henson JE, Walport MJ, Henson PM, Haslett C. Macrophage phagocytosis of aging neutrophils in inflammation. Programmed cell death in the neutrophil leads to its recognition by macrophages, The Journal of clinical investigation. 1989;**83**:865-875

[18] Silva MT, Silva MN, Appelberg R. Neutrophil-macrophage cooperation in the host defence against mycobacterial infections. Microbial Pathogenesis. 1989;**6**:369-380

[19] Scott HM, Flynn JL. Mycobacterium tuberculosis in chemokine receptor 2-deficient mice: Influence of dose on disease progression. Infection and Immunity. 2002;**70**:5946-5954

[20] Gonzalez-Juarrero M, Shim TS, Kipnis A, Junqueira-Kipnis AP, Orme IM. Dynamics of macrophage cell populations during murine pulmonary tuberculosis. The Journal of Immunology. 2003;**171**:3128-3135

[21] Tsai MC, Chakravarty S, Zhu G, Xu J, Tanaka K, Koch C, et al. Characterization of the tuberculous granuloma in murine and human lungs: Cellular composition and relative tissue oxygen tension. Cellular Microbiology. 2006;**8**:218-232

[22] Torrado E, Fraga AG, Castro AG, Stragier P, Meyers WM, Portaels F, et al. Evidence for an intramacrophage growth phase of mycobacterium ulcerans. Infection and Immunity. 2007;**75**: 977-987

[23] Altimira J, Prats N, Lopez S, Domingo M, Briones V, Dominguez L, et al. Repeated Oral dosing withListeria monocytogenesin mice as a model of central nervous system listeriosis in man. Journal of Comparative Pathology. 1999;**121**:117-125

[24] Tam MA, Rydström A, Sundquist M, Wick MJ. Early cellular responses to salmonella infection: Dendritic cells, monocytes, and more. Immunological Reviews. 2008;**225**:140-162

[25] Brieland J, Freeman P, Kunkel R, Chrisp C, Hurley M, Fantone J, et al. Replicative legionella pneumophila lung infection in intratracheally inoculated a/J mice. A murine model of human Legionnaires' disease, The American journal of pathology. 1994;**145**:1537

[26] Tournay C, Courtoy J, Marodi L, Totté P, Jacquet A, Garcia-Quintana L, et al. Uptake of recombinant myeloperoxidase, free or fused to fc, by macrophage enhances killing activity toward micro-organisms. DNA and Cell Biology. 1996;**15**:617-624

[27] Maródi L, Tournay C, Káposzta R, Johnston RB Jr, Moguilevsky N. Augmentation of human macrophage candidacidal capacity by recombinant human myeloperoxidase and granulocytemacrophage colony-stimulating factor. Infection and Immunity. 1998;**66**:2750-2754

[28] Couto MA, Liu L, Lehrer RI, Ganz T. Inhibition of intracellular histoplasma capsulatum replication by murine macrophages that produce human defensin. Infection and Immunity. 1994;**62**:2375-2378

[29] Lima M, Kierszenbaum F. Lactoferrin effects on phagocytic cell function. I. Increased uptake and killing of an intracellular parasite by murine macrophages and human monocytes. The Journal of Immunology. 1985;**134**:4176-4183

[30] Xu Y, Liu Y, Yang C, Kang L, Wang M, Hu J, et al. Macrophages transfer antigens to dendritic cells by releasing exosomes containing dead-cell-associated antigens partially through a ceramide-dependent pathway to enhance CD 4+ T-cell responses. Immunology. 2016;**149**:157-171

[31] Miyake K, Karasuyama H. Emerging roles of basophils in allergic inflammation. Allergology International. 2017;**66**:382-391

[32] Cohen M, Giladi A, Gorki A-D, Solodkin DG, Zada M, Hladik A, et al. Lung single-cell signaling interaction map reveals basophil role in macrophage imprinting. Cell. 2018;**175**:1031-1044.e1018

[33] Smith-Garvin JE, Koretzky GA, Jordan MS. T cell activation. Annual Review of Immunology. 2009;**27**:591-619

[34] Nakayama T, Yamashita M. The TCR-mediated signaling pathways that control the direction of helper T cell differentiation, in. Seminars in Immunology. 2010;**22**:303-309

[35] Boise LH, González-García M, Postema CE, Ding L, Lindsten T, Turka LA, et al. Bcl-x, a bcl-2-related gene that functions as a dominant regulator of apoptotic cell death. Cell. 1993;**74**:597-608

[36] Cho H, Kang H, Lee HH, Kim CW. Programmed cell death 1 (PD-1) and cytotoxic T lymphocyte-associated antigen 4 (CTLA-4) in viral hepatitis. International Journal of Molecular Sciences. 2017;**18**:1517

[37] Chen L, Flies DB. Molecular mechanisms of T cell co-stimulation and co-inhibition. Nature Reviews Immunology. 2013;**13**:227-242

[38] Sharpe AH, Pauken KE. The diverse functions of the PD1 inhibitory pathway. Nature Reviews Immunology. 2018;**18**:153-167

[39] Swain SL, McKinstry KK, Strutt TM. Expanding roles for CD4+ T cells in immunity to viruses. Nature Reviews Immunology. 2012;**12**:136-148

[40] Guerriero JL. Macrophages: Their untold story in T cell activation and function. International Review of Cell and Molecular Biology. 2019;**342**:73-93

[41] Afonina IS, Cullen SP, Martin SJ. Cytotoxic and non-cytotoxic roles of the CTL/NK protease granzyme B. Immunological Reviews. 2010;**235**:105-116

[42] Thiery J, Lieberman J. Perforin: A key pore-forming protein for immune control of viruses and cancer, MACPF/CDC Proteins-Agents of Defence, Attack and Invasion. Sub-cellular Biochemistry. 2014;**80**:197-220

[43] Rosales C, Uribe-Querol E. Phagocytosis: A fundamental process in immunity. BioMed Research International. 2017;**2017**:9042851

[44] Kumar V. Phagocytosis: Phenotypically simple yet a mechanistically complex process: Phagocytosis is a very complex but crucial process playing a pivotal role in embryonic development and host defense to maintain immune homeostasis.

International Reviews of Immunology. 2020;**39**:118-150

[45] Rosales C. Fc receptor and integrin signaling in phagocytes. Signal Transduction. 2007;7:386-401

[46] Bajno L, Peng X-R, Schreiber AD, Moore H-P, Trimble WS, Grinstein S. Focal exocytosis of VAMP3-containing vesicles at sites of phagosome formation. The Journal of Cell Biology. 2000;**149**:697-706

[47] Roos D. The involvement of oxygen radicals in microbicidal mechanisms of leukocytes and macrophages. Klinische Wochenschrift. 1991;**69**:975-980

[48] Akaki T, Sato K, Shimizu T, Sano C, Kajitani H, Dekio S, et al. Effector molecules in expression of the antimicrobial activity of macrophages against Mycobacterium avium complex: Roles of reactive nitrogen intermediates, reactive oxygen intermediates, and free fatty acids. Journal of Leukocyte Biology. 1997;**62**:795-804

[49] Klebanoff SJ. Myeloperoxidase-halide-hydrogen peroxide antibacterial system. Journal of Bacteriology. 1968;**95**:2131-2138

[50] Hiemstra P. Defensins and cathelicidins in inflammatory lung disease: Beyond antimicrobial activity. Biochemical Society Transactions. 2006;**34**:276-278

[51] Bohlson SS, O'Conner SD, Hulsebus HJ, Ho M-M, Fraser DA. Complement, c1q, and c1q-related molecules regulate macrophage polarization. Frontiers in Immunology. 2014;**5**:402

[52] Cole FS, Matthews W, Marino JT, Gash DJ, Colten HR. Control of complement synthesis and secretion in bronchoalveolar and peritoneal macrophages. The Journal of Immunology. 1980;**125**:1120-1124

[53] Hartung H, Hadding U. Synthesis of complement by macrophages and modulation of their functions through complement activation. Seminars in Immunopathology. 1983;**6**:283-326

[54] De Ceulaer C, Papazoglou S, Whaley K. Increased biosynthesis of complement components by cultured monocytes, synovial fluid macrophages and skynovial membrane cells from patients with rheumatoid arthritis. Immunology. 1980;**41**:37

[55] Rabs U, Martin H, Hitschold T, Golan MD, Heinz HP, Loos M. Isolation and characterization of maerophage-derived C1q and its similarities to serum C1q. European Journal of Immunology. 1986;**16**:1183-1186

[56] Laufer J, Boichis H, Farzam N, Passwell J. IgA and IgG immune complexes increase human macrophage C3 biosynthesis. Immunology. 1995;**84**:207

[57] van Kooten C, Fiore N, Trouw LA, Csomor E, Xu W, Castellano G, et al. Complement production and regulation by dendritic cells: Molecular switches between tolerance and immunity. Molecular Immunology. 2008;**45**:4064-4072

[58] Kurita-Taniguchi M, Hazeki K, Murabayashi N, Fukui A, Tsuji S, Matsumoto M, et al. Molecular assembly of CD46 with CD9, alpha3–beta1 integrin and protein tyrosine phosphatase SHP-1 in human macrophages through differentiation by GM-CSF. Molecular Immunology. 2002;**38**:689-700

[59] Wetsel RA. Structure, function and cellular expression of complement

anaphylatoxin receptors. Current Opinion in Immunology. 1995;**7**:48-53

[60] Gasque P, Singhrao SK, Neal JW, Wang P, Sayah S, Fontaine M, et al. The receptor for complement anaphylatoxin C3a is expressed by myeloid cells and nonmyeloid cells in inflamed human central nervous system: Analysis in multiple sclerosis and bacterial meningitis. The Journal of Immunology. 1998;**160**:3543-3554

[61] Vijayan S, Asare Y, Grommes J, Soehnlein O, Lutgens E, Shagdarsuren G, et al. High expression of C5L2 correlates with high proinflammatory cytokine expression in advanced human atherosclerotic plaques. The American Journal of Pathology. 2014;**184**:2123-2133

[62] Merle NS, Church SE, Fremeaux-Bacchi V, Roumenina LT. Complement system part I–molecular mechanisms of activation and regulation. Frontiers in Immunology. 2015;**6**:262

[63] Helmy KY, Katschke KJ Jr, Gorgani NN, Kljavin NM, Elliott JM, Diehl L, et al. Van Lookeren Campagne, CRIg: A macrophage complement receptor required for phagocytosis of circulating pathogens. Cell. 2006;**124**:915-927

[64] He JQ, Wiesmann C, van Lookeren Campagne M. A role of macrophage complement receptor CRIg in immune clearance and inflammation. Molecular Immunology. 2008;**45**:4041-4047

[65] Mège J-L, Mehraj V, Capo C. Macrophage polarization and bacterial infections. Current Opinion in Infectious Diseases. 2011;**24**:230-234

[66] Patel U, Rajasingh S, Samanta S, Cao T, Dawn B, Rajasingh J. Macrophage polarization in response to epigenetic modifiers during infection and inflammation. Drug Discovery Today. 2017;**22**:186-193

[67] Weiss G, Schaible UE. Macrophage defense mechanisms against intracellular bacteria. Immunological Reviews. 2015;**264**:182-203

[68] Atri C, Guerfali FZ, Laouini D. Role of human macrophage polarization in inflammation during infectious diseases. International Journal of Molecular Sciences. 2018;**19**:1801

[69] Biswas SK, Mantovani A. Orchestration of metabolism by macrophages. Cell Metabolism. 2012;**15**:432-437

[70] Kaufmann SH. Immunopathology of mycobacterial diseases. Seminars in Immunopathology. 2016;**38**:135-138

[71] Moraco AH, Kornfeld H. Cell death and autophagy in tuberculosis. Seminars in Immunology. 2014;**26**:497-511

[72] Divangahi M, King IL, Pernet E. Alveolar macrophages and type I IFN in airway homeostasis and immunity. Trends in Immunology. 2015;**36**:307-314

[73] Huang Z, Luo Q, Guo Y, Chen J, Xiong G, Peng Y, et al. Mycobacterium tuberculosis-induced polarization of human macrophage orchestrates the formation and development of tuberculous granulomas in vitro. PLoS One. 2015;**10**:e0129744

[74] Marino S, Cilfone NA, Mattila JT, Linderman JJ, Flynn JL, Kirschner DE. Macrophage polarization drives granuloma outcome during mycobacterium tuberculosis infection. Infection and Immunity. 2015;**83**:324-338

[75] Mattila JT, Ojo OO, Kepka-Lenhart D, Marino S, Kim JH, Eum SY, et al. Microenvironments in tuberculous

granulomas are delineated by distinct populations of macrophage subsets and expression of nitric oxide synthase and arginase isoforms. The Journal of Immunology. 2013;**191**:773-784

[76] Quiding-Järbrink M, Raghavan S, Sundquist M. Enhanced M1 macrophage polarization in human helicobacter pylori-associated atrophic gastritis and in vaccinated mice. PLoS One. 2010;**5**:e15018

[77] Fehlings M, Drobbe L, Moos V, Renner Viveros P, Hagen J, Beigier-Bompadre M, et al. Comparative analysis of the interaction of helicobacter pylori with human dendritic cells, macrophages, and monocytes. Infection and Immunity. 2012;**80**:2724-2734

[78] Thompson LJ, Dunstan SJ, Dolecek C, Perkins T, House D, Dougan G, et al. Transcriptional response in the peripheral blood of patients infected with salmonella enterica serovar typhi. Proceedings of the National Academy of Sciences. 2009;**106**:22433-22438

[79] Burdo TH, Walker J, Williams KC. Macrophage polarization in AIDS: Dynamic interface between anti-viral and anti-inflammatory macrophages during acute and chronic infection. J. Clin. Cell. Immunol. 2015;**6**:4612489

[80] Alfano M, Graziano F, Genovese L, Poli G. Macrophage polarization at the crossroad between HIV-1 infection and cancer development. Arteriosclerosis, Thrombosis, and Vascular Biology. 2013;**33**:1145-1152

[81] Cassol E, Cassetta L, Alfano M, Poli G. Macrophage polarization and HIV-1 infection. Journal of Leukocyte Biology. 2010;**87**:599-608

[82] Shi C, Pamer EG. Monocyte recruitment during infection and inflammation. Nature Reviews Immunology. 2011;**11**:762-774

[83] Brockman MA, Kwon DS, Tighe DP, Pavlik DF, Rosato PC, Sela J, et al. IL-10 is up-regulated in multiple cell types during viremic HIV infection and reversibly inhibits virus-specific T cells, blood, the journal of the American society of. Hematology. 2009;**114**:346-356

[84] Flynn JK, Dore GJ, Hellard M, Yeung B, Rawlinson WD, White PA, et al. Early IL-10 predominant responses are associated with progression to chronic hepatitis C virus infection in injecting drug users. Journal of Viral Hepatitis. 2011;**18**:549-561

[85] Zhang Q, Wang Y, Zhai N, Song H, Li H, Yang Y, et al. HCV core protein inhibits polarization and activity of both M1 and M2 macrophages through the TLR2 signaling pathway. Scientific Reports. 2016;**6**:1-12

[86] Saha B, Kodys K, Szabo G. Hepatitis C virus-induced monocyte differentiation into polarized M2 macrophages promotes stellate cell activation via TGF-β. Cellular and Molecular Gastroenterology and Hepatology. 2016;**2**:302-316.e308

[87] Chan G, Nogalski MT, Yurochko AD. Human cytomegalovirus stimulates monocyte-to-macrophage differentiation via the temporal regulation of caspase 3. Journal of Virology. 2012;**86**:10714-10723

[88] Avdic S, Cao JZ, McSharry BP, Clancy LE, Brown R, Steain M, et al. Human cytomegalovirus interleukin-10 polarizes monocytes toward a deactivated M2c phenotype to repress host immune responses. Journal of Virology. 2013;**87**:10273-10282

[89] Martinez FO, Helming L, Gordon S. Alternative activation of macrophages:

An immunologic functional perspective. Annual Review of Immunology. 2009;**27**: 451-483

[90] Nair MG, Herbert DBR. Immune polarization by hookworms: Taking cues from T helper type 2, type 2 innate lymphoid cells and alternatively activated macrophages. Immunology. 2016;**148**:115-124

[91] Tundup S, Srivastava L, Harn J. Donald a, polarization of host immune responses by helminth-expressed glycans. Annals of the New York Academy of Sciences. 2012;**1253**: E1-E13

[92] Lackey DE, Olefsky JM. Regulation of metabolism by the innate immune system, nature reviews. Endocrinology. 2016;**12**:15-28

[93] Chua CLL, Brown G, Hamilton JA, Rogerson S, Boeuf P. Monocytes and macrophages in malaria: Protection or pathology? Trends in Parasitology. 2013;**29**:26-34

[94] Beschin A, De Baetselier P, Van Ginderachter JA. Contribution of myeloid cell subsets to liver fibrosis in parasite infection. The Journal of Pathology. 2013;**229**:186-197

[95] Mantovani A, Biswas SK, Galdiero MR, Sica A, Locati M. Macrophage plasticity and polarization in tissue repair and remodelling. The Journal of Pathology. 2013;**229**:176-185

[96] Wager CL, Wormley F. Classical versus alternative macrophage activation: The Ying and the Yang in host defense against pulmonary fungal infections. Mucosal Immunology. 2014;**7**:1023-1035

[97] Wagener J, MacCallum DM, Brown GD, Gow NA. Candida albicans chitin increases arginase-1 activity in human macrophages, with an impact on macrophage antimicrobial functions. MBio. 2017;**8**:e01820-e01816

Chapter 4

Lung Macrophages: Pivotal Immune Effector Cells Orchestrating Acute and Chronic Lung Diseases

Stephan F. van Eeden and Don D. Sin

Abstract

Macrophages are key immune cells, where they play a pivotal role in host defense and tissue homeostasis. The lungs have two major subsets, alveolar macrophages (AMs) found in airspaces and interstitial macrophages (IMs) found in lung tissues. Lung macrophages (LM) are highly heterogeneous and have high levels of plasticity. A long-lasting population of LM with self-renewal ability populate the lung during embryogenesis and monocyte-derived macrophages recruited during infection, inflammation, or tissue repair, which are more short lived. AMs have been the main focus of research due in part to their abundance, accessibility, and ease of isolation compared with IMs. With advances in multichannel flow cytometry and single-cell sequencing, the importance of IMs has been recently appreciated. LM's functions in the lungs include maintenance of homoeostasis, immune surveillance, removal of cellular debris, tissue repair, clearance of pathogens, and the resolution of inflammation. They also activate the adaptive immune response by functioning as antigen-presenting cells. LMs are pivotal in the pathogenesis of acute and chronic inflammatory lung conditions including lung cancer. This chapter will discuss the ontology, phenotypic heterogeneity, and functions of LM's and how these characteristics orchestrate and impact common acute and chronic lung conditions.

Keywords: alveolar macrophages, interstitial macrophages, macrophage phenotypes, lung infections, asthma, lung cancer, lung fibrosis

1. Introduction

Macrophages are immune effector cells that are present in most organs and tissues, are highly phagocytic in nature and produce large amounts of a wide variety of mediators. They are either resident in tissues or are recruited and as part of the innate immune effector system, are activated to mount an appropriate immune response to neutralize harmful insults [1].

The lungs are continuously challenged by a variety of foreign inhaled substances which include allergens, microbial pathogens, chemicals, particulates matter and noxious gasses. These insults require an exquisite capacity to appropriately calibrate inflammatory responses in the airways and lung tissues to maintain physiologic homeostasis (e.g., gas exchange). The lung macrophages have all the properties to orchestrate and calibrate such inflammatory responses given their location in the lungs, their large abundance in tissue and their high degree of functional plasticity and ability to communicate with neighboring cells. Research over the past three decades has shed light on the origins of lung macrophages, their ability to adapt to the local microenvironment, their plasticity, and their functional responses to maintain tissue homeostasis. In addition, their pivotal role in orchestrating the innate immune response and activating adaptive immunity when airways are challenged with pathogenic insults has also been elucidated [1, 2].

1.1 Macrophage populations in the lung

Two well-studied populations of lung macrophages have been defined: (1) alveolar macrophages (AMs), which are predominantly located on alveolar epithelial surfaces and can be harvested from the lungs by bronchoalveolar lavage (BAL) and (2) interstitial macrophages (IMs), which are located within alveolar walls or interstitial lung tissue and can be harvested directly from lung tissue specimens through biopsy or surgical resections [3]. Two less well-defined populations of macrophages are airway macrophages, which are found on mucosal surfaces of the airways and intravascular macrophages, which reside on capillary blood vessel walls. Limited data suggest that airway macrophages are phenotypically and functionally very similar to AMs and may represent AMs that have migrated up the tracheobronchial tree [4]. Airway macrophages are usually grouped with AMs because of their phenotypic similarity and their ability to be captured by BAL. The intravascular macrophages are located on the inner side of capillaries, suggesting that they fight against blood-borne pathogens. Limited (older) data suggest that their function is comparable to that of AMs and that they may reflect an intermediate stage of differentiation between blood monocytes and AMs [5, 6].

It was previously thought that resident lung macrophages originate primarily from blood monocytes, which are produced and released from the bone marrow [7, 8]. The last decade this paradigm has been turned on its head as research has shown that most resident macrophages in different tissues throughout the body, including lung macrophages, arise predominantly from embryonic precursors. These macrophages are produced before birth, become colonized in the lungs in the prenatal period and are maintained throughout life by local proliferation [9–11]. Resident alveolar macrophages originate as erythromyeloid progenitors (EMPs) in the yolk sac on embryonic day (E) 8.5. EMPs colonize the fetal liver by E10.5, and then give rise to fetal monocytes, which migrate to the lungs by E12.5 [12]. The maturation of fetal monocytes to alveolar macrophages occurs in the presence of granulocyte-monocyte colony stimulating factor (GM-CSF) and is fully completed by the third postnatal day (**Figure 1**).

These resident lung macrophages are the primary "janitors" of the lung, protecting the lungs from inhaled environmental insults. In contrast to resident alveolar macrophages, recruited monocytes, which enter airspaces 24-72 hrs after the onset of an inflammatory stimulus in the lung, differentiate into macrophages in the tissues where they initially take on a pro-inflammatory phenotype (by promoting inflammation) and later assumes a regulatory role by suppressing the inflammatory process. Classically, the initial phenotype has been described as M1 macrophages and the regulatory phenotype as M2 macrophages.

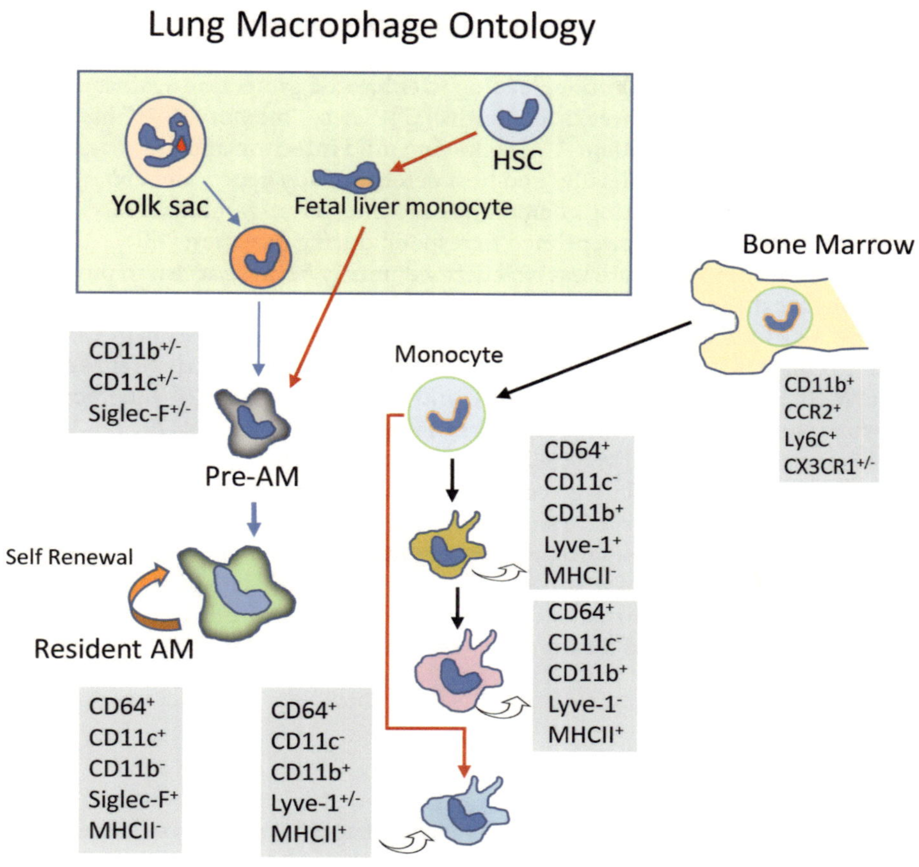

Figure 1.
The origin of alveolar (AM) and interstitial (IM) macrophages in mice. Resident AMs, derived from the embryo (yolk sac and/orfetal liver), are capable of self-replicating during homeostasis and when challenge in lung. IMs are derived from bone marrow monocytes and there are three unique IMs in murine lung in homeostasis: IM1, IM2 and IM3 (Gibbings et al.). During steady state, the maintenance of AM pool does not need the contribution of bone marrow -derived monocytes, but in the circumstance of inflammation, monocytes are strongly recruited to areas of inflammatory alveoli and differentiated into recruited monocyte-derived AMs. IM3 are originated from BM-derived monocytes and play different roles in diseases such as pulmonary fibrosis (Chakarov et al.).

While M1 macrophages promote inflammation, M2 macrophages induce efferocytosis (phagocytosis of apoptotic and dead cells) to enable inflammatory clearance, and secrete anti-inflammatory cytokines such as IL-10 and soluble (decoy) IL-1R [13].

Studies in animal models have shown that resident AMs can be replaced by IMs or be derived from circulating monocytes [8, 14, 15], underlining the adaptability of macrophage kinetics and function. Schneider and co-workers have shown that the nuclear receptor peroxisome proliferator-activated receptor gamma (PPAR-γ) is essential for the differentiation of AMs and that PPAR-γ deletion in the myeloid lineage cells prevents the formation of mature AMs, resulting in impaired microbial clearance and development of a clinical condition called pulmonary alveolar proteinosis, which is characterized by excess surfactant accumulation in lungs [16]. PPAR-γ expression requires GM-CSF, which is produced largely by type II alveolar epithelial cells. A lack of GM-CSF leads to a loss of mature AMs, accumulation of surfactant and ultimately alveolar proteinosis [9]. Recently the interesting concept of innate immune memory resulting from resetting of the cell's epigenetic program and functional state after infection, leading to enhanced protection against a secondary infection in the ensuing weeks to months [17]. These "memory AMs" have been shown to originate from resident AMs following mild infection and are characterized by a high level of MHCII molecules and host defense-ready genes, and enhanced production of neutrophil attracting chemokines and interferon-gamma (IFN-γ) derived from effector T cells, which are primed to respond during infection [18].

Interstitial macrophages are less well defined mostly because access to pure populations are difficult in humans. Studies in laboratory animals suggest that there are at least 3 different populations of IM: IM1, IM2 and IM3. Expression of CD11c and MHCII on IMs at a steady state classifies these population into three subsets, IM1 ($CD11c^{lo}MHCII^{lo}$), IM2 ($CD11c^{lo}MHCII^{hi}$), and IM3 ($CD11c^{hi}MHCII^{hi}$) in mice [19]. At least two of these three populations have been identified in humans [20, 21]. Whether these IMs are resident, long lived cells possessing self-renewal properties similar to resident AMs, or represent derived cells from blood monocytes is still unclear.

Macrophages in the lungs have a range of function, including maintenance of homeostasis, immune surveillance, repair, removal of cellular debris and surfactant clearance, and elimination of microbes, allergens and particulate matter, and resolution of inflammation. These distinct functions are linked to the different subsets of macrophages, ontogeny, and location of the macrophages and influence of the local microenvironment.

2. Macrophage phenotypes

Similar to T helper 1/2 (Th1/Th2) cells, macrophages are categorized as either classically activated M1 macrophages or alternatively activated M2 macrophages. The classical or M1 macrophages are activated by microbial products and/or IFN-γ. MI cells are pro-inflammatory and possess anti-microbial functions, and ability destroy tumor cells [22]. Signal transducer and activator of transcription 1 (STAT1), interferon regulatory factor (IRF)3, IRF5, and nuclear factor-κβ (NF-κβ) are key molecules that become activated in M1 macrophages to generate pro-inflammatory mediators such as tumor necrosis factor-α (TNF-α), Interleukin-1 (IL-1), IL- 12 and IL- 23, [23], nitric oxide (NO), and reactive oxygen intermediates (ROI). They also promote increased expression of major histocompatibility complex (MHC) molecules (**Figure 2**). Over the inflammatory period, the microenvironment changes and Th2 cytokines, including IL- 4 and IL- 13, stimulate monocytes or macrophages to transform into a M2 phenotype. M2 macrophages promote resolution of the inflammatory process and stimulate wound healing, favoring a milieu of angiogenesis and tissue remodeling. IL-10, glucocorticoid hormones and IL-1R may also induce M2 macrophage polarization.

The M2 macrophage phenotype is not homogenous and consists of several subtypes including M2a, M2b, M2c and M2d (**Figure 3**). The M2a macrophages are produced by exposure to cytokine such as IL-4 or IL-13. They can also be induced by fungal and helminth infections. They are characterized by expression of high levels of the mannose receptor (CD 206), CD209, IL-4R and FcεR, secreting transforming growth factor β1 (TGF-β1) and insulin-like growth factor. Functionally M2a macrophages contribute towards wound healing and tissue repair [24]. In contrast,

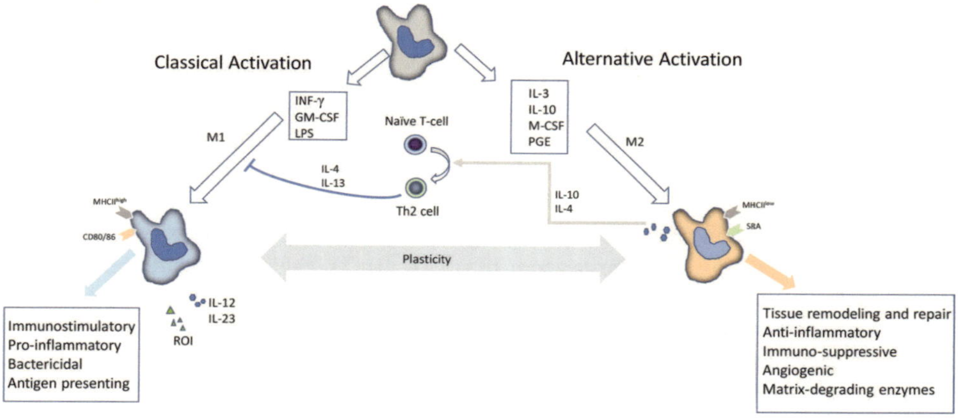

Figure 2.
Paradigm of macrophage phenotypes. Naïve macrophages are activated to either a M1 phenotype (classical activation) or to M2 phenotype (alternatively activated) dependent on their microenvironment milieau. Macrophages are polarized to an M1 (or T-helper type 1 cell [Th1]) phenotype in response to IFN-g, granulocyte–macrophage colony–stimulating factor (GM-CSF), and bacterial products (e.g., LPS). They are characterized by a high production of the proinflammatory cytokines IL-12 and IL-23, and with high expression of major histocompatibility complex class II (MHCII) molecules and coactivation proteins (CD80 and CD86) are considered excellent antigen-presenting cells that can activate an adaptive immune response and fight foreign insults through the production of toxic intermediates such as reactive oxygen intermediates [ROI]). Macrophages are polarized to an M2 (or Th2) phenotype in response to macrophage colony–stimulating factor (M-CSF), IL-3 and IL-10 and antiinflammatoryfactors. They produce a variety of antiinflammatorycytokines, immunosuppressive mediators, and matrix-degrading enzymes, and promote angiogenesis and are involved in tissue remodeling and repair.

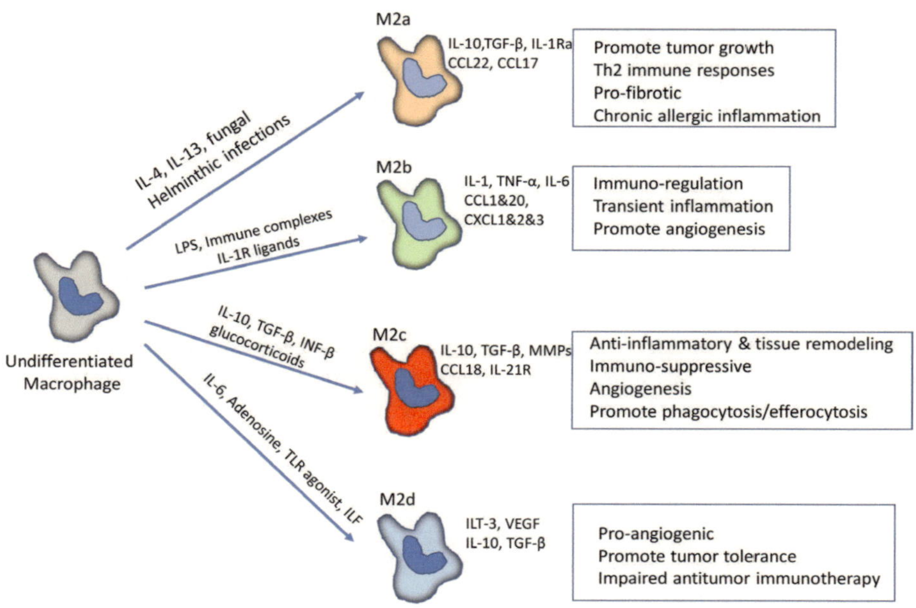

Figure 3.
Different M2 macrophage phenotypes are generated by different microenvironments and stimuli. The functional responses of the four different M2 sub-phenotypes are determine by them producing different mediators.

M2b macrophages are induced by immune complexes, IL-1β and lipopolysaccharide (LPS) exposure, and secrete abundance of IL-10, IL-1β, IL-6 and TNF-α, that have predominantly anti-inflammatory properties [25]. The M2c macrophages are induced cytokines such as IL-10, TGF-β and glucocorticoids and have increased expression of receptor for advance glycation and end products (RAGE), CD163 and CD206. M2c macrophages are thought to be involved in immunosuppression, tissue repair and matrix remodeling [26, 27]. Lastly, M2d macrophages, are activated by leukocyte inhibitory factor, toll like receptor (TLR) ligands and adenosine. They express low levels of CD206, and produce large amounts of IL-10, TGF-β and vascular endothelial growth factor (VEGF) which facilitate immunosuppression and angiogenesis [28].

A unique characteristic of macrophages is their plasticity and their ability to differentiate into several phenotypes and also to de-differentiate. For example, M2 macrophages may revert to M1 macrophages under certain conditions. This switch in polarization is dynamic and induced predominantly by their microenvironment. The distinct M1 and M2 subtypes is an overly simplification of macrophage polarization, for example, 5% of the macrophages in lung cancer specimens express both M1 and M2 markers [29], and mixed macrophage polarization have been described in other lung conditions [29, 30]. With the advent of genetic analysis and specifically single cell RNA sequencing technology, the basic macrophage characterization of M1 and M2 phenotypes has been challenged and may change in the near future [31].

3. Macrophages in lung infections

Airspace or resident AMs represent the first line of defense and play a central role in protecting the lungs against a range of respiratory pathogens. Yet, pulmonary immune responses need to be contained and refined to avoid excessive tissue damage and safeguard gas exchange. Resident AMs (ResAM) are less responsive than recruited monocyte-derived macrophages in the context of infection in the lung [32]. As resident AMs are predominantly involved in lung tissue homeostasis, resident AMs are generally "anti-inflammatory", which in part is linked to their production of type I interferons (IFNs) [33]. Notably Type I IFNs negatively regulate IL-1 production and positively regulate IL-10 production in monocyte-derived macrophages [34]. AMs have low expression of complement-associated genes such as *C1qa*, *C1qb*, *C1qc*, *C2*, *C4b* and *C3ar1* [19], in contrast to macrophages isolated from other tissues. Epigenetic profiling of AMs during inflammation has shown that while the *C1q* locus is inaccessible in ResAMs, complement genes are highly accessible in inflammatory AMs (InfResAMs) that arise in the AM pool during influenza infection [35]. With human SARS-CoV-2 infection, recruited macrophages were more $C1q^{hi}$ compared with the ResAMs, which were more $C1q^{lo}$, suggesting that repression of the complement-associated genes in ResAMs is conserved in humans [36]. Importantly, the overt activation of complements has been linked to coronavirus 2019 (COVID-19) severity [37, 38]. It is reasonable to suggest that the sharp drop in ResAMs and their replacement by recruited macrophages expressing high levels of the complement-associated genes during SARS-CoV-2 infection may fuel the complement cascade and actively participate in the COVID-19 pathogenesis. Furthermore, it could be that repression of these complement genes in ResAMs is the result of evolutionary pressure to protect the lungs from complement-mediated collateral damage during infections.

Kinetic studies have shown that bone marrow derived monocytes are recruited into alveolar space within 24 hrs following a focal instillation of *Streptococcus pneumoniae* into the lung [15]. These monocyte derived macrophages become the dominant immune cells in the airspaces during the resolution phase of pneumonia. Bacteria have developed strategies to take advantage of hypo-responsive ResAMs by enhancing their survival and promoting spread [39]. An example of this concept is the relocation of *Mycobacterium tuberculosis*-infected AMs into pulmonary tissues, which is a pivotal preparatory step for bacterial dissemination in the host [40]. Furthermore, following viral infection such as influenza, the resident AM population are depleted and subsequently restored by monocyte recruitment from the bloodstream which differentiate into long-lived InfResAMs and partially replace the resident AM [41, 42]. These newly recruited monocytes replace the resident macrophages and the extend of this replacement is linked to the dose and/or virulence of the pathogen. The reduction of resident macrophages by viral infections renders the host more susceptible to other microbial infections until the resident macrophages recover their numbers via self-renewal [43]. InfResAMs that develop during a viral infection have been shown to differ functionally from the ResAMs that were present before the infection [16, 42]. For example, InfResAMs that developed during influenza infection are more responsive to TLR ligands and subsequent *S. pneumoniae* infection compared with ResAMs. The InfResAMs acquired innate memory qualities via enhanced IL-6 production that provides protection against subsequent bacterial infections such as *S. pneumoniae* infection. Comparing the epigenetic signature of these ResAMs and InfResAMs shows that monocytes recruited by the virus infection have an epigenetic profile similar to tissue residency, but addition also acquire a more inflammatory signature induced by the viral infection. For example, the IL-6 enhancer regions are more accessible in InfResAMs that are recruited during an influenza lung infection compared with ResAMs. This altered epigenetic signature is still evident 1 month after the viral infection but started to alter at 2 months post-infection (**Figure 4**).

Long-term memory cells, which are characterized by altered gene expression, metabolism and antimicrobial responsiveness, have been proposed as a subset of ResAMs [44]. These cells have reduced phagocytic capacity by over-expressing signal regulatory protein α [45]. Similarly, InfResAMs that develop during an infection can acquire innate memory, thus altering their responses to subsequent infections. However, these InfResMacs show increased epigenetic plasticity. Much less is known about the impact of viral infections on resident IMs and their plasticity after an infectious insult. These cells have a significantly shorter half-life compared with ResAMs and robust fate-mapping systems have not been developed for IM.

Our ability to separate lung ResMacs from InfResMacs has shown that InfResMacs are more strongly imprinted across a range of infectious stimuli. This imprinting has the capacity to generate long-lasting innate immune memory cells that alter macrophage function during subsequent challenges. Multiple lung infectious challenges may therefore allow the engraftment of many waves of InfResMacs into lungs. However, over time and in a steady state, InfResMac may lose their unique genetic or epigenetic signature, leading to a loss in memory. Recurrent infections or inflammatory stimuli, on the other hand, could revive the memory of these InfResMacs. Innate memory in InfResMacs may be beneficial in some cases and may confer resistance to subsequent infections, but could also exacerbate tissue inflammation and injury during subsequent infections [46]. This has been proposed as a potential reason for the difference in severity of Covid-19 infection in older versus younger subjects and the generally mild inflammatory response seen in children. Therefore, the duration

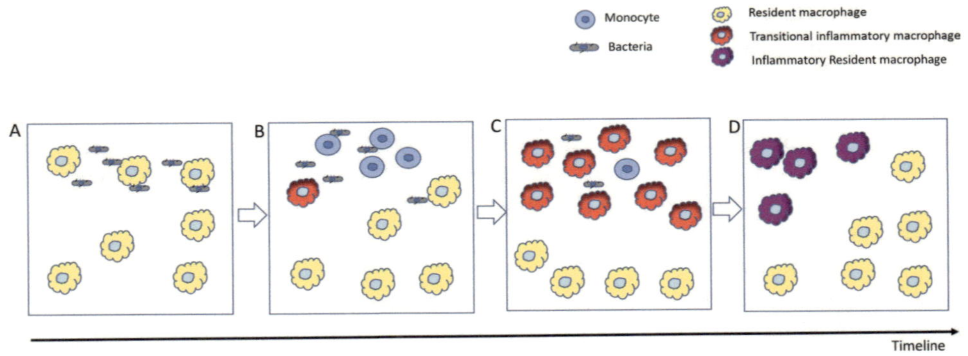

Figure 4.
Inflammation and/or infection in the lung and subsequent resolution reshape the composition of the pulmonary macrophage pool. A) An infectious episode in the lung results in the resident macrophages (ResMac) send signals for recruitment of monocytes from the blood. B) Monocytes from the blood are recruited into alveolar spaces to help dealing with the infection. C) these monocytes change intotransitional inflammatory macrophages that help clearing the infection. D) some of these transitional macrophages change intoinflammatory resident macrophages (InfResMac), the rest disappear. The InfResMacremain in the airspaces for months and ResMacproliferate to slowly replace them over time.

of residence in a homeostatic environment such as the lung, becomes a key factor determining lung macrophage biology [47, 48].

4. Macrophages and COPD

Chronic Obstructive Pulmonary Disease (COPD) is a chronic inflammatory lung disease caused by the long-term exposure to toxic particles and gasses. Worldwide, tobacco cigarette smoke is the main culprit, though biomass exposure may be a more important cause of COPD in some parts of the developing world [49]. These exposures elicit a persistent innate and eventually an adaptive immune response in the airways and lung tissues, which is characterized by overproduction of mucus in the central airways, fibrosis and obstruction of small airways and eventual destruction of the lung parenchyma leading to emphysema [50]. There is also evidence for impaired tissue repair responses and altered tissue remodeling that contribute to a progressive disease phenotype [51].

Lung macrophages are key immune effector cells in the pathogenesis of COPD. Airspace macrophages are directly exposed to inhaled antigens, pathogens and noxious particles and gasses, and several studies have shown an increase in their numbers in subjects with COPD compared to controls [52–54]. Cigarette smoking is still the major cause of COPD in developed countries, but biomass exposure is a more important cause of COPD in the developing world [49]. For both of these exposure types, lung macrophages play a pivotal role in processing and clearing these particles from the lungs. Due to the chronicity of these exposures in COPD, functional responses of lung macrophages to these exposures are thought to participate in the development of COPD. There is a significant increase in macrophages in induced sputum and BAL fluid (BALF) samples in COPD patients [55], supporting this notion [54]. In COPD, lung macrophages also secrete large amounts of potential tissue damaging enzymes such as elastase, matrix metalloproteinases (MMPs) MMP-2, MMP-9, MMP-12 and cathepsin S in response to exposure to cigarette smoke, ambient particulate matter or micro-organisms [55, 56]. In addition, continuous exposure to cigarette smoke or biomass markedly depletes intracellular anti-oxidants such as glutathione, causing excessive oxidative stress, which suppresses macrophage bacterial phagocytosis and efferocytosis [57]. Therefore, macrophages in COPD generate a more pro-inflammatory milieu that promotes tissue injury. They also demonstrate defective immune surveillance and protective (phagocytic) functions that collectively contribute to the progression of COPD. The majority of acute exacerbations of COPD are triggered by either viral or bacterial respiratory infections that could alter the airway microbiome and cause frequent exacerbations [58], a clinical phenotype that is associated with a poor long-term outcome [51].

In COPD, M1 macrophages demonstrate enhanced pro-inflammatory capacity producing more TNF-α and MMPs [59], leading to increased extracellular matrix (ECM) deposition, elastin breakdown and excessive accumulation of collagen in the lung parenchyma. In contrast, Stout and co-workers [60] showed that M2 macrophages have a lower pro-inflammatory capacity (TNF-α, IL-1β, and IL-6), when stimulated. Morphological studies have shown that macrophages accumulate in areas of persistent inflammation in lung tissues of COPD including airway walls that lead to airway narrowing and obstruction and destructive changes in lung parenchyma [50, 61]. Several studies have shown phenotypic shifts in lung macrophages in COPD airways. Dewhurst and co-workers showed that the total number of macrophages in the airspaces of COPD subjects increased and morphologically became predominantly larger macrophages, which produced fewer pro-inflammatory cytokines and demonstrated reduced phagocytic ability [62]. Berenson and co-workers showed that macrophages from patients with COPD have impaired phagocytosis of respiratory pathogens which strongly correlated with COPD severity (FEV1% predicted) [63]. Studies from our laboratory recently showed that the majority of airspace macrophages in COPD do not express either M1 or M2 markers and that these "non-polarized" macrophages have significantly reduced phagocytic capacity compared to polarized (M1 or M2) macrophages [30]. In this study, airspace macrophages could be divided into 4 distinct groups using surface markers, as either M1, M2, dual positive for M1 & M2 (double polarized) or negative for both M1 & M2 markers (non-polarized). Using the phagocytosis of opsonized *Staphylococcus aureus* as a readout, we showed that the double polarized macrophages had the best phagocytic function while the non-polarized macrophages had the worst (**Figure 5**). These data highlight the importance of macrophage micro-environment that impacts polarization and ultimately function.

The inability of macrophages to polarize may render the airways in COPD more vulnerable for colonization with pathogens and subsequent infection resulting in COPD exacerbation. The presence of large numbers of non-polarized macrophages in COPD may collectively reduce phagocytosis of pathogens and noxious particles, and in certain cases promote a pro-inflammatory milieu that contributes to airway and lung tissue injury and remodeling.

The air spaces have their own unique microbiome shown by next-generation sequencing technologies, such as 16 s RNA gene measurement, and studies in COPD cohorts have shown alterations in this microbiome that vary with the severity of COPD, during and after an acute COPD exacerbations, and with the use of inhaled steroids and/or antimicrobial treatment [64]. Alterations in the lung microbiome may contribute to the pathogenesis of COPD by impacting inflammatory and/or immune processes in the lungs. Lung macrophages play a central role in clearing harmful bacteria such as *Haemophilus influenzae, Moraxella catarrhalis* and *S. pneumoniae,* from the lungs, and this macrophage function deteriorates as the disease progresses

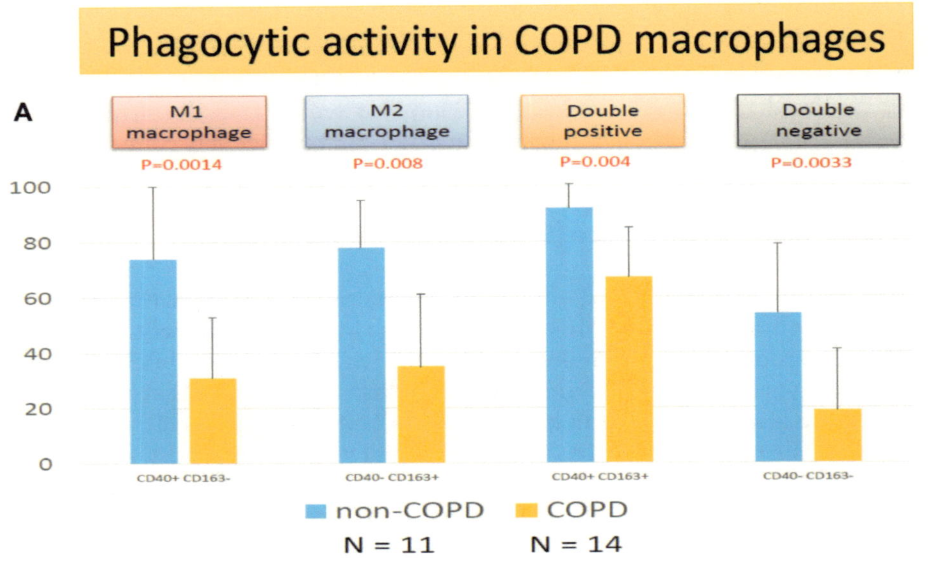

Figure 5.
Phagocytic activity of airspace macrophages, harvested from bronchial alveolar lavage, in subjects with COPD. CD40 was used to label M1 and CD163 to label M2 macrophages. The phagocytosis of flourescentlabelled StapholococcusAureas was measured using flow cytometry. Phagocytosis was reduced in COPD subjects compared to control subjects in all the different macrophage populations but was particular lowin the most abundant non-labeled or double negative cells.

[63] leading to colonization of airspaces and exacerbations of COPD [65]. Therefore, the defective phagocytic function of macrophages in COPD could contribute to the colonization of the airways with various bacteria, specifically those known to cause acute exacerbations and pneumonia during COPD.

One of the key functions of lung macrophages is to remove and clear cellular debris as well as dead or damage cells following an inflammatory insult to the lungs. This process, which is termed efferocytosis, is defective in subjects with COPD [66]. In most subjects with COPD, there are an access of neutrophils in the airspaces (as measured by bronchial alveolar lavage), which further increase during acute COPD exacerbations. Defective clearance of these recruited neutrophils results in the accumulation of necrotic neutrophils that indiscriminately release toxic granule proteins containing neutrophil elastase and proteases that has been associated with tissue damage and COPD progression [67]. Since LMs are the primary "janitors" of the lungs, dysfunctional processing and clearance of apoptotic and necrotic cells and cellular debris could contribute to ongoing lung tissue inflammation in subjects with COPD, even long after they stop smoking [68].

Lung macrophages are primary responsible for processing and removing of inhaled irritants and particulate matter from the lungs. In this process they release proinflammatory mediators that could also inflict damage to lung tissues, promoting a dysregulated inflammatory response, which may lead to dysfunctional tissue repair and a persistent state of chronic low-grade lung inflammation, a hallmark of COPD. Studies that unravel the mechanisms promoting macrophage anti-inflammatory and reparative functions could contribute to the development of more targeted therapeutic interventions to reduce the destructive inflammatory response induced by cigarette smoke and environmental exposures that eventually lead to COPD.

5. Macrophages and lung cancer

The majority of lung cancers (~80%) are diagnosed at an advanced stage with >50% in older subjects who are ineligible for surgery [69, 70] leaving chemotherapy as their primary treatment modality. A better understanding of tumor immunology and our body's natural immune response to combat cancer over the last two decades have highlighted the key role macrophages play in containing the progression and metastasis of tumor cells. The tumor microenvironment (TME), characterized by low levels of nutrients, hypoxia and acidity, promotes tumor growth, invasion and metastasis [71]. The most abundant immune cells in or surrounding lung tumors are "tumor-associated macrophages" (TAMs), and the functions of these macrophages are determined by the TME [72].

The tumor microenvironment recruits both innate and adaptive immune cells to the tumor site, with macrophages abundant at all stages of tumorigenesis. Evidence suggests that TAMs originate predominantly from blood monocytes, and are recruited to tumor sites by tumor-derived chemotactic signals, including monocyte chemo-attractant protein-1 (MCP-1), which is also known as CCL 2 [73]. Initially these macrophages have an M1-like phenotype, activated by interferon-γ (IFN-γ), demonstrating pro-inflammatory functions with the capacity to facilitate tumor cell destruction. They are also characterized by a high production of nitric oxide (NO) and reactive oxygen intermediates (ROI), and pro-inflammatory cytokines, including TNF-α, IL- 1, IL- 12 and IL- 23 and MHC molecules [74]. These mediators recruit cytotoxic CD8+ T and NK cells that destroy the tumor cells [72] (**Figure 6**).

With tumor progression the TME changes to a milieu that converts macrophages to a more M2-like phenotype macrophages, which suppress anti-tumor immune responses. This in turn promotes cell proliferation, angiogenesis and ultimately

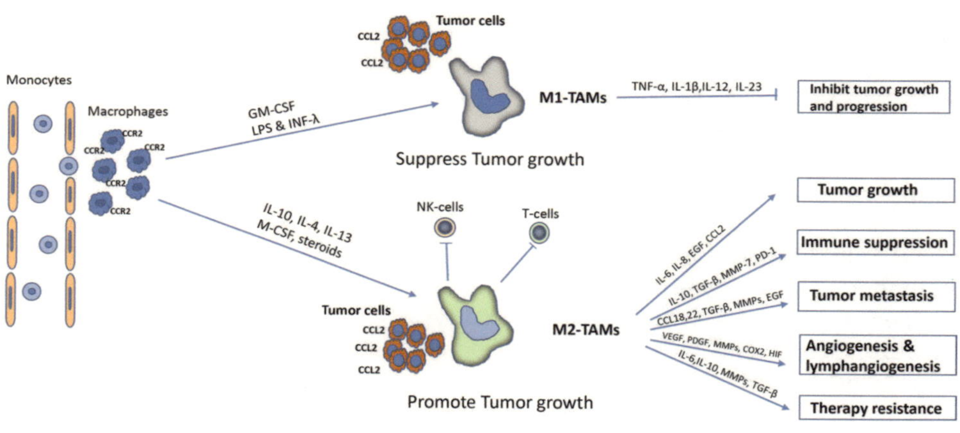

Figure 6.
The effects of tumor associated macrophages (TAMs) on tumor growth, progression and metastasis. The immune response elicited by lung cancer cells included recruitment of monocytes from the blood (via CCL2/CCR2 interaction) that convert to macrophages and are recruited tothe tumor niche where they become either M1 type TAMs under the influence of mediators such as GM-CSF and INF-λand inhibit tumor growth via secreting mediators such as TNF-α, IL-1β, IL-12 and 23. Mediators such as IL-10, IL-4 and M-CSF will change the macrophages to a more M2 type TAMs that promote tumor growth via immuno-suppressive properties that include blocking NK-cell and other T-cells tumorcidaleffects. The M2-TAMsenvironment will also promote angiogenesis via mediators such as VEGF and PDGF and tumor invasion and metastasis via mediators such as MMPs and TGF-B. other mediators in the tumor environment produced by M2 macropahagessuch as IL-6, TGF-βand MMPs have also been shown to elicit chemotherapy resistance of tumors.

metastasis. Damage-associated molecular patterns (DAMPs) from dead or dying cells in the tumor microenvironment promote polarization of macrophages to immunosuppressive TAM [75]. These M2-like TAM have a similar phenotype as LPS-tolerant macrophages and is thought to contribute to the immunosuppression in the tumor microenvironments. They express a variety of mediators that inhibit the host anti-tumor immune responses. These include cell surface receptors, cytokines, chemokines and a variety of enzymes. This anti-tumor immune response is via inhibition of direct cell-to-cell contact between TAM receptors and their ligand counterpart death/ inhibitory receptors expressed by the target immune effector cells. For example, TAMs express the ligand receptors for PD-1 and CTLA-4 that upon activation suppress cytotoxic functions of T- cell and NK cells. They also express the ligand for the death receptors FAS and TRAIL that triggers T-cells and induce caspase dependent apoptosis of tumor cells. The TAMs produce TGF-β that impedes the cytotoxicity of NK cells, and promotes expression of PD-L1 that impedes the anti-tumor activity of T cells [76]. They also secrete cytokines IL-10 that inhibit T cells effector functions and chemokines such as CCL5, CCL20, CCL22 that recruit Treg cells that are immunosuppressive.

The density of macrophages, in particular M2 phenotypes, has been associated with a poor prognosis in almost all human cancer types including lung cancers in clinical trials [77]. The $CD68^+CD163^+$ or $CD68^+CD206^+$ markers on TAM are used to identify M2-like macrophages and these macrophages are associated with more dense peritumoral lymphatic microvessels, a pathological feature that relate to poor patients' prognoses in subjects with lung cancer [78]. Furthermore, an increased density of $CD68^+CD163^+$ macrophages in tumor nests and stroma was associated with lymph node metastases [78] and Cao *et al* showed expression levels of CD 68^+CD163^+on M2 macrophages were inversely correlated with overall survival, and disease free survival in non-small cell lung cancer (NSCLC) [77].

The overwhelming evidence that TAMs and especially M2 macrophages promote tumorigenesis has made TAMs a target for a novel anti-tumor strategy in lung cancer. Several strategies that have been explored include blockade of the CCL2-CCR 2 interaction and the CSF1-CSF1R recruitment of monocyte pathways that decrease TAM infiltration, thereby reversing their immunosuppressive effects [73]. Mu and co-workers have suggested that reprogramming TAM macrophages can be a promising approach to address immunosuppressive failure in the cancer environment [79]. Re-educating TAMs to a M1 phenotype or switching M2 to M1 macrophages with several drugs has also shown promise including the use of BTH1677 (a yeast β-glucan immunomodulator), hydroxychloroquine, and celecoxib [80, 81]. Another approach is to block the levels of critical TAM-secreted cytokines involved in tumor biology such as CCL18, CCL 22, and MIP-3α, which are mainly produced by M2-type macrophages, and promote malignant behavior of tumors [82, 83]. Furthermore, nanoparticles or nanoparticle-based drug delivery are more reliable and effective in regulating the macrophage phenotype by ensuring that the drug reaches the cancer site without off-target activities [84, 85]. In addition, materials used in nanoparticle production, including TiO2 and Ag, may preferentially polarize TAMs towards an M1 phenotype [86, 87].

6. Macrophages and their role in asthma

Asthma is characterized by chronically inflamed airways, leading to remodeling and constriction in response to a wide variety of stimuli. One of the prototypical traits of asthma is airway hyperresponsiveness. Typical triggers of bronchoconstriction are aero-allergens and viral pathogens but non-specific stimuli such as irritating chemicals, cold air, and exercise (increase flow) can also trigger this response. Airway inflammation is characterized by increased mucus secretion, thickening of all the components of the airway wall and luminal narrowing, leading to symptoms of shortness of breath, chest tightness, wheezing, and cough [88]. The inflammatory response in the airways is typically type 2 (Th2) in which allergens are detected by pattern recognition receptors (PRRs) on epithelial cells, which, upon activation, secrete alarmins such as interleukin (IL)-33, IL-25 and thymic stromal lymphopoietin (TSLP) and cytokines such as GM-CSF. These mediators induce type 2 inflammation by activating dendritic cells (DCs) and type 2 innate lymphoid cells (ILC2s) and differentiating naïve T cells into T helper (Th) 2 cells, which produce IL-4, IL-5, and IL-13 [88, 89]. These type 2 cytokines are involved in producing IgE and recruiting eosinophils into the airways. A classic type 2 inflammatory response can be suppressed by treatment with corticosteroids. In adults a substantial subset of patients with non-atopic asthma may be driven by a Th1 response, which is characterized by infiltration of neutrophils. Th1 inflammation is more difficult to treat, as it is often resistant to corticosteroids [90].

Macrophages are the most abundant leukocytes found in alveoli, and in small as well as conducting airways, suggesting that they have an important role in providing protection against foreign inhaled particulate matter including allergens, pathogens and noxious gasses. Links between lung macrophages and airway inflammation, including eosinophilic inflammation and airway remodeling are well documented in asthma [91–95]. However, it is not still unclear whether macrophages have a predominant pro-inflammatory or regulatory role in asthma.

As discussed previously, macrophages have the ability to adapt to their microenvironment (plasticity). In asthmatic lung inflammation this plasticity of macrophage function is most likely responsible for their apparent dual or contrasting roles as pro-inflammatory versus immunosuppressive effector immune cells. Zaslona and co-workers showed that during allergic inflammation, resident alveolar macrophages proliferate locally and exert a protective effect on allergic inflammation, whereas recruited monocytes/macrophages aggravate allergic inflammation [96]. These recruited monocytes are also involved in the characteristic chronic remodeling of airways [97]. When circulating monocytes were depleted by intravenous injection of clodronate, there was significant attenuation of allergic inflammation in the airways and when clodronate was administered via the intratracheal route to deplete resident airspace macrophages, eosinophilic inflammation was enhanced [97]. Collectively, these data suggest that resident macrophages serve to maintain lung homeostasis by suppressing inflammatory responses, while recruited monocytes primarily promote allergic inflammation. The picture that emerges is one of rapid recruitment of monocytes to fight the perceived dangers of the allergen by mounting an inflammatory response and then subsequently expanding the pool of suppressive AMs in an attempt to restore homeostasis (**Figure 7**). The dominant macrophages in allergic asthma are alternatively activated AMs, which respond to IL-4/IL-13. Although the presence of these macrophages correlates well with the severity of airway inflammation, it is not clear whether these macrophages significantly contribute to the allergic inflammatory response or are the downstream consequence of the allergic inflammation [98–100]. This issue has been addressed in several experimental studies using transgenic murine models of asthma [101–103]. Together, these studies have shown distinct differences between resident and recruited macrophages in contributing to asthmatic

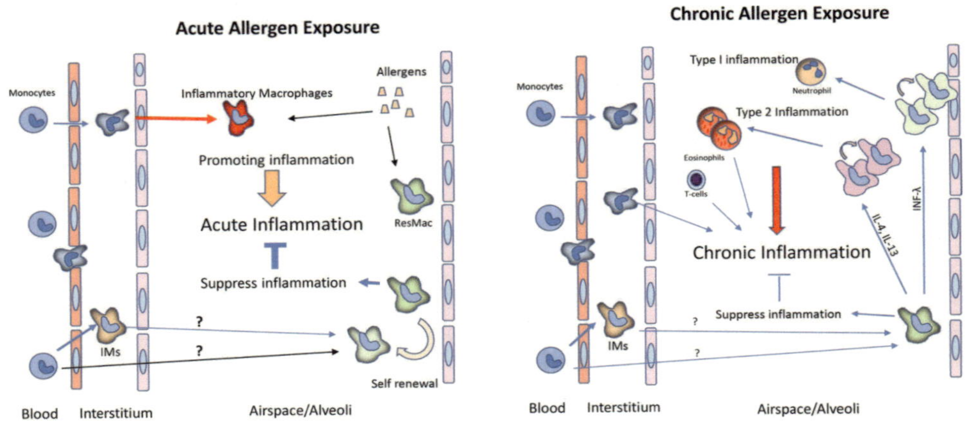

Figure 7.
After allergen exposure, there is rapid recruitment of monocytes from the blood that become inflammatory macrophages that predominantly promote acute inflammatory responses in the airspace. Resident macrophages (ResMac), which are largely self-replicating, act to suppress the acute inflammation in an attempt torestore homeostasis. It is as yetunclear whether ResMaccan arise directly from recruited monocytes or from IMs as intermediate progenitors. These newly recruited monocyte-derived cells appear to oppose the suppressive actions of resident AMs. **b** *inflammation becomes chronic after repeated exposures to allergen with the increased recruitment of immune cells and consequent elevated levels of cytokines such as IL-4, IL-13, and IFNγ. In response to these signals, ResMaccan polarize across a continuum of activation phenotypes, losing their suppressive functions and gaining pathogenic functions. IL-4/IL-13-induced AMs promote type 2/eosinophilic inflammation, and IFNγ-induced AMs are associated with type I/neutrophilic inflammation. It is as yetunclear whether these activated phenotypes can arise from recruited monocytes directly or from IMs as an intermediate progenitor.*

inflammation. However, as there may be significant differences between mice and humans, these findings should be interpreted cautiously. Recent studies have shown that there is a mixed population of macrophage phenotypes in both human and mouse models of allergic inflammation [101–103] with functional studies showing that IFNγ-stimulated macrophages (M1) prevent the development of allergic inflammation in mice by suppressing DC maturation [104]. However in human studies of subjects with established asthma, there is a higher number of macrophages expressing the IFNγ-activated transcription factor, interferon regulatory factor 5 (IRF5), in airways which in turn correlates with the severity of airflow obstruction [102]. These studies highlight the potential dual role of classically activated macrophages (M1) in asthma.

The presence of type 1 cytokines, such as IL-6, would be expected during host responses to viruses and to a variety of exogenous and endogenous ligands that trigger asthma exacerbations [88, 105]. Infections with common respiratory viruses such as rhinovirus are a major trigger of asthma exacerbations and in these virus-induced exacerbations, there is direct interaction of the rhinovirus with airspace macrophages [105]. Asthma models in mice, support the role of macrophages in viral induced exacerbations, but interestingly, the pathogenic macrophage phenotype involved varies with the underlying inflammatory milieu. In mice with a predominant type 2 inflammatory response, viral infection induces activation of alternative AMs, which amplifies eosinophil recruitment into the airways. However, mice with predominantly type 1 inflammation demonstrate mostly classical activation of AMs, skewing the phenotype to a more neutrophilic inflammation upon virus infection [106].

The role of lung macrophages in allergic asthma is still evolving. Current paradigms suggest that macrophages of different origins or phenotypes have the potential to be either protective and/or harmful in different stages of allergic airway disease. In asthma, macrophages may have a dual role: with induction of the allergic inflammatory response they may be predominantly regulatory to resolve the inflammation but when persistently activated, they may contribute to chronic inflammation and further damage of the airways (**Figure 7**). The role of resident and recruited macrophages as well as the macrophage phenotypes in the pathogenesis of allergic airways disease requires additional studies.

7. Macrophages in interstitial lung disease

Chronic and aberrant lung repair responses that lead to irreversible scarring and remodeling of the airways and lung parenchyma are hallmarks of pulmonary fibrotic diseases. These diseases are characterized by excessive deposition of ECM leading to fibrotic remodeling of lungs and irreversible lung dysfunction [107]. Alveolar macrophages have been shown to be involved in ECM processing by secreting matrix metalloproteinases (MMPs) such as MMP9, a type IV collagenase known to degrade extracellular matrix, and numerous non-matrix protein, which have been demonstrated in a murine model of lung fibrosis induced by bleomycin [108, 109] These macrophages also endocytose collagen and produce soluble mediators required for collagen-degradation, and enhance the activity of fibroblast-specific protein-1 (FSP-1) that increases the proliferation and production of ECM by lung fibroblasts [110]. Recent animal studies have shown that the AMs involved in the bleomycin murine lung fibrosis model are monocyte derived and not resident AMs. Depletion of resident AMs by intratracheal instillation of liposomal clodronate before bleomycin administration does not alter the fibrotic response, indicating that resident AMs are dispensable for the development of fibrosis [111]. To support this concept, deletion of the anti-apoptotic protein c-Flip in circulating monocytes (the precursors of monocyte-derived AMs) in mice showed that the number of monocyte-derived AMs decreased, which was accompanied by a reduction in lung fibrosis with bleomycin injury [112] Gene expression studies of resident AMs and monocyte-derived AMs also indicate that only monocyte-derived AMs have a profibrotic gene profile in bleomycin induced model of lung fibrosis [112] Single cell transcriptomic studies support these findings [113]. Transgenic reporter mice that marked the Cx3cr1-expressing transitional macrophages showed that these macrophages localize to fibrotic niches suggesting that these transitional macrophages arise from monocytes and interact with fibroblasts to drive fibrosis, in concordance to studies of Misharin et al. and McCubbrey et al. [111, 112].

In human interstitial lung diseases, AMs show greater heterogeneity compared with healthy lungs. In subjects with idiopathic pulmonary fibrosis, lung tissues have a higher proportions of AMs lacking CD71, a transferrin receptor. These CD71 negative macrophages were also more immature and showed impaired phagocytosis and enhanced expression of profibrotic genes [114]. Single cell RNA sequencing analysis from eight normal compared to eight lungs from advanced lung fibrosis subjects (from patients undergoing lung transplantation) supports the idea of increased heterogeneity of macrophages in fibrotic lungs and subsets of AMs that were enriched with pro-fibrotic genes [115]. Together these studies suggest lung macrophages contribute significantly to the pathogenesis of interstitial fibrotic lung disease. However, it is still unclear whether these macrophages are from the resident pool or newly recruited into the lung, what signals attract these macrophages or whether they are just secondary to the change in microenvironment, and lastly, what their contribution is to progression of the disease [116].

Interstitial macrophages (IMs) are ideally positioned to participate in the lung fibrotic processes. In a radiation-induced lung fibrosis (RIF) mouse models, IMs have acquired a pro-fibrotic phenotype, and express high levels of CD206, a marker of alternatively activated M2 macrophages [117]. Interstitial macrophages isolated from RIF lungs promote fibrosis by inducing the differentiation myocytes to myofibroblasts. Myofibroblasts have been shown to be key players in the initiation and progression of lung fibrosis [118]. Depletion of IMs in the RIF mouse model with CSF1-R specific mAb exerts an anti-fibrotic effect, while the depletion of AMs by intranasal administration of clodronate liposomes has no effects on RIF [117]. Recent studies showed that lung fibrosis was exacerbated after depletion of $Lyve1_{hi}MHCII_{lo}$ IM1s during the induction of fibrosis, which suggested that these IM1 might have an early antifibrotic role. This is in keeping with expression of high levels of genes associated with wound healing, repair, and fibrosis in this subset of IMs [20].

8. Conclusion

It is clear that lung macrophages have an essential role in both lung homeostasis and in disease states. Here we have highlighted the specific origins, unique phenotypes and functions of the two main populations of lung macrophages, AMs and IMs, and emphasized the distinct roles in common lung diseases. It is still not clear if lung macrophages derived from circulating monocytes eventually become indistinguishable from embryonically derived resident AMs in chronic lung diseases or if they are long lived in the lungs with a slightly different genomic and functional profile thereby changing the lung macrophage landscape. There is still a lack of knowledge of IMs in terms of how they are maintained and their importance in lung conditions. With the increasing power of phenotyping and genomic techniques, there will be opportunities to better characterize the origin, subtypes and functions of AMs and IMs in both health and disease. There is a pressing need to focus strongly on macrophage function, especially in regards to mechanisms of their role in inflammatory and anti-inflammatory pathways, their turnover and survival during the immune response, and their interactions with recruited macrophages in promoting wound healing. Refining our understanding of macrophage plasticity and the role of distinct populations of macrophages in various pulmonary diseases will lead to the identification of novel macrophage-targeted therapies.

Acknowledgements

This work was grant supported by Canadian Institute of Health Research, the British Columbia Lung Association, and the Providence Airway Centre. Stephan F. van Eeden is the Canadian Institute for Health Research/Glaxo Smith Kline (CIHR/GSK) Professor in Chronic Obstructive Pulmonary Disease and Don D. Sin holds a Tier 1 Canada Research Chair in COPD and the HLI De Lazzari Family Chair.

Author details

Stephan F. van Eeden[1,2]* and Don D. Sin[1,2]

1 Department of Medicine (Respirology), University of British Columbia, Vancouver, BC, Canada

2 Centre for Heart Lung Innovation, St. Paul's Hospital, Vancouver, BC, Canada

*Address all correspondence to: stephan.vaneeden@hli.ubc.ca

References

[1] Wynn TA, Chawla A, Pollard JW. Origins and hallmarks of macrophages: Development, homeostasis, and disease. Nature. 2013;**496**:445-455

[2] Epelman S, Lavine KJ, Randolph GJ. Origin and functions of tissue macrophages. Immunity. 2014;**41**:21-35

[3] Shi T, Denney L, An H, Ho L-P, Zheng Y. Alveolar and lung interstitial macrophages: Definitions, functions, and roles in lung fibrosis. Journal of Leukocyte Biology. 2021;**110**:107-114

[4] Lehnert BE, Valdez YE, Sebring RJ, Lehnert NM, Saunders GC, Steinkamp JA. Airway intraluminal macrophages: Evidence of origin and comparisons to alveolar macrophages. American Journal of Respiratory Cell and Molecular Biology. 1990;**3**:377-391

[5] Warner AE, Molina RM, Brain JD. Uptake of bloodborne bacteria by pulmonary intravascular macrophages and consequent inflammatory responses in sheep. The American Review of Respiratory Disease. 1987;**136**:683-690

[6] Dehring DJ, Wismar BL. Intravascular macrophages in pulmonary capillaries of humans. The American Review of Respiratory Disease. 1989;**139**:1027-1029

[7] van Furth R, Cohn ZA. The origin and kinetics of mononuclear phagocytes. The Journal of Experimental Medicine. 1968;**128**:415-435

[8] Landsman L, Jung S. Lung macrophages serve as obligatory intermediate between blood monocytes and alveolar macrophages. Journal of Immunology. 2007;**179**:3488-3494

[9] Guilliams M, De Kleer I, Henri S, Post S, Vanhoutte L, De Prijck S, et al. Alveolar macrophages develop from fetal monocytes that differentiate into long-lived cells in the first week of life via GM-CSF. The Journal of Experimental Medicine. 2013;**210**:1977-1992

[10] Hashimoto D, Chow A, Noizat C, Teo P, Beasley MB, Leboeuf M, et al. Tissue resident macrophages self-maintain locally throughout adult life with minimal contribution from circulating monocytes. Immunity. 2013;**38**:792-804

[11] Hoeffel G, Wang Y, Greter M, See P, Teo P, Malleret B, et al. Adult Langerhans cells derive predominantly from embryonic fetal liver monocytes with a minor contribution of yolk sac-derived macrophages. The Journal of Experimental Medicine. 2012;**209**:1167-1181

[12] Gomez Perdiguero E, Klapproth K, Schulz C, Busch K, Azzoni E, Crozet L, et al. Tissue-resident macrophages originate from yolksac- derived erythro-myeloid progenitors. Nature. 2015;**518**(7540):547-551

[13] Aggarwal NR, King LS, D'Alessio FR. Diverse macrophage populations mediate acute lung inflammation and resolution. American journal of Physiology, Lung Cellular and Molecular Physiology. 2014;**306**(8):L709-L725

[14] Cai Y, Sugimoto C, Arainga M, Alvarez-Hernandez X, Didier ES, Kuroda MJ. In vivo characterization of alveolar and interstitial lung macrophages in rhesus macaques: Implications for understanding lung disease in humans. Journal of Immunology. 2014;**192**:2821-2829

[15] Goto Y, Hogg JC, Whalen B, Shih CH, Ishii H, Van Eeden SF.

Monocyte recruitment into the lungs in pneumococcal pneumonia. American Journal of Respiratory Cell and Molecular Biology. 2004;**30**(5):620-626. DOI: 10.1165/rcmb.2003-0312OC

[16] Schneider C, Nobs SP, Kurrer M, et al. Induction of the nuclear receptor PPAR- gamma by the cytokine GM-CSFis critical for the differentiation of fetal monocytes into alveolar macrophages. Nature Immunology. 2014;**15**:1026-1037

[17] Gourbal B, Pinaud S, Beckers GJM, et al. Innate immune memory: An evolutionary perspective. Immunological Reviews. 2018;**283**:21-40

[18] Yao Y, Jeyanathan M, Haddadi S, et al. Induction of autonomous memory alveolar macrophages requires T cell help and is critical to trained immunity. Cell. 2018;**175**:1634-1650

[19] Gibbings SL, Thomas SM, Atif SM, et al. Three unique interstitial macrophages in the murine lung at steady state. American Journal of Respiratory Cell and Molecular Biology. 2017;**57**:66-76

[20] Chakarov S, Lim HY, Tan L, et al. Two distinct interstitial macrophage populations coexist across tissues in specific subtissular niches. Science. 2019;**363**:eaau0964

[21] Lambrechts D, Wauters E, Boeckx B, et al. Phenotype molding of stromal cells in the lung tumor microenvironment. Nature Medicine. 2018;**24**:1277-1289

[22] Biswas SK, Mantovani A. Macrophage plasticity and interaction with lymphocyte subsets: Cancer as a paradigm. Nature Immunology. 2010;**11**:889-896

[23] Biswas SK, Gangi L, Paul S, Schioppa T, Saccani A, Sironi M, et al. A distinct and unique transcriptional program expressed by tumor-associated macrophages (defective NF-kappaB and enhanced IR F-3/STAT1 activation). Blood. 2006;**107**:2112-2122

[24] Nelson MP, Christmann BS, Dunaway CW, Morris A, Steele C. Experimental pneumocystis lung infection promotes M2a alveolar macrophage-derived MMP12 production. American Journal of Physiology. Lung Cellular and Molecular Physiology. 2012;**303**:L469-L475

[25] Zhang W, Xu W, Xiong S. Blockade of Notch1 signaling alleviates murine lupus via blunting macrophage activation and M2b polarization. Journal of Immunology. 2010;**184**:6465-6478

[26] Koscsó B, Csóka B, Kókai E, Németh ZH, Pacher P, Virág L, et al. Adenosine augments IL-10-induced STAT3 signaling in M2c macrophages. Journal of Leukocyte Biology. 2013;**94**:1309-1315

[27] Olmes G, Buttner-Herold M, Ferrazzi F, Distel L, Amann K, Daniel C. CD 163+ M2c-like macrophages predominate in renal biopsies from patients with lupus nephritis. Arthritis Research & Therapy. 2016;**18**:90

[28] Wang Q, Ni H, Lan L, Wei X, Xiang R, Wang Y. Fra-1 protooncogene regulates IL-6 expression in macrophages and promotes the generation of M2d macrophages. Cell Research. 2010;**20**:701-712

[29] Helm O, Held-Feindt J, Grage-Griebenow E, Reiling N, Ungefroren H, Vogel I, et al. Tumor-associated macrophages exhibit pro- and anti-inflammatory properties by which they impact on pancreatic tumorigenesis. International Journal of Cancer. 2014;**135**:843-861

[30] Akata K, Yamasaki K, Filho FSL, Yang CX, Takiguchi H, Sahin B, et al. Abundance of non-polarized lung macrophages with poor phagocytic function in chronic obstructive pulmonary disease (COPD). Biomedicine. 2020;**8**(10):398. DOI: 10.3390/biomedicines 8100398

[31] Baßler K, Fujii W, Kapellos TS, Horne A, Reiz B, Dudkin E, et al. Alterations of multiple alveolar macrophage states in chronic obstructive pulmonary disease. bioRxiv. **2020**. DOI: 10.1101/2020.05.28.121541

[32] Naessens T et al. Innate imprinting of murine resident alveolar macrophages by allergic bronchial inflammation causes a switch from hypo-inflammatory to hyper-inflammatory reactivity. The American Journal of Pathology. 2012;**181**:174-184

[33] Kumagai Y et al. Alveolar macrophages are the primary interferon-α producer in pulmonary infection with RNA viruses. Immunity. 2007;**27**:240-252

[34] Guarda G et al. Type I interferon inhibits interleukin-1 production and inflammasome activation. Immunity. 2011;**34**:213-223

[35] Aegerter H et al. Influenza-induced monocyte-derived alveolar macrophages confer prolonged antibacterial protection. Nature Immunology. 2020;**21**(2):145-157. DOI: 10.1038/s41590-019-0568-x

[36] Bost P et al. Host–viral infection maps reveal signatures of severe COVID-19 patients. Cell. 2020;**181**:1475-1488.e12

[37] Gao T et al. Highly pathogenic coronavirus N protein aggravates lung injury by MASP-2-mediated complement over-activation. medRxiv. 2020. DOI: 10.1101/2020.03.29.20041962

[38] Carvelli J et al. Association of COVID-19 inflammation with activation of the C5a–C5aR1 axis. Nature. 2020;**588**:146-150

[39] Knapp S et al. Alveolar macrophages have a protective anti-inflammatory role during murine pneumococcal pneumonia. American Journal of Respiratory and Critical Care Medicine. 2003;**167**:171-179

[40] Cohen SB et al. Alveolar macrophages provide an early *Mycobacterium tuberculosis* niche and initiate dissemination. Cell Host & Microbe. 2018;**24**:439-446. e4

[41] Misharin AV et al. Monocyte-derived alveolar macrophages drive lung fibrosis and persist in the lung over the life span. The Journal of Experimental Medicine. 2017;**214**:2387-2404

[42] Machiels B et al. A gamma-herpesvirus provides protection against allergic asthma by inducing the replacement of resident alveolar macrophages with regulatory monocytes. Nature Immunology. 2017;**18**:1310-1320

[43] Ghoneim HE, Thomas PG, McCullers JA. Depletion of alveolar macrophages during influenza infection facilitates bacterial superinfections. Journal of Immunology. 2013;**191**:1250-1259

[44] Yao Y et al. Induction of autonomous memory alveolar macrophages requires T cell help and is critical to trained immunity. Cell. 2018;**175**:1634-1650. e17

[45] Roquilly A et al. Alveolar macrophages are epigenetically altered

after inflammation, leading to long-term lung immune-paralysis. Nature Immunology. 2020;**21**:636-648

[46] Goulding J et al. Respiratory infections: Do we ever recover? Proceedings of the American Thoracic Society. 2007;**4**:618-625

[47] Blériot C, Chakarov S, Ginhoux F. Determinants of resident tissue macrophage identity and function. Immunity. 2020;**52**:957-970

[48] Kulikauskaite J, Wack A. Teaching old dogs new tricks? The plasticity of lung alveolar macrophage subsets. Trends in Immunology. 2020;**41**:864-877

[49] Eisner MD, Anthonisen N, Coultas D, Kuenzli N, Perez-Padilla R, Postma D, et al. An official American Thoracic Society public policy statement: Novel risk factors and the global burden of chronic obstructive pulmonary disease. American Journal of Respiratory and Critical Care Medicine. 2010;**182**(5):693-718

[50] Hogg JC, Chu F, Utokaparch S, Woods R, Elliott WM, Buzatu L, et al. The nature of small-airway obstruction in chronic obstructive pulmonary disease. The New England Journal of Medicine. **2004**;**350**:2645-2653

[51] Hogg JC, Paré PD, Hackett TL. The contribution of small airway obstruction to the pathogenesis of chronic obstructive pulmonary disease. Physiological Reviews. 2017;**97**(2):529-552

[52] Ando M, Sugimoto M, Nishi R, Suga M, Horio S, Kohrogi H, et al. Surface morphology and function of human pulmonary alveolar macrophages from smokers and non-smokers. Thorax. 1984;**39**:850-856

[53] Finkelstein R, Fraser RS, Ghezzo H, Cosio MG. Alveolar inflammation and its relation to emphysema in smokers. American Journal of Respiratory and Critical Care Medicine. 1995;**152**:1666-1672

[54] Barnes PJ. Alveolar macrophages as orchestrators of COPD. COPD: Journal of Chronic Obstructive Pulmonary Disease. 2004;**1**:59-70

[55] Russell RE, Culpitt SV, DeMatos C, Donnelly L, Smith M, Wiggins J, et al. Release and activity of matrix metalloproteinase-9 and tissue inhibitor of metalloproteinase-1 by alveolar macrophages from patients with chronic obstructive pulmonary disease. American Journal of Respiratory Cell and Molecular Biology. 2002;**26**(5):602-609

[56] Nakajima T, Nakamura H, Owen CA, Yoshida S, Tsuduki K, Chubachi S, et al. Plasma cathepsin S and cathepsin S/cystatin C ratios are potential biomarkers for COPD. Disease Markers. 2016;**2016**:4093870

[57] Donnelly LE, Barnes PJ. Defective phagocytosis in airways disease. Chest. 2012;**141**(4):1055-1062

[58] Zakharkina T, Koczulla AR, Mardanova O, Hattesohl A, Bals R. Detection of microorganisms in exhaled breath condensate during acute exacerbations of COPD. Respirology. 2011;**16**(6):932-938

[59] Eurlings IM, Dentener MA, Mercken EM, et al. A comparative study of matrix remodeling in chronic models for COPD; mechanistic insights into the role of TNF-α. American Journal of Physiology. Lung Cellular and Molecular Physiology. 2014;**307**(7):557-565

[60] Stout RD, Suttles J. Functional plasticity of macrophages:

Reversible adaptation to changing microenvironments. Journal of Leukocyte Biology. 2004;**76**(3):509-513

[61] Stewart JI, Criner GJ. The small airways in chronic obstructive pulmonary disease: Pathology and effects on disease progression and survival. Current Opinion in Pulmonary Medicine. 2013;**19**(2):109-115

[62] Dewhurst JA, Lea S, Hardaker E, et al. Characterization of lung macrophage subpopulations in COPD patients and controls. Scientific Reports. 2017;**7**(1):7143

[63] Berenson CS, Kruzel RL, Eberhardt E, et al. Phagocytic dysfunction of human alveolar macrophages and severity of chronic obstructive pulmonary disease. The Journal of Infectious Diseases. 2013;**208**(12):2036-2045

[64] Mammen MJ, Sethi S. COPD and the microbiome. Respirology. 2016;**21**:590-599

[65] Naito K, Yamasaki K, Yatera K, Akata K, Noguchi S, Kawanami T, et al. Bacteriological incidence in pneumonia patients with pulmonary emphysema: A bacterial floral analysis using the 16S ribosomal RNA gene in bronchoalveolar lavage fluid. International Journal of Chronic Obstructive Pulmonary Disease. 2017;**12**:2111-2120

[66] Kirkham PA, Spooner G, Rahman I, Rossi AG. Macrophage phagocytosis of apoptotic neutrophils is compromised by matrix proteins modified by cigarette smoke and lipid peroxidation products. Biochemical and Biophysical Research Communications. 2004;**318**:32-37

[67] Pandey KC, De S, Mishra PK. Role of proteases in chronic obstructive pulmonary disease. Frontiers in Pharmacology. 2017;**8**:512

[68] Hodge S, Hodge G, Holmes M, Reynolds PN. Increased airway epithelial and T-cell apoptosis in COPD remains despite smoking cessation. The European Respiratory Journal. 2005;**25**:447-454

[69] American Cancer Society. Cancer facts and figures. 2015. Available from: http://www.cancer.org/research/cancerfactsstatistics/cancerfactsfigures2015/ [Accessed: July 13, 2015]

[70] Gridelli C, Perrone F, Monfardini S. Lung cancer in the elderly. European Journal of Cancer. 1997;**33**:2313-2314

[71] Goswami KK, Ghosh T, Ghosh S, Sarkar M, Bose A, Baral R. Tumor promoting role of anti-tumor macrophages in tumor microenvironment. Cellular Immunology. 2017;**316**:1-10

[72] Mosser DM, Edwards JP. Exploring the full spectrum of macrophage activation. Nature Reviews. Immunology. 2008;**8**:958-969

[73] Li X, Yao W, Yuan Y, Chen P, Li B, Li J, et al. Targeting of tumour-infiltrating macrophages via CCL 2/CCR 2 signalling as a therapeutic strategy against hepatocellular carcinoma. Gut. 2017;**66**:157-167

[74] Biswas SK, Mantovani A. Macrophage plasticity and interaction with lymphocyte subsets: Cancer as a paradigm. Nature Immunology. 2010;**11**:889-896

[75] Ostuni R, Kratochvill F, Murray PJ, Natoli G. Macrophages and cancer: From mechanisms to therapeutic implications. Trends in Immunology. 2015;**36**:229-239. DOI: 10.1016/j.it.2015.02.004

[76] Sumitomo R, Hirai T, Fujita M, Murakami H, Otake Y, Huang CL.

PD-L1 expression on tumor-infiltrating immune cells is highly associated with M2 TAM and aggressive malignant potential in patients with resected non-small cell lung cancer. Lung Cancer. 2019;**136**:136-144

[77] Cao L, Che X, Qiu X, Li Z, Yang B, Wang S, et al. M2 macrophage infiltration into tumor islets leads to poor prognosis in non-small-cell lung cancer. Cancer Management and Research. 2019;**11**:6125-6138

[78] Zhang B, Yao G, Zhang Y, Gao J, Yang B, Rao Z, et al. M2-polarized tumor-associated macrophages are associated with poor prognoses resulting from accelerated lymphangiogenesis in lung adenocarcinoma. Clinics (São Paulo, Brazil). 2011;**66**:1879-1886

[79] Mu Q, Najafi M. Modulation of the tumor microenvironment (TME) by melatonin. European Journal of Pharmacology. 2021;**907**:174365

[80] Li Y, Cao F, Li M, Li P, Yu Y, Xiang L, et al. Hydroxychloroquine induced lung cancer suppression by enhancing chemo-sensitization and promoting the transition of M2-TAMs to M1-like macrophages. Journal of Experimental & Clinical Cancer Research. 2018;**37**:259

[81] Brandão RD, Veeck J, Van de Vijver KK, Lindsey P, de Vries B, van Elssen CH, et al. A randomised controlled phase II trial of pre-operative celecoxib treatment reveals anti-tumour transcriptional response in primary breast cancer. Breast Cancer Research. 2013;**15**:R29

[82] Zhu B, Zou L, Cheng X, Lin Z, Duan Y, Wu Y, et al. Administration of MIP-3alpha gene to the tumor following radiation therapy boosts anti-tumor immunity in a murine model of lung carcinoma. Immunology Letters. 2006;**103**:101-107

[83] Zhou Z, Peng Y, Wu X, Meng S, Yu W, Zhao J, et al. CCL 18 secreted from M2 macrophages promotes migration and invasion via the PI3K/Akt pathway in gallbladder cancer. Cellular Oncology (Dordrecht). 2019;**42**:81-92

[84] Han S, Wang W, Wang S, Wang S, Ju R, Pan Z, et al. Multifunctional biomimetic nanoparticles loading baicalin for polarizing tumor-associated macrophages. Nanoscale. 2019;**11**:20206-20220

[85] Cao M, Yan H, Han X, Weng L, Wei Q, Sun X, et al. Ginseng-derived nanoparticles alter macrophage polarization to inhibit melanoma growth. Journal for Immunotherapy of Cancer. 2019;**7**:326

[86] Zhang J, Song W, Guo J, Zhang J, Sun Z, Li L, et al. Cytotoxicity of different sized TiO2 nanoparticles in mouse macrophages. Toxicology and Industrial Health. 2013;**29**:523-533

[87] Park J, Lim DH, Lim HJ, Kwon T, Choi JS, Jeong S, et al. Size dependent macrophage responses and toxicological effects of Ag nanoparticles. Chemical Communications. 2011;**47**:4382-4384

[88] Holgate ST. Pathogenesis of asthma. Clinical and Experimental Allergy. 2008;**38**:872-897

[89] Licona-Limon P, Kim LK, Palm NW, Flavell RA. TH2, allergy and group 2 innate lymphoid cells. Nature Immunology. 2013;**14**:536-542

[90] Peters SP. Asthma phenotypes: Nonallergic (intrinsic) asthma. The Journal of Allergy and Clinical Immunology. In Practice. 2014;**2**:650-652

[91] Arjomandi M et al. Repeated exposure to ozone increases alveolar macrophage recruitment into asthmatic airways. American Journal of Respiratory and Critical Care Medicine. 2005;**172**:427-432

[92] Gordon S. Alternative activation of macrophages. Nature Reviews. Immunology. 2003;**3**:23-35

[93] Leung TF, Wong GW, Ko FW, Lam CW, Fok TF. Increased macrophage-derived chemokine in exhaled breath condensate and plasma from children with asthma. Clinical and Experimental Allergy. 2004;**34**:786-791

[94] Mautino G et al. Increased expression of tissue inhibitor of metalloproteinase-1 and loss of correlation with matrix metalloproteinase-9 by macrophages in asthma. Laboratory Investigation. 1999;**79**:39-47

[95] Moon KA et al. Allergen-induced CD11b+ CD11c(int) CCR3+ macrophages in the lung promote eosinophilic airway inflammation in a mouse asthma model. International Immunology. 2007;**19**:1371-1381

[96] Zasłona Z, Przybranowski S, Wilke C, van Rooijen N, Teitz-Tennenbaum S, Osterholzer JJ, et al. Resident alveolar macrophages suppress, whereas recruited monocytes promote, allergic lung inflammation in murine models of asthma. Journal of Immunology. 2014;**193**:4245-4253

[97] Lee YG, Jeong JJ, Nyenhuis S, Berdyshev E, Chung S, Ranjan R, et al. Recruited alveolar macrophages, in response to airway epithelial-derived monocyte chemoattractant protein 1/CCl2, regulate airway inflammation and remodeling in allergic asthma. American Journal of Respiratory Cell and Molecular Biology. 2015;**52**:772-784

[98] Chung S, Lee TJ, Reader BF, Kim JY, Lee YG, Park GY, et al. FoxO1 regulates allergic asthmatic inflammation through regulating polarization of the macrophage inflammatory phenotype. Oncotarget. 2016;**7**:17532-17546

[99] Nieuwenhuizen NE, Kirstein F, Jayakumar J, Emedi B, Hurdayal R, Horsnell WGC, et al. Allergic airway disease is unaffected by the absence of IL-4Rα-dependent alternatively activated macrophages. The Journal of Allergy and Clinical Immunology. 2012;**130**:743-750

[100] Gundra UM, Girgis NM, Ruckerl D, Jenkins S, Ward LN, Kurtz ZD, et al. Alternatively activated macrophages derived from monocytes and tissue macrophages are phenotypically and functionally distinct. Blood. 2014;**123**:e110-e122

[101] Draijer C, Robbe P, Boorsma CE, Hylkema MN, Melgert BN. Characterization of macrophage phenotypes in three murine models of house-dust-mite-induced asthma. Mediators of Inflammation. 2013;**2013**:632049

[102] Draijer C, Boorsma CE, Robbe P, Timens W, Hylkema MN, Ten Hacken NHT, et al. Human asthma is characterized by more IRF5+ M1 and CD206+ M2 macrophages and less IL10+ M2-like macrophages around airways compared to healthy airways. The Journal of Allergy and Clinical Immunology. 2016;**140**(1):280-283

[103] Kim Y-K, Oh S-Y, Jeon SG, Park H-W, Lee S-Y, Chun E-Y, et al. Airway exposure levels of lipopolysaccharide determine type 1 versus type 2 experimental asthma. Journal of Immunology. 2007;**178**:5375-5382

[104] Bedoret D, Wallemacq H, Marichal T, Desmet C, Quesada

Calvo F, Henry E, et al. Lung interstitial macrophages alter dendritic cell functions to prevent airway allergy in mice. The Journal of Clinical Investigation. 2009;**119**:3723-3738

[105] Karta MR, Wickert LE, Curran CS, Gavala ML, Denlinger LC, Gern JE, et al. Allergen challenge in vivo alters rhinovirus-induced chemokine secretion from human airway macrophages. The Journal of Allergy and Clinical Immunology. 2014;**133**:1227-1230.e4

[106] Hong JY, Chung Y, Steenrod J, Chen Q, Lei J, Comstock AT, et al. Macrophage activation state determines the response to rhinovirus infection in a mouse model of allergic asthma. Respiratory Research. 2014;**15**:63

[107] Chanda D, Otoupalova E, Smith SR, et al. Developmental pathways in the pathogenesis of lung fibrosis. Molecular Aspects of Medicine. 2019;**65**:56-69

[108] Dancer RC, Wood AM, Thickett DR. Metalloproteinases in idiopathic pulmonary fibrosis. The European Respiratory Journal. 2011;**38**:1461-1467

[109] Craig VJ, Zhang L, Hagood JS, et al. Matrix metalloproteinases as therapeutic targets for idiopathic pulmonary fibrosis. American Journal of Respiratory Cell and Molecular Biology. 2015;**53**:585-600

[110] Zhang W, Ohno S, Steer B, et al. S100a4 is secreted by alternatively activated alveolar macrophages and promotes activation of lung fibroblasts in pulmonary fibrosis. Frontiers in Immunology. 2018;**9**:1216

[111] Misharin AV, Morales-Nebreda L, Reyfman PA, et al. Monocyte derived alveolar macrophages drive lung fibrosis and persist in the lung over the life span. The Journal of Experimental Medicine. 2017;**214**:2387-2404

[112] McCubbrey AL, Barthel L, Mohning MP, et al. Deletion of c-FLIP from CD11b(hi) macrophages prevents development of bleomycin-induced lung fibrosis. American Journal of Respiratory Cell and Molecular Biology. 2018;**58**:66-78

[113] Aran D, Looney AP, Liu L, et al. Reference-based analysis of lung single-cell sequencing reveals a transitional profibrotic macrophage. Nature Immunology. 2019;**20**:163-172

[114] Allden SJ, Ogger PP, Ghai P, et al. The transferrin receptor CD71 delineates functionally distinct airway macrophage subsets during idiopathic pulmonary fibrosis. American Journal of Respiratory and Critical Care Medicine. 2019;**200**:209-219

[115] Reyfman PA, Walter JM, Joshi N, et al. Single-cell transcriptomic analysis of human lung provides insights into the pathobiology of pulmonary fibrosis. American Journal of Respiratory and Critical Care Medicine. 2019;**199**:1517-1536

[116] Shi T, Denney L, An H, Ho L-P, Zheng Y. Alveolar and lung interstitial macrophages: Definitions, functions, and roles in lung fibrosis. Journal of Leukocyte Biology. 2021;**110**:107-114

[117] Meziani L, Mondini M, Petit B, et al. CSF1R inhibition prevents radiation pulmonary fibrosis by depletion of interstitial macrophages. The European Respiratory Journal. 2018;**51**:1702120

[118] Wynn TA, Barron L. Macrophages: Master regulators of inflammation and fibrosis. Seminars in Liver Disease. 2010;**30**:245-257

Chapter 5

Macrophages in the Smooth Muscle Layers of the Gastrointestinal Tract

Gianluca Cipriani and Suraj Pullapantula

Abstract

Muscularis macrophages are a newly discovered population of immune cells populating the smooth muscle layers of the gastrointestinal tract. Beyond their well-established role in modulating innate immunity, these cells are emerging for their ability to communicate with cells required for gastrointestinal motility. This chapter will describe the factors contributing to muscularis macrophages' phenotype and the functional connections these cells established with different cell types.

Keywords: macrophages, gut, enteric neurons, enteric glia, gastrointestinal motility

1. Introduction

The gut is home to the body's largest population of immune cells [1, 2]. Beyond the frontline defenses against unparalleled exposure to foreign antigens, gut macrophages (MΦ) also constantly communicate with an intricate network of cell types orchestrating gastrointestinal (GI) functions [3, 4]. By now, the plasticity of MΦ in different organs of the body (inter-diversity) and within tissue layers (intra-diversity) has been established. While the M1/M2 dogma has served to advance the field of Immunology and understand MΦ phenotype and function [5, 6], immunologists now generally agree that there is a spectrum of phenotypes between the two classifications [7–9]. This chapter will outline the phenotype and function of a population of MΦ in the GI tract, called muscularis macrophages (MMΦ). As the name states, MMΦ resides in the muscularis layers of the GI tract, called muscularis propria. MMΦ fulfills multiple functions across development, adulthood, and under disease conditions. This chapter will report the factors contributing to MMΦ' phenotype heterogeneity and describe the functional interaction MMΦ establish with cells populating the same environment.

2. Identification of MMΦ: a new population of macrophages

Mikkelsen and colleagues first identified "macrophage-like" cells in the muscularis propria of the small intestine using combination of electron microscopy and immunohistochemistry [10]. Subsequent studies by the same group confirmed these cells to be MMΦ after endocytosis of FITC-dextran and F4/80 labeling co-labeled. In addition to the identification of MMΦ by immunohistochemistry, electron microscopy analysis revealed distinct morphological features based on location within the muscularis

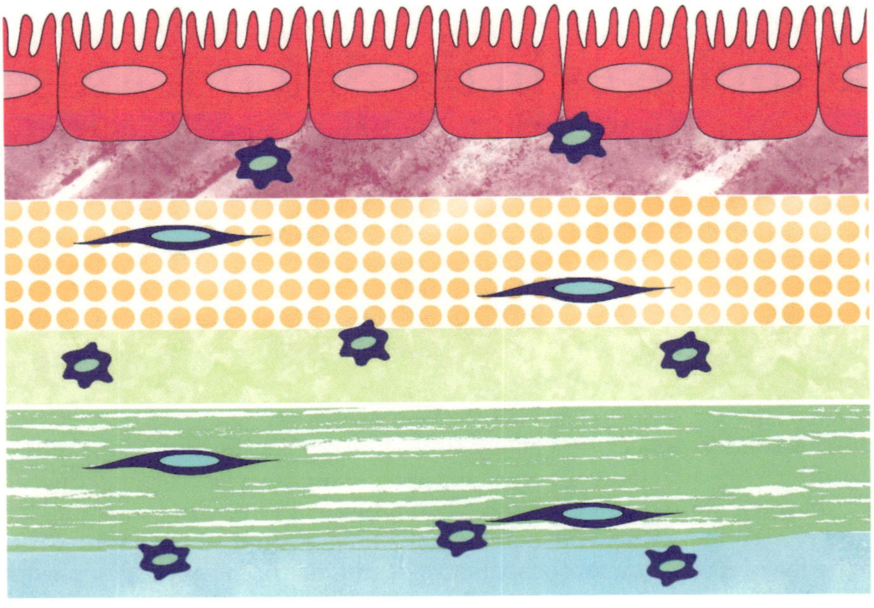

Figure 1.
Different regions of the gastrointestinal tract along with the varying morphologies of MΦ.

propria. These cells were noted to contain a nucleus, Golgi bodies, smooth and rough endoplasmic reticulum, and enveloped by the processes of interstitial cells of Cajal (ICC). The GI muscularis propria (**Figure 1**) is separated from the external environment by the mucosa, which is in constant contact with ingested food along with the gut microbes and other pathogens.

The primary function of the mucosa is to absorb the dietary nutrients and protect against the different external stimuli [11–13]. On the other hand, the muscularis propria is mainly responsible for coordinating contractions for proper food movement through the GI tract. The cellular anatomy of the muscularis propria is complex and characterized by different regions. The two muscular layers are called longitudinal and circular, respectively, based on their orientation. The myenteric plexus, also known as the Auerbach plexus, contains a significant number of enteric neurons (ENs) and pace-making ICC, which regulate peristalsis between the two muscle regions [14–17] (**Figure 1**). Advanced technologies further demonstrated MMΦ's heterogeneity within the muscularis propria, as recent studies described differences in MMΦ distribution and phenotype within different regions of the GI muscularis propria. Current understanding revolves around MMΦ acquiring distinct phenotypes upon exposure to intrinsic GI cues. However, emerging evidence suggests that MMΦ display differences in their functions and phenotypes that are not exclusively driven by the GI milieu but also by their ontogeny.

3. MMΦ heterogeneity: ontogeny vs. environmental cues

For the longest time, the origin of MΦ was attributed entirely to circulating blood monocytes, which after engrafting the tissue, acquired tissue-resident MΦ resemblance [18–20]. However, studies in the late 2010s challenged this paradigm as scientists theorized that populations of resident MΦ in homeostatic tissues also derived from embryonic progenitors of the yolk sac and fetal liver [21–23]. After this finding, there is now a consensus on the double origin of tissue-resident MΦ in multiple organs, where monocyte-derived- and embryonic MΦ coexist [24]. Embryonic MΦ are established before birth and their number is maintained by cell division, independently of circulating monocytes' recruitment. On the other hand, a population of MΦ is continuously replenished by a monocyte waterfall wherein circulating adult monocytes ingress into tissues and differentiate to tissue-resident MΦ [24].

While MMΦ ontogeny in homeostatic condition has been recently studied [25], most of the research in the last couple of decades has primarily been focused on disease models. Like microglia in the central nervous system (CNS), MMΦ contains populations of different origins, as cells of both embryonic and circulating monocyte origin constitute the entire pool of tissue-resident MMΦ. MMΦ as microglia in the brain express the high level of CX3CR1 as a canonical marker of tissue-resident cells.

Using a lineage tracing mouse model, CX3CR1 MMΦ were followed from the embryonic stage to adulthood. This population represents the totality of tissue-resident MMΦ at the embryonic stage and declines with time. This decline starts between 4 and 20 weeks after birth and stops after this timepoint. Consequently, the population that remains seeded has come to be known as long-lived MMΦ. Importantly, this population of embryonic MMΦ has a different transcriptional profile compared with monocyte-derived MMΦ. In fact, a population of tissue-resident MMΦ expresses high levels of CX3CR1, also known as $CX3CR1^{hi}$. $CX3CR1^{low}$ MMΦ, on the contrary—as the name suggests—express low levels of CX3CR1 and highly express C-C chemokine receptor 2 (CCR2). CCR2 is involved in monocyte homing in response to inflammation in the local tissue environment [26, 27]. Resident MMΦ exhibits a general anti-inflammatory phenotype at steady-state conditions compared to the more inflammatory phenotype of mucosal MΦ. This is underscored by the expression of their wound healing and tissue-protective genes.

Long-lived MMΦ express genes responsible for cell-to-cell adhesion, cytoskeletal anchoring, and neuron development, suggesting their anatomical association with ENs. In addition, 26% of the genes enriched in a subpopulation of long-lived MMΦ is unique compared to the data set from tissue-resident MΦ populating other tissues. However, most of this population express gene previously associated with microglia in the brain, such as Fc receptor-like scavenger (*FCRLS*), cystatin C (*CST3*), platelet factor 4 (*PF4*), apolipoprotein E (*ApoE*), and disabled-2 (*Dab2*). Although a subtype of MMΦ is maintained by cell division, most tissue-resident MMΦ are continuously replenished by circulating monocytes. In fact, bone marrow transplanted $CX3CR1^{EGFP}$ cells engrafted into the muscle layers, and within 4 weeks of transplantation, they re-established the number of tissue-resident MMΦ [28].

A study aimed at differentiating between long-lived MΦ and monocyte-derived MΦ used Tim4 and CD4 as surface markers to separate the two populations [29]. Long-lived MΦ were $Tim\text{-}4^{+}/CD4^{+}$ as evidenced by the slower rate of turnover compared to $Tim\text{-}4^{-}/CD4^{-}$ cells as expressed by chimerism of cells post-irradiation. Although the total pool of small bowel MΦ was considered, this segregation is largely driven by mucosal tissue-resident MΦ in commensal-rich areas as noted in the study due to the higher rate of monocyte-macrophage turnover. Interestingly, Tim-4 is as an important apoptotic cell uptake receptor indicating that these long-lived MΦ might be playing a crucial role in efferocytosis, a process which has been shown to resolve inflammation in the brain by microglia [30], and other tissue types [31].

A new population of embryonic MMΦ called perivascular (PVMs) was recently identified in anatomical association with blood vessels within the muscularis propria of the ileum and small intestine [32]. The authors identified a gene—musculoaponeurotic fibrosarcoma (*Maf*)—which is required for the development of this subpopulation in white adipose tissue (WAT). This population, named vasculature-associated macrophages (VAMs), existed in all organs in proximity to blood vessels. This commonality led them to understand the effect of *Maf* regulation in the muscularis propria of the ileum and small intestine since they harbor MMΦ expressing similar markers to VAMs, specifically, VAM2. Furthermore, when the *Maf* gene was deleted, there was a total loss of CD206+ MMΦ in the small and large intestines, implicating its critical role in their phenotype and function.

All these data suggest the bivalent origin of tissue-resident MMΦ with the coexistence of monocyte- and embryonic-derived MMΦ. This level of heterogeneity has been recently described in the single-cell transcriptomic analysis of colonic MMΦ. Colonic MMΦ can be divided into three different populations, including "transient" monocyte-like MMΦ expressing high levels of calprotectin (heterodimer of S100A8 and S100A9) and long-lived calprotectin-negative MΦ expressing a TRM phenotype [33, 34].

Further investigation is needed to outline the key similarities and differences between murine and human MMΦ distribution, morphology, and composition. Although the murine monocyte waterfall in the intestine depicts a detailed transition of $Ly6C^{hi}$ $CX3CR1^{int}$ monocytes to $CX3CR1^{hi}$ $MHC\text{-}II^{hi}$ CD64+ MMΦ, information on human MMΦ is sparse, generally relied upon immunohistochemistry and morphological studies.

Another study by Bernardo and colleagues tracked the transition phenotype of human monocytes to tissue-resident MΦ [35]. It was found that $CD14^{+}$ monocytes differentiated into inflammatory monocyte-like cells upon entering healthy and inflamed colonic mucosa. These cells, identified by $CD11c^{hi}$ $CCR2^{hi}$ $CX3CR1^{+}$ expression, then transitioned through an intermediate phenotype of $CD11c^{dim}$ $CCR2^{low}$ $CX3CR1^{low}$ before finally becoming tissue-resident—or tolerogenic—MΦ with a $CD11c^{-}$ $CCR2^{-}$ $CX3CR1^{-}$ signature. As is true in the mouse model, CCR2 remains critical in recruiting monocytes in humans. Furthermore, the authors found that homing was abrogated when it was blocked on monocytes before migration. Whether this is true in MMΦ is yet to be elucidated. Changes to monocyte-derived or long-lived embryonic MMΦ can alter the total MMΦ number in diseases where homeostasis is challenged. For example, in diabetic and diabetic gastroparetic mice [36], there is an increase in MMΦ which is linked to the recruitment of inflammatory circulating monocytes.

MMΦ phenotype depends on regional distribution across the muscularis propria and the interaction MMΦ established with other cell types populating the same environment. MMΦ have a different morphology [37] in the different regions of the muscularis propria. MMΦ located in the myenteric plexus and serosal regions is multipolar, with many branches originating from the main body (**Figure 1**).

On the other hand, MMΦ distributed within the muscular layers have a bipolar shape that follows muscle cells' orientation. Further data are needed to understand if morphological differences between these diverse MMΦ populations translate into functional changes. Such differences have been easier to study in the brain since the various CNS regions are accessible and can be separated. Whereas this has enabled the study of microglial phenotype residing in each area, it is more complicated to get the same type of information from the muscularis layers of the GI tract due to the technical difficulties in separating the different regions.

Long-lived MMΦ occupy a specific anatomical niche within the GI muscularis propria. De Schepper and colleagues [25] identified this MMΦ population as essential for maintaining ENs, located within the myenteric plexus region where they interact with ENs. The critical role of the environmental cue in shaping MMΦ phenotype is evident as embryonic MΦ are also present in the mucosa, but they have an overall distinct phenotype compared to long-lived MMΦ. Interestingly, another population of embryonic MMΦ does not express CX3CR1, but in this case, it appeared to be anatomically coupled with blood vessels [32].

Another essential feature contributing to MMΦ heterogeneity is the location of MMΦ in different regions of the muscularis propria. Whereas in the small intestine MMΦ are mostly concentrated in the myenteric plexus, gastric MMΦ are evenly distributed between the myenteric plexus and smooth muscle layers [38]. Further studies are needed to understand if this difference in MMΦ distribution is also responsible for functional changes. Phenotypically, at resting, gastric MMΦ do not express high levels of CD206 as MMΦ from the small intestine does. MMΦ density also differs between the small intestine and colon in young mice, with a reduction of MMΦ density observed in the colon [39]. However, this type of difference was no longer observed in adult mice. It also appeared that MMΦ in the different gut regions responds to external stimuli differently, suggesting a possible intrinsic phenotypic difference. For example, in diabetes, gastric MMΦ change their phenotype leading to gastric dysfunction, whereas, in the context of the same disease, MMΦ in the small intestine are unchanged [36].

Although we have a clearer picture of MMΦ distribution in different smooth muscle layers at steady-state conditions, we have only partial information about their distribution in states of altered homeostasis and disease. In aging, clusters of CD163-IR immune cells are visualized in proximity to sympathetic hyperinnervation in the jejunum of rats [40]. In a mouse model of diabetic gastroparesis, an increased number of MMΦ has been described with the onset of diabetes, but no changes in the MMΦ distribution have been reported [41].

More studies are needed to understand the differences between the populations of MMΦ residing in the different gut regions looking at (1) phenotypic changes, (2) changes in response to inflammation/stimuli, and (3) origin.

4. MMΦ: new players of gastrointestinal motility

As anticipated in the previous section of the chapter, the muscularis propria contains numerous ENs that work in concert with the CNS to control digestive function. The enteric nervous system (ENS) has 200–600 million ENs distributed in thousands of small ganglia [15, 16]. Importantly, the ENS can function independently from the CNS to control digestive function. The GI tract is innervated by intrinsic ENs and the CNS axons of extrinsic sympathetic and parasympathetic neurons.

Since some MMΦ are closely associated with ENs, this raises the following questions: Do these MMΦ functionally interact with enteric nerves, and what does such communication entail?

4.1 Functional interaction between MMΦ and intrinsic innervation

MMΦ-ENs functional interaction has been studied extensively in the homeostatic and diseased gut. Muller and colleagues showed for the first time an active interaction between MMΦ and ENs in 2014 [42]. In this study, the investigators showed that MMΦ expresses a high level of bone morphogenetic protein 2 (BMP2) compared to mucosal MΦ. Notably, certain ENs express the receptor (BMP2r) that, upon interaction with

BMP2, respond by a pSMAD1/5/8 related mechanism. This type of functional interaction is regulated by microbiota, as microbiota-free mice have reduced BMP2 expression. Depletion of MMΦ results in poorly coordinated colonic contractions in an ex vivo model and abnormal colonic transit time in vivo. Adding exogenous BMP2 to the colonic rings from MMΦ -deficient mice decreases stretch-induced contractions. Enteric neuron number results from a dynamic balance between the ENs dying by apoptosis and the continuous production of new ENs by neurogenesis. As microglia in the CNS, MMΦ played an essential role in clearing cellular debris resulting from neuronal death. In vitro models have shown the bidirectionality of this interaction. Oxytocin (OT) is traditionally considered a nonapeptide hormone synthesized in the hypothalamus that is released from the posterior pituitary into circulation and is involved in milk let-down and uterine contraction. Polarized pro-inflammatory MMΦ regulate the expression of OT and its receptor, OTR in cultured enteric neurons via STAT3 or NF-κB pathway [43].

On the other hand, TGF-β released by anti-inflammatory MMΦ induces the upregulation of OT/OTR [44]. Interestingly higher levels of pro-inflammatory cytokines correlated with a lower level of OT/OTR in DSS-colitis. In the colon, ENS is reduced by pro-inflammatory MMΦ via the GK1-FOXO3 pathway.

Most studies described a close association between MMΦ and nerve fibers. However, recently a paper for the first time also describes a rare population of MMΦ distributed within the ganglia [45, 46], which house the bodies of the ENs. In their study, the authors demonstrated that this population of MMΦ, called intra ganglionic macrophages (IGMs), has processes in this region of mouse colon, suggesting phagocytic capability. Colitis-induced mouse models are characterized by an increased level of pro-inflammatory MMΦ and associated with a reduction of IGMs. Notably, the loss of IGMs in colitis is associated with enteric neuroinflammation, characterized by neuronal hypertrophy.

A series of studies questioned the role of MMΦ in regulating the total number and the genetic coding of ENs. CX3CR1 MMΦ [25] of embryonic origin persisted with aging and remained primarily associated with ENs in the myenteric plexus region. The conditional removal of this population of MMΦ during development results in the overall reduction of ENs, leading to GI dysfunction. Csf1$^{op/op}$ mice, which do not have MMΦ from birth, have an abnormal myenteric plexus and more ENs than control mice [41, 42]. Although the number of nitrergic ENs is increased in Csf1$^{op/op}$ mice [47], the number of cholinergic ENs is not altered, suggesting that MMΦ may regulate different subtypes of ENs (**Figure 2**).

In the same animal model, Cipriani and colleagues also showed that the absence of MMΦ from birth is associated with more ENs sharing cholinergic and nitrergic phenotypes, indicative of a more undifferentiated population of ENs. A reduced number of anti-inflammatory MMΦ in aged mice is linked to ENs loss [48, 49].

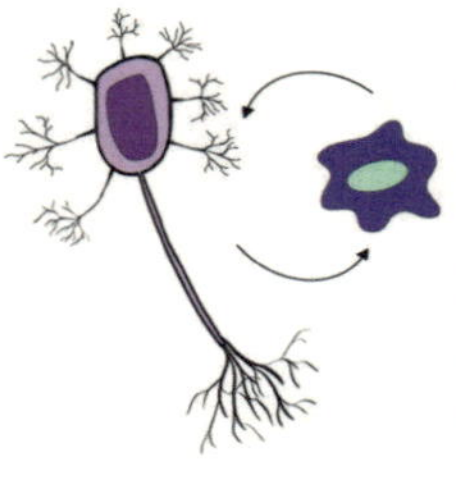

Homeostasis	Disease
1) MMΦ clear cellular debris as a result of neuronal apoptosis maintaining EN balance 2) MMΦ confer anti-inflammatory effects such as HO-1 release which are neuroprotective 3) B2AR mediated sympathetic innervation of MMΦ induces neuroprotection	1) Vagal nerve perturbation from surgery/inflammation leads to EN loss from pro-inflammatory MMΦ 2) Vagal nerve stimulation can alleviate inflammation in muscularis propria 3) Vagotomy results in mice results in severe colitis and IBD related issues

Figure 2.
Bidirectional interactions between EN and MMΦ comparing homeostasis and disease.

To further understand this intimate relationship between MMΦ and the ENS, papers understanding their dynamics during development have shed some light on this. MMΦ colonize the gut independently of ENs at E9.5. Although they engraft into the muscularis propria, tissue-resident MMΦ are not close to ENs but are closer to other cells populating the same environment during this period [50]. The investigators identified a plausible explanation for this observation as the absence of CSF1 release by ENs during this period, contrary to adulthood where ENs represent the primary source of CSF1. An increasing number of MMΦ engraft into the muscularis propria during development, where they occupy a distinct niche compared to mucosal MΦ and establish an intimate connection with neuronal processes [51]. Conditional depletion of *irf8*, a gene enriched in this population of MMΦ, leads to impaired intestinal GI motility. More studies are needed to dissect further the possible role of MMΦ in orchestrating ENs differentiation and distribution.

4.2 Functional interaction between MMΦ and extrinsic innervation

The amount of data describing the functional interaction between tissue MMΦ, and peripheral nerves is limited, mainly because the number of MMΦ is minimal compared to the total number of tissue MΦ. For example, MMΦ expressing CX3CR1 are closely associated with sympathetic nerve fibers of adipose tissue [52]. Precise extrinsic afferent (visceral sensory) and efferent (sympathetic and parasympathetic) innervation of the gut is fundamental for gut-brain cross talk. While the extrinsic nerves do not directly modulate gut motility, they can affect it by regulating other cell types within the ENS [53]. Interactions between MMΦ and extrinsic innervation and the effect of sympathetic and catecholaminergic signaling in the immune cells' modulation of multiple organs have been extensively studied in the past [54]. However, their possible involvement in modulating MMΦ polarization phenotype in the gut has been described only recently. In their study, Gabanyi and colleagues [37] suggest the regulation of MMΦ activation by the β-adrenergic receptor β-2AR receptor (β2AR). B2AR$^+$ MMΦ resides near neuronal cell bodies or processes of the myenteric ganglia. Because of this interaction, MMΦ expresses higher levels of β2AR, a neuropeptide receptor, than lamina propria MΦ. Notably, adrenergic signaling through this receptor reduces ENs loss following infection [55].

Acetylcholine (Ach) represents the primary parasympathetic neurotransmitter released by preganglionic nerve fibers and the vagus nerve. Ach has been studied for its anti-inflammatory effects in the periphery, as its stimulation is sufficient to suppress systemic inflammation in response to endotoxin. Cholinergic neuronal release during vagal nerve stimulation (VNS) induces an anti-inflammatory MMΦ phenotype activation via the alpha7 nAChR (α7nAChR), ameliorating muscular inflammation [56]. In addition, vagal manipulation leads to an increased number of gastric MHCII+ MMΦ, resulting in delayed gastric emptying [57].

The vagal nerve represents the longest nerve in the body and the main component of parasympathetic innervation. It is well established that the vagal nerve innervating the GI tract originates from 2 central regions of the CNS: the ambiguous nucleus and the dorsal motor nucleus of the vagus. This indeed represents one of the most studied roots to access the ENS from the CNS [58]. VNS mediates MMΦ anti-inflammatory phenotype activation in a model of inflammation induced by mechanical stimulation of the mucosa. This pathway is independent of vagal stimulation from the spleen as vagus denervation from the spleen did not prevent MMΦ activation. In this mouse model, the activation of anti-inflammatory MMΦ through VNS reduced the overall level of inflammation in the tissue. It appeared that this type of pathway is effective through the α7nAChR since MMΦ from α7nAChR knockout mice did not respond to VNS [56]. Extrinsic vagal innervation is involved in regulating contractions generated by the stomach. Preclinical studies underlined this pathway's involvement and its possible therapeutic role in preventing muscularis propria inflammation in inflammatory bowel disease (IBD). Mice in which the vagus is resected develop severe colitis associated with increased pro-inflammatory cytokine levels such as IL-1β, IL-6, and TNF-α [59].

Interestingly, patients with depression and psychological stress are typically associated with adverse and worst forms of ulcerative colitis. This important association also translates into animal models of depression, which are more prone to develop forms of colitis [60]. Notably, the beneficial effect of antidepressant drug application is abolished after vagotomy. Although this mechanism is not entirely understood, the transfer of MΦ from animal models with depression made the recipient mice more susceptible to developing forms of colitis [61].

Gastroparesis is a disease that affects the stomach and is associated with impaired motility and increased pro-inflammatory MMΦ. VNS stimulation in patients with gastroparesis induced anti-inflammatory MMΦ activation and an incremental improvement in symptom scores [62]. In addition, VNS prevents gastroparesis by inducing anti-inflammatory MMΦ through STAT3-JAK2 mediated mechanism. Abdominal surgery is often associated with pro-inflammatory MMΦ activation leading to an overall inflammation of the muscularis propria and affected gastric motility, which VNS3 abolishes [63].

It appears that this interaction is bidirectional, as ENs can also affect MMΦ phenotype, differentiation, and maintenance. In an animal model in which pharmaceutical and genetic sympathetic innervation is deprived, there is an increase of circulating monocytes that ingress into the muscularis propria compared to controls [64]. In addition, isolated MMΦ from sympathetic-deprived mice have anti-inflammatory phenotype and concomitant increment of pro-inflammatory phenotype that led to accelerated GI transit time. Intestinal manipulation in postoperative ileus (POI) promoted an increased level of anti-inflammatory ED1 MMΦ [65] in the colon blocked by an anti-α7nAChR antibody. The authors proposed a mechanism in which ENs released acetylcholine upon intestinal manipulation that binds its receptor (α7nAChR) on the surface [56]. This represents a mechanism that could be targeted to prevent POI. A mouse model of post-infectious irritable bowel syndrome (IBS) is associated with subtype-specific neuronal loss via NRLP6 and caspase 11 mechanism and dysmotility. Notably, in this model, β2-AR signaling depletion in MMΦ resulted in increased loss of ENs in the post-infectious IBS model. These results indicate that, while short-term depletion of MMΦ does not impact intrinsic enteric-associated neurons (iEANs) survival in the unperturbed state, MMΦ may play an iEAN-protective role during enteric infection [56].

5. MMΦ interactions with non-neuronal cells

5.1 MMΦ-ICC

The GI tract represents a highly heterogeneous system where multiple cell types coexist and contribute to GI contractility. Similar to the pacemaker cells of the heart, the gut contains cells called ICC that set up the GI contractility pattern. ICC was described more than 100 years ago by Ramon y Cajal. For many years these cells were characterized only by non-specific histological stains and later, more reliably, by electron microscopy. The ultrastructural features and the ICC's anatomical distributions

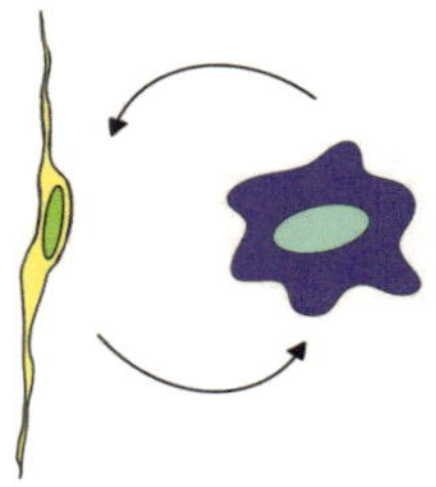

Homeostasis	Disease
1) Needs to be further elucidated	1) Injurious cytokines such as TNF-a, IL-6 result in injury to ICC
2) MMΦ do not make direct cell contacts with ICCs	2) Decrease in CD206+ MMΦ skews tissue profile towards pro-inflammation
3) Separated by 300 microns	

Figure 3.
Bidirectional interactions between ICC and MMΦ in homeostasis and disease.

suggested their critical physiological roles: (1) they are pacemaker cells and propagate slow waves [66, 67], (2) they mediate both inhibitory and excitatory neurotransmission [68–70], (3) they work as mechanosensory cells.

Limited data describe MMΦ-ICC interaction in homeostatic conditions in the ENS. Electron microscopy and immunofluorescence analysis showed that MMΦ populations are closely associated with ICC [10, 14], suggesting a potential functional role for this type of interaction. Ji and colleagues [38] recently demonstrated that despite their close association, MMΦ rarely touches ICC, but they are separated by a space of 300 microns. In Csf1$^{op/op}$ mice, that do not have MΦ from birth, ICC appears to have a normal distribution, and the level of expression of kit, a specific ICC marker, is not different from controls (**Figure 3**).

The information relative to MMΦ-ICC functional interaction in GI disease is more extensive. Blockade of IL-17A signal reduced ICC loss in sepsis by affecting the overall number of pro-inflammatory MMΦ [71]. Numerous MMΦ are observed closely associated with ICC in the antiinflammation model compared to controls at ultrastructural level [72]. In the same model with the progression of inflammation, MMΦ has large phagosomes and lysosomes in the proximity of injured ICC, suggesting a possible ongoing phagocytic activity. During development, ICC releases CSF1 in the small intestine, thus contributing to MMΦ migration and survival during this period. IL-6 released by MMΦ during GI surgery promotes upregulation of miR-19a responsible for ICC depletion [73]. An increase of pro-inflammatory cytokines produced by MMΦ is associated with decreased c-kit positive ICC in the dilated colon of Hirschsprung disease (HSCR) associated with enterocolitis [74].

Most of the information acquired in recent years describing a functional interaction between MMΦ and ICC has been produced in the context of diabetic gastroparesis, a functional disease affecting the stomach. One of the main cellular changes observed in both mice and patients with diabetic gastroparesis is ICC depletion and changes to MMΦ composition. Conditioned media from pro-inflammatory activated MMΦ reduces kit positive ICC *in-vitro* [75]. The ineffectiveness of the same conditional media in the presence of a TNF-alpha neutralizing antibody suggests this cytokine's implication in regulating kit expression. Patients with diabetic gastroparesis have fewer CD206^{+}, anti-inflammatory MΦ. This reduction correlates with ICC loss, suggesting a protective role of anti-inflammatory MMΦ on ICC, that is impaired in diabetic gastroparesis [76]. Anti-inflammatory MMΦ also secrete interleukin 10 (IL-10) to induce heme oxygenase (HO1) expression [77], an enzyme that has a protective effect on ICC. Mice with delayed gastric emptying treated with exogenous IL-10 return to regular gastric emptying with higher levels of HO1 and better connected, more organized, and evenly distributed ICC networks [78]. Thus, treatment to promote MMΦ polarization to an anti-inflammatory phenotype may be a viable treatment for diabetic gastroparesis. Progression of diabetes and development of delayed gastric emptying is associated with increased levels of pro-inflammatory MMΦ and reduced anti-inflammatory MMΦ.

A small number of data suggest the contribution of MMΦ-ICC functional interaction in the development of other GI diseases. For example, Crohn's disease is associated with ICC injury and changes to MMΦ morphology [79]. In Achalasia, ICC closely related to immune cells are preserved [80]. Cytokines released by MMΦ have been considered responsible for ICC network disruption in endothelin-B receptor null rat, a model of Hirschsprung's disease [81]. Other functional diseases, such as slow transit constipation, are associated with ICC loss. In this disease, ICC loss depends on the release of exosome miR-34c-5p from MMΦ [82].

5.2 MMΦ/smooth muscle cells and fibroblast-like cells

Although MMΦ exists in the muscle layers of the gut, the limited research surrounding their spatiotemporal dynamics with smooth muscle cells (SMCs) has hampered their full understanding. Only recently has their spatial interactions with SMCs been characterized in a paper. In it, MMΦ establishes membrane-to-membrane contacts with SMCs forming structures akin to peg-and-socket joints observed using Transmission Electron Microscopy [38] (TEM) in both humans and mice. Due to this tight interaction, it is speculated that chemokines/cytokines that are released by SMCs and vice versa maybe be pertinent for the maintenance of homeostasis in the local environment and ensure proper gut motility (**Figure 4**).

In fact, a study revealed a transient receptor potential vanilloid 4 receptor (TRPV4) mediated interaction between MMΦ and SMCs in the colon of mice [83]. TRPV4 is a biosensor that can detect mechanical, thermal, and chemical cues and has been implicated in various GI disorders. However, because its effect on gut motility was not established, the authors sought to determine its role, specifically in colonic motility. Using TRPV4−/− and TRPV4+/+ as comparisons, they found various indications of impaired colonic motility. For example, they found that TRPV4−/− mice had a significantly increased number of pellets retained in the colons as opposed to their WT controls. This led to the identification of a subtype of MMΦ expressing the TRPV4 channel responsible for colonic contractions independent of ENS input. This independence was confirmed by optogenetic stimulation of the same MMΦ while applying tetrodotoxin (TTX) which resulted in prostaglandin E2 release leading to spontaneous contractions.

Postoperative ileus (POI) is a common abdominal complication almost after every intra-abdominal surgery characterized by a prolonged absence of bowel movement. This leads to symptoms such as a distended abdomen, nausea, vomiting, and other

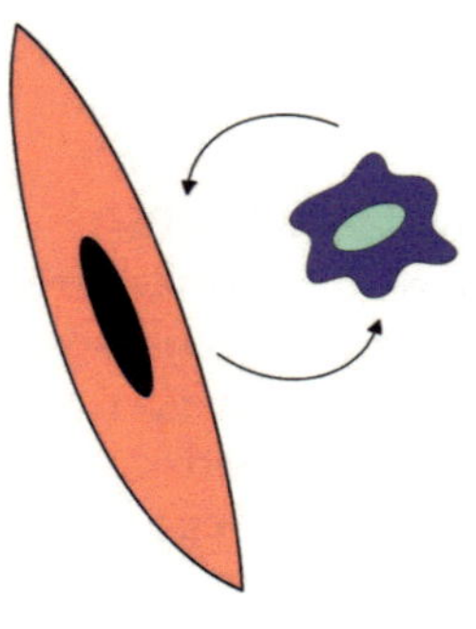

Homeostasis	Disease
1) MMΦ expressing TRPV4 are responsible for colonic contractions independent of ENS input 2) SMCs and MMΦ establish peg-and-socket type connections 3) Further studies warranted to elucidate mechanistic interactions	1) POI caused by MMΦ recruiting monocytes, neutrophils and other lymphocytes 2) In Crohn's, differentiation of monocytes in tissue is halted in pro-inflammatory state. 3) TNF-a and IL-23 release promotes injury to SMCs

Figure 4.
Bidirectional interactions between SMC and MMΦ comparing homeostasis and disease.

complications that prolong patients' stay in the hospital, furthering the epidemiological burden for all parties involved. Shortly after intestinal manipulation in mice, the MMΦ network in the muscularis propria evokes a localized inflammatory response that recruits neutrophils and mast cells. The extravasation of leukocytes in tandem with MMΦ [84] results in the synthesis of prostaglandins and nitric oxide which directly impair SMCs contractility leading to POI. In the inflammatory cascade that ensues initially, there is an upregulation of MIP-1a, IL-1B, IL-6, ICAM-1, and MCP-1 compared to WT controls, indicating that MMΦ recruits monocytes, which then become resident-MΦ, and subsequently attract more monocytes. The cytokines and chemokine released are injurious to the SMCs resulting in impaired contractility depletion of this MMΦ network has been shown to decrease overall inflammation and prevent POI completely [85].

Crohn's disease is an inflammatory bowel disease (IBD) characterized by persistent inflammation that typically affects both terminal ileum and colon. Due to simplicity, reproducibility, and commonalities associated with humans, TNBS-colitis in the murine model is used to study Crohn's disease [86]. In this model, MCP-1 RNA and protein levels are upregulated in the muscularis layer of the gut [46]. Similarly, in humans, inflammation resulting from Crohn's is associated with an increased number of pro-inflammatory MMΦ, neutrophils, and other immune cells recruited in the smooth muscle layers via a CCL2 and MCP-1 dependent mechanism [87]. Consequently, prolonged inflammation and hypertrophy of the surrounding smooth muscle layers have been observed [88]. Further studies are required to properly understand how MMΦ contribute to the pathogenesis of Crohn's disease.

In the process of characterizing ICC at the ultrastructural level, cells with morphological similarities to ICC were discovered [89]. These fibroblast-like cells were shown to contain gap junctions with SMCs in mice, rats, and guinea pigs indicating their potential involvement in GI motility. Years later, they came to be known as PDGFRα positive cells/telocytes (TC) since they were positive for the platelet-derived growth factor receptor alpha (PDGFRα) and negative for c-kit thus differentiating them from ICC. These cells are located all throughout the GI tract but specifically in the muscularis propria, as they can be found encircled around muscle bundles and ganglia. Their long processes form an intricate mesh-like network interacting with ICC networks, once again highlighting their importance in motility and function—specifically, purinergic motor transmission (**Figure 5**) [90].

Recently, it has been shown that MMΦ establishes cell-to-cell contacts with PDGFRα-positive cells using TEM. Due to the close association of PDGFRα-positive cells with SMCs and the connections made with MMΦ, it has further bolstered the notion that MMΦ contributes to homeostasis and GI motility in some fashion that has yet to be elucidated in greater detail.

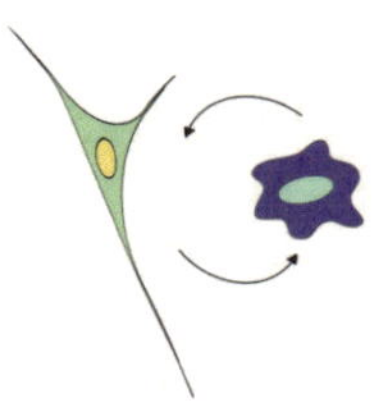

Homeostasis	Disease
1) Cell to cell contacts established with MMΦ 2) Contribute to purinergic motor transmission 3) Further studies required for deeper understanding	1) Relationship with MMΦ needs to be established

Figure 5.
Bidirectional interactions between PDGFRα-positive/TC and MMΦ comparing homeostasis and disease.

5.3 MMΦ: enteric glial cells

Enteric glial cells (EGCs) are found in the muscularis propria surrounding the ENs, sharing similar features with the brain macroglia, represented by astrocytes and oligodendrocytes. As oligodendrocytes in the brain, EGCs contribute significantly to ENs maintenance, survival, and function [91–94]. As previously described, a subpopulation of MMΦ is specifically situated in this space, making the two cell types sharing the same anatomical space and a functional interaction possible.

EGCs as astrocytes in the brain can shift the phenotype in disrupted homeostasis conditions, such as inflammation. They actively mediate acute and chronic inflammation in the gut by regulating circulating monocyte recruitment during inflammation and the expression of pro-inflammatory cytokines. In vivo and in vitro studies demonstrate that EGCs secrete several cytokines and chemokines, including interferon-γ (IFN-γ), chemokine ligand 20, TNF-α, and prostaglandin D2 [95, 96].

The increased number of CD68 MMΦ during inflammation, partially due to circulating monocyte extravasation, is reduced after conditional depletion of connexin 43 (*Cx43*)—a gene which encodes for gap junctions—from EGCs. IL-1B level, which is increased in inflammation, binds to its receptor on EGCs and regulates CSF1 expression by a Cx43 dependent mechanism [97].

A similar mechanism involving EGCs-MMΦ crosstalk was also observed in POI, which is associated with an increased level of IL-1β. Intraperitoneal injection of IL-1β promoted the expression of pro-inflammatory genes, and deficient mice for IL-1R1, a receptor for IL-1β, are protected from POI. Interestingly, immunohistochemistry study showed that IL-1R1 in POI co-labeled with EGC labeled with GFAP. Culture enteric glial stimulated with 10 ng/mL of IL1-β for 24 h expressed a high level of MCP-1, suggesting the possible involvement of these cells on circulating monocyte recruitment [98].

Another study showed that EGCs, after inflammation, express CCL2, which promotes monocyte recruitment upon binding with its receptor CCR2 [99]. Another study on POI described the activation of ATP, which through the P2x receptor triggered IL6 production, which is selectively blocked by the P2x2 antagonist ambroxol [100].

In colitis induced by *Heligmosomoides polygyrus* infection, transcriptome analysis of isolated MMΦ revealed the enrichment of IFNγ in the colon. This data is consistent with an enrichment of IFNγ from EGC from patients with undergoing inflammation. Interestingly IFNγ drives a feedback effect on EGC by eliciting chemokine interferon-γ inducible protein 10 kDa (CXCL10) and guanylate-binding protein 10 (GBP10) expression through STAT1, leading to reduced proliferation of EGC. CXCL10 and GBP10 are involved in host defense and mediate immune responses with regards to anti-bacterial immunity and cancer, respectively [101, 102]. In addition to directly impacting ECs, the IFNγ-EGC-Cxcl10 signaling axis regulates tissue repair after helminthes infection through MMΦ via CCL8, CCL7, CXCL2, and CCL2 activation [102].

α-Synuclein (α-Syn) aggregates are found in the brain of patients with Alzheimer's disease. Most patients with this disease suffered from GI functional disorders, however, the mechanism is not understood. Application of α-synuclein (α-Syn) aggregates into the muscularis propria promotes the expansion of EGCs and overall tissue inflammation. Although it is not directly tested, it is possible that in this context, EGCs orchestrate the overall α-Syn mediated inflammation by talking with MMΦ, as multiple genes expressed following EGCs expansion are associated with MMΦ (**Figure 6**) [103].

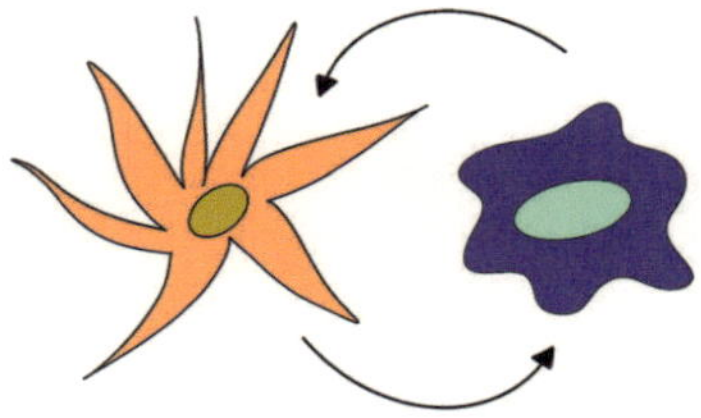

Homeostasis	Disease
1) Bi-directional communication involves maintaining gut homeostasis 2) Release of TNF-a and IL1-B by MMΦ results in expression of nerve growth factor 3) Enteric nerves secrete CSF-1 necessary for MMΦ development	1) EGCs mediate acute and chronic inflammation 2) MMΦ can induce a pro-inflammatory phenotype in EGCs secretory molecules

Figure 6.
Bidirectional interactions between EGC and MMΦ comparing homeostasis and disease.

Pro-inflammatory MMΦ products, such as IL-1, IL-4, and TNF-α, promote EGCs activation like reactive gliosis in the CNS. It is also evident that MMΦ products can affect EGCs phenotype during inflammation. Esposito and colleagues showed that upon LPS treatment, EGCs acquire an activated phenotype that coordinates the inflammatory response in the ENS. Inhibiting the NF-κB pathway on EGCs ameliorated the overall inflammatory response in colitis and in-vitro models. On the other hand, treatment of EGCs in vitro with LPS promoted the expression of genes associated with an anti-inflammatory response [104].

As in the CNS, EGCs play a role in maintaining gut homeostasis by interacting with ENs. By interacting with EGC, MMΦ can potentially contribute to ENs maintenance. In fact, the application of TNF-α and IL-1β, 2 cytokines produced by pro-inflammatory MMΦ, can induce the expression of nerve growth factor (NGF), which is implicated in neuronal outgrowth.

6. Conclusion and future directions for MMΦ in the GI tract

MMΦ are specialized phagocytic cells that fulfill an important role in regulating GI homeostasis and disease. They contain different subpopulations whose phenotype depends on their GI tract location and origin. These unique MMΦ, compared to mucosal MΦ, share an anti-inflammatory phenotype. It is evident now that MMΦ has a dual origin. The MMΦ pool is maintained by both monocytes derived- and embryonic-derived MMΦ. Although there is evidence suggesting the involvement of embryonic-derived MMΦ in regulating ENs, no information supports the possible contribution of circulating monocytes to tissue homeostasis. Depending on their location, MMΦ can interact functionally with cells that are important for GI physiology. Further studies are needed to elucidate the underlying mechanisms regulating this type of interactions.

Author details

Gianluca Cipriani* and Suraj Pullapantula
Enteric Neuroscience Program, Mayo Clinic, Rochester, Minnesota,
United States of America

*Address all correspondence to: gianluca.cipriani@mayo.edu

References

[1] Wu HJ, Wu E. The role of gut microbiota in immune homeostasis and autoimmunity. Gut Microbes. 2012;**3**(1):4-14. DOI: 10.4161/gmic.19320

[2] Vighi G, Marcucci F, Sensi L, Di Cara G, Frati F. Allergy and the gastrointestinal system. Clinical and Experimental Immunology. 2008;**153**(Suppl. 1):3-6. DOI: 10.1111/j.1365-2249.2008.03713.x

[3] Shi N, Li N, Duan X, et al. Interaction between the gut microbiome and mucosal immune system. Military Medical Research. 2017;**4**:14. DOI: 10.1186/s40779-017-0122-9

[4] Maloy K, Powrie F. Intestinal homeostasis and its breakdown in inflammatory bowel disease. Nature. 2011;**474**:298-306. DOI: 10.1038/nature10208

[5] Mills CD, Kincaid K, Alt JM, Heilman MJ, Hill AM. M-1/M-2 macrophages and the Th1/Th2 paradigm. Journal of Immunology. 2000;**164**:6166-6173

[6] Mills CD, Shearer J, Evans R, Caldwell MD. Macrophage arginine metabolism and the inhibition or stimulation of cancer. Journal of Immunology. 1992;**149**:2709-2714

[7] Xue J, Schmidt SV, Sander J, Draffehn A, Krebs W, Quester I, et al. Transcriptome-based network analysis reveals a spectrum model of human macrophage activation. Immunity. 2014;**40**(2):274-288. DOI: 10.1016/j.immuni.2014.01.006

[8] Gosselin D, Link VM, Romanoski CE, Fonseca GJ, Eichenfield DZ, Spann NJ, et al. Environment drives selection and function of enhancers controlling tissue-specific macrophage identities. Cell. 2014;**159**(6):1327-1340. DOI: 10.1016/j.cell.2014.11.023

[9] Gautier E, Shay T, Miller J, et al. Gene-expression profiles and transcriptional regulatory pathways that underlie the identity and diversity of mouse tissue macrophages. Nature Immunology. 2012;**13**:1118-1128. DOI: 10.1038/ni.2419

[10] Rumessen JJ, Thuneberg L, Mikkelsen HB. Plexus muscularis profundus and associated interstitial cells. II. Ultrastructural studies of mouse small intestine. The Anatomical Record. 1982;**203**(1):129-146

[11] Caspary WF. Physiology and pathophysiology of intestinal absorption. The American Journal of Clinical Nutrition. 1992;**55**(1):299S-308S. DOI: 10.1093/ajcn/55.1.299s

[12] Blikslager AT, Moeser AJ, Gookin JL, Jones SL, Odle J. Restoration of barrier function in injured intestinal mucosa. Physiological Reviews. 2007;**87**(2):545-564. DOI: 10.1152/physrev.00012.2006

[13] Macpherson AJ, Geuking MB, McCoy KD. Immune responses that adapt the intestinal mucosa to commensal intestinal bacteria. Immunology. 2005;**115**(2):153-162. DOI: 10.1111/j.1365-2567.2005.02159.x

[14] Costa M, Brookes SJ, Hennig GW. Anatomy and physiology of the enteric nervous system. Gut. 2000;**47**(Suppl. 4):iv15-iv19; discussion iv26. DOI: 10.1136/gut.47.suppl_4.iv15

[15] Furness JB. The enteric nervous system and neurogastroenterology. Nature Reviews. Gastroenterology

& Hepatology. 2012;**9**(5):286-294. DOI: 10.1038/nrgastro.2012.32

[16] Furness JB, Callaghan BP, Rivera LR, Cho HJ. The enteric nervous system and gastrointestinal innervation: Integrated local and central control. Advances in Experimental Medicine and Biology. 2014;**817**:39-71. DOI: 10.1007/978-1-4939-0897-4_3

[17] Faussone-Pellegrini MS, Pantalone D, Cortesini C. Smooth muscle cells, interstitial cells of Cajal and myenteric plexus interrelationships in the human colon. Acta Anatomica. 1990;**139**(1):31-44

[18] Gordon S, Taylor PR. Monocyte and macrophage heterogeneity. Nature Reviews. Immunology. 2005;**5**(12):953-964. DOI: 10.1038/nri1733

[19] van oud Alblas AB, van Furth R. Origin, Kinetics, and characteristics of pulmonary macrophages in the normal steady state. The Journal of Experimental Medicine. 1979;**149**(6):1504-1518. DOI: 10.1084/jem.149.6.1504

[20] Bain C, Bravo-Blas A, Scott C, et al. Constant replenishment from circulating monocytes maintains the macrophage pool in the intestine of adult mice. Nature Immunology. 2014;**15**:929-937

[21] Ginhoux F, Greter M, Leboeuf M, Nandi S, See P, Gokhan S, et al. Fate mapping analysis reveals that adult microglia derive from primitive macrophages. Science. 2010;**330**(6005):841-845. DOI: 10.1126/science.1194637. Epub 2010 Oct 21

[22] Gomez Perdiguero E, Klapproth K, Schulz C, et al. Tissue-resident macrophages originate from yolk-sac-derived erythro-myeloid progenitors. Nature. 2015;**518**:547-551

[23] Schulz C, Gomez Perdiguero E, Chorro L, Szabo-Rogers H, Cagnard N, Kierdorf K, et al. A lineage of myeloid cells independent of Myb and hematopoietic stem cells. Science. 2012;**336**:86-90

[24] Guilliams M, Thierry GR, Bonnardel J, Bajenoff M. Establishment and maintenance of the macrophage niche. Immunity. 2020;**52**(3):434-451

[25] De Schepper S, Verheijden S, Aguilera-Lizarraga J, Viola MF, Boesmans W, Stakenborg N, et al. Self-maintaining gut macrophages are essential for intestinal homeostasis. Cell. 2019;**176**(3):676

[26] Zigmond E, Varol C, Farache J, Elmaliah E, Satpathy AT, Friedlander G, et al. Ly6C hi monocytes in the inflamed colon give rise to proinflammatory effector cells and migratory antigen-presenting cells. Immunity. 2012;**37**(6):1076-1090

[27] Honda M, Surewaard BGJ, Watanabe M, et al. Perivascular localization of macrophages in the intestinal mucosa is regulated by Nr4a1 and the microbiome. Nature Communications. 2020;**11**:1329. DOI: 10.1038/s41467-020-15068-4

[28] Batra A, Bui TM, Rehring JF, Yalom LK, Muller WA, Sullivan DP, et al. Experimental colitis enhances temporal variations in CX3CR1 cell colonization of the gut and brain following irradiation. The American Journal of Pathology. Feb 2022;**192**(2):295-307. DOI: 10.1016/j.ajpath.2021.10.013. Epub 2021 Nov 10. PMID: 34767810

[29] Shaw TN, Houston SA, Wemyss K, Bridgeman HM, Barbera TA, Zangerle-Murray T, et al. Tissue-resident macrophages in the intestine are long lived and defined by Tim-4 and CD4

expression. The Journal of Experimental Medicine. 2018;**215**(6):1507-1518

[30] Mazaheri F, Breus O, Durdu S, et al. Distinct roles for BAI1 and TIM-4 in the engulfment of dying neurons by microglia. Nature Communications. 2014;**5**:4046

[31] Yanagihashi Y, Segawa K, Maeda R, Nabeshima YI, Nagata S. Mouse macrophages show different requirements for phosphatidylserine receptor Tim4 in efferocytosis. Proceedings of the National Academy of Sciences of the United States of America. 2017;**114**(33):8800-8805

[32] Moura Silva H, Kitoko JZ, Queiroz CP, Kroehling L, Matheis F, Yang KL, et al. c-MAF-dependent perivascular macrophages regulate diet-induced metabolic syndrome. Science Immunology. 2021;**6**(64):eabg7506. DOI: 10.1126/sciimmunol.abg7506. Epub 2021 Oct 1

[33] Domanska D, Majid U, Karlsen VT, Merok MA, Beitnes AR, Yaqub S, et al. Single-cell transcriptomic analysis of human colonic macrophages reveals niche-specific subsets. Journal of Experimental Medicine. 9 Feb 2022;**219**(3):e20211846. DOI: 10.1084/jem.20211846. Epub 2022 Feb 9. PMID: 35139155

[34] Bujko A, Atlasy N, Landsverk OJB, Richter L, Yaqub S, Horneland R, et al. Transcriptional and functional profiling defines human small intestinal macrophage subsets. The Journal of Experimental Medicine. 2018;**215**(2):441-458

[35] Bernardo D, Marin AC, Fernández-Tomé S, et al. Human intestinal pro-inflammatory CD11c(high) CCR2(+)CX3CR1(+) macrophages, but not their tolerogenic CD11c(−)CCR2(−) CX3CR1(−) counterparts, are expanded in inflammatory bowel disease. Mucosal Immunology. 2018;**11**:1114-1126

[36] Choi KM, Kashyap PC, Dutta N, Stoltz GJ, Ordog T, Shea Donohue T, et al. CD206-positive M2 macrophages that express heme oxygenase-1 protect against diabetic gastroparesis in mice. Gastroenterology. 2010;**138**(7):2399-409, 2409.e1

[37] Gabanyi I, Muller PA, Feighery L, Oliveira TY, Costa-Pinto FA, Mucida D. Neuro-immune interactions drive tissue programming in intestinal macrophages. Cell. 2016;**164**(3):378-391

[38] Ji S, Traini C, Mischopoulou M, Gibbons SJ, Ligresti G, Faussone-Pellegrini MS, et al. Muscularis macrophages establish cell-to-cell contacts with telocytes/PDGFRα-positive cells and smooth muscle cells in the human and mouse gastrointestinal tract. Neurogastroenterology and Motility. 2021;**33**(3):e13993

[39] Mikkelsen HB, Garbarsch C, Tranum-Jensen J, Thuneberg L. Macrophages in the small intestinal muscularis externa of embryos, newborn and adult germ-free mice. Journal of Molecular Histology. 2004;**35**(4):377-387. DOI: 10.1023/b:hijo.0000039840.86420.b7

[40] Phillips RJ, Hudson CN, Powley TL. Sympathetic axonopathies and hyperinnervation in the small intestine smooth muscle of aged Fischer 344 rats. Autonomic Neuroscience. 2013;**179**(1-2):108-121

[41] Cipriani G, Gibbons SJ, Miller KE, Yang DS, Terhaar ML, Eisenman ST, et al. Change in populations of macrophages promotes development of delayed gastric emptying in mice. Gastroenterology. 2018;**154**(8):2122-2136.e12

[42] Muller PA, Koscsó B, Rajani GM, Stevanovic K, Berres ML, Hashimoto D, et al. Crosstalk between muscularis macrophages and enteric neurons

regulates gastrointestinal motility. Cell. 2014;**158**(2):300-313

[43] Shi Y, Li S, Zhang H, Zhu J, Che T, Yan B, et al. The effect of macrophage polarization on the expression of the oxytocin signalling system in enteric neurons. Journal of Neuroinflammation. 2021;**18**(1):261. DOI: 10.1186/s12974-021-02313-w

[44] Sanjabi S, Zenewicz LA, Kamanaka M, Flavell RA. Anti-inflammatory and pro-inflammatory roles of TGF-beta, IL-10, and IL-22 in immunity and autoimmunity. Current Opinion in Pharmacology. 2009;**9**(4):447-453

[45] Dora D, Arciero E, Hotta R, Barad C, Bhave S, Kovacs T, et al. Intraganglionic macrophages: A new population of cells in the enteric ganglia. Journal of Anatomy. 2018;**233**(4):401-410. DOI: 10.1111/joa.12863. Epub 2018 Jul 18

[46] Dora D, Ferenczi S, Stavely R, Toth VE, Varga ZV, Kovacs T, et al. Evidence of a myenteric plexus barrier and its macrophage-dependent degradation during murine colitis: Implications in enteric neuroinflammation. Cellular and Molecular Gastroenterology and Hepatology. 2021;**12**(5):1617-1641. DOI: 10.1016/j.jcmgh.2021.07.003. Epub 2021 Jul 8

[47] Cipriani G, Terhaar ML, Eisenman ST, Ji S, Linden DR, Wright AM, et al. Muscularis propria macrophages alter the proportion of nitrergic but not cholinergic gastric myenteric neurons. Cellular and Molecular Gastroenterology and Hepatology. 2019;**7**(3):689-691.e4

[48] Becker L, Spear ET, Sinha SR, Haileselassie Y, Habtezion A. Age-related changes in gut microbiota alter phenotype of muscularis macrophages and disrupt gastrointestinal motility. Cellular and Molecular Gastroenterology and Hepatology. 2019;**7**(1):243-245.e2

[49] Becker L, Nguyen L, Gill J, Kulkarni S, Pasricha PJ, Habtezion A. Age-dependent shift in macrophage polarisation causes inflammation-mediated degeneration of enteric nervous system. Gut. 2018;**67**(5):827-836

[50] Avetisyan M, Rood JE, Huerta Lopez S, Sengupta R, Wright-Jin E, Dougherty JD, et al. Muscularis macrophage development in the absence of an enteric nervous system. Proceedings of the National Academy of Sciences of the United States of America. 2018;**115**(18):4696-4701

[51] Earley AM, Graves CL, Shiau CE. Critical role for a subset of intestinal macrophages in shaping gut microbiota in adult zebrafish. Cell Reports. 2018;**25**(2):424-436

[52] Wolf YS, Boura-Halfon N, Cortese Z, Haimon H, Sar Shalom Y, Kuperman V, et al. Brown-adipose-tissue macrophages control tissue innervation and homeostatic energy expenditure. Nature Immunology. 2017;**18**:665-674

[53] Jacobson A, Yang D, Vella M, Chiu IM. The intestinal neuro-immune axis: Crosstalk between neurons, immune cells, and microbes. Mucosal Immunology. 2021;**14**(3):555-565. DOI: 10.1038/s41385-020-00368-1. Epub 2021 Feb 4

[54] Phillips RJ, Powley TL. Macrophages associated with the intrinsic and extrinsic autonomic innervation of the rat gastrointestinal tract. Autonomic Neuroscience. 2012;**169**(1):12-27. DOI: 10.1016/j.autneu.2012.02.004. Epub 2012 Mar 20

[55] Matheis F, Muller PA, Graves CL, Gabanyi I, Kerner ZJ, Costa-Borges D, et al. Adrenergic signaling in muscularis

macrophages limits infection-induced neuronal loss. Cell. 2020;**180**(1):64-78.e16

[56] Matteoli G, Gomez-Pinilla PJ, Nemethova A, Di Giovangiulio M, Cailotto C, van Bree SH, et al. A distinct vagal anti-inflammatory pathway modulates intestinal muscularis resident macrophages independent of the spleen. Gut. 2014;**63**(6):938-948

[57] Lu KH, Cao J, Oleson S, et al. Vagus nerve stimulation promotes gastric emptying by increasing pyloric opening measured with magnetic resonance imaging. Neurogastroenterology and Motility. 2018;**30**(10):e13380

[58] Travagli RA, Anselmi L. Vagal neurocircuitry and its influence on gastric motility. Nature Reviews. Gastroenterology & Hepatology. 2016;**13**(7):389-401

[59] Payne SC, Furness JB, Burns O, Sedo A, Hyakumura T, Shepherd RK, et al. Anti-inflammatory effects of abdominal vagus nerve stimulation on experimental intestinal inflammation. Frontiers in Neuroscience. 2019;**13**:418. DOI: 10.3389/fnins.2019.00418

[60] Filipovic BR, Filipovic BF. Psychiatric comorbidity in the treatment of patients with inflammatory bowel disease. World Journal of Gastroenterology. 2014;**20**(13):3552-3563

[61] Ghia JE, Park AJ, Blennerhassett P, Khan WI, Collins SM. Adoptive transfer of macrophage from mice with depression-like behavior enhances susceptibility to colitis. Inflammatory Bowel Diseases. 2011 Jul;**17**(7):1474-1489. DOI: 10.1002/ibd.21531. Epub 2011 Jan 18

[62] Gottfried-Blackmore A, Adler EP, Fernandez-Becker N, Clarke J, Habtezion A, Nguyen L. Open-label pilot study: Non-invasive vagal nerve stimulation improves symptoms and gastric emptying in patients with idiopathic gastroparesis. Neurogastroenterology & Motility. 2020;**32**(4):e13769. DOI: 10.1111/nmo.13769. Epub 2019 Dec 5

[63] de Jonge WJ, van der Zanden EP, The FO, Bijlsma MF, van Westerloo DJ, Bennink RJ, et al. Stimulation of the vagus nerve attenuates macrophage activation by activating the Jak2-STAT3 signaling pathway. Nature Immunology. 2005;**6**(8):844-851. DOI: 10.1038/ni1229. Epub 2005 Jul 17. Erratum in: Nature Immunology. 2005;**6**(9):954

[64] Willemze RA, Welting O, van Hamersveld P, Verseijden C, Nijhuis LE, Hilbers FW, et al. Loss of intestinal sympathetic innervation elicits an innate immune driven colitis. Molecular Medicine. 2019;**25**(1):1

[65] Kalff JC, Schraut WH, Simmons RL, Bauer AJ. Surgical manipulation of the gut elicits an intestinal muscularis inflammatory response resulting in postsurgical ileus. Annals of Surgery. 1998;**228**(5):652-663

[66] Sanders KM, Stevens R, Burke E, Ward SW. Slow waves actively propagate at submucosal surface of circular layer in canine colon. The American Journal of Physiology. 1990;**259**(2 Pt 1): G258-G263

[67] Dickens EJ, Hirst GD, Tomita T. Identification of rhythmically active cells in guinea-pig stomach. Journal of Physiology. 1999;**514**(Pt 2):515-531

[68] Lies B, Gil V, Groneberg D, Seidler B, Saur D, Wischmeyer E, et al. Interstitial cells of Cajal mediate nitrergic inhibitory neurotransmission in the murine gastrointestinal tract. American Journal of Physiology. Gastrointestinal and Liver Physiology. 2014;**307**(1):G98-G106

[69] Ward SM, Sanders KM. Involvement of intramuscular interstitial cells of Cajal in neuroeffector transmission in the gastrointestinal tract. The Journal of Physiology. 2006;**576**(Pt 3):675-682

[70] Burns AJ, Lomax AE, Torihashi S, Sanders KM, Ward SM. Interstitial cells of Cajal mediate inhibitory neurotransmission in the stomach. Proceedings of the National Academy of Sciences of the United States of America. 1996;**93**(21):12008-12013

[71] Li J, Kong P, Chen C, Tang J, Jin X, Yan J, et al. Targeting IL-17A improves the dysmotility of the small intestine and alleviates the injury of the interstitial cells of Cajal during sepsis. Oxidative Medicine and Cellular Longevity. 2019;**2019**:1475729

[72] Wang XY, Berezin I, Mikkelsen HB, Der T, Bercik P, Collins SM, et al. Pathology of interstitial cells of Cajal in relation to inflammation revealed by ultrastructure but not immunohistochemistry. The American Journal of Pathology. 2002;**160**(4):1529-1540

[73] Deng J, Yang S, Yuan Q, Chen Y, Li D, Sun H, et al. Acupuncture ameliorates postoperative ileus via IL-6-miR-19a-KIT axis to protect interstitial cells of Cajal. The American Journal of Chinese Medicine. 2017;**45**:737-755

[74] Chen X, Meng X, Zhang H, Feng C, Wang B, Li N, et al. Intestinal proinflammatory macrophages induce a phenotypic switch in interstitial cells of Cajal. The Journal of Clinical Investigation. 2020;**130**(12):6443-6456

[75] Eisenman ST, Gibbons SJ, Verhulst PJ, Cipriani G, Saur D, Farrugia G. Tumor necrosis factor alpha derived from classically activated "M1" macrophages reduces interstitial cell of Cajal numbers. Neurogastroenterology & Motility. Apr 2017;**29**(4):12984. DOI: 10.1111/nmo.12984. Epub 2016 Oct 25. PMID: 27781339; PMCID: PMC5367986

[76] Grover M, Bernard CE, Pasricha PJ, Parkman HP, Gibbons SJ, Tonascia J, et al. NIDDK Gastroparesis Clinical Research Consortium (GpCRC). Diabetic and idiopathic gastroparesis is associated with loss of CD206-positive macrophages in the gastric antrum. Neurogastroenterology & Motility. Jun 2017;**29**(6):13018. DOI: 10.1111/nmo.13018. Epub 2017 Jan 9. PMID: 28066953; PMCID: PMC5423829

[77] Kashyap PC, Choi KM, Dutta N, Linden DR, Szurszewski JH, Gibbons SJ, et al. Carbon monoxide reverses diabetic gastroparesis in NOD mice. American Journal of Physiology. Gastrointestinal and Liver Physiology. 2010;**298**(6):G1013-G1019

[78] Choi KM, Gibbons SJ, Sha L, Beyder A, Verhulst PJ, Cipriani G, et al. Interleukin 10 restores gastric emptying, electrical activity, and interstitial cells of Cajal networks in diabetic mice. Cellular and Molecular Gastroenterology and Hepatology. 2016;**2**(4):454-467

[79] Wang XY, Zarate N, Soderholm JD, Bourgeois JM, Liu LW, Huizinga JD. Ultrastructural injury to interstitial cells of Cajal and communication with mast cells in Crohn's disease. Neurogastroenterology and Motility. 2007;**19**:349-364

[80] Zarate N, Wang XY, Tougas G, Anvari M, Birch D, Mearin F, et al. Intramuscular interstitial cells of Cajal associated with mast cells survive nitrergic nerves in achalasia. Neurogastroenterology and Motility. 2006;**18**:556-568

[81] Suzuki T, Won KJ, Horiguchi K, Kinoshita K, Hori M, Torihashi S, et al.

Muscularis inflammation and the loss of interstitial cells of Cajal in the endothelin ETB receptor null rat. American Journal of Physiology. Gastrointestinal and Liver Physiology. 2004;**287**:G638-G646

[82] Xu S, Zhai J, Xu K, et al. M1 macrophages-derived exosomes miR-34c-5p regulates interstitial cells of Cajal through targeting SCF. Journal of Biosciences. 2021;**46**:90

[83] Luo J, Qian A, Oetjen LK, Yu W, Yang P, Feng J, et al. TRPV4 channel signaling in macrophages promotes gastrointestinal motility via direct effects on smooth muscle cells. Immunity. 2018;**49**(1):107-119.e4

[84] Iizuka Y, Kuwahara A, Karaki S. Role of PGE2 in the colonic motility: PGE2 generates and enhances spontaneous contractions of longitudinal smooth muscle in the rat colon. The Journal of Physiological Sciences: JPS. 2014;**64**(2):85-96

[85] Wehner S, Behrendt FF, Lyutenski BN, Lysson M, Bauer AJ, Hirner A, et al. Inhibition of macrophage function prevents intestinal inflammation and postoperative ileus in rodents. Gut. 2007;**56**(2):176-185

[86] Antoniou E, Margonis GA, Angelou A, Pikouli A, Argiri P, Karavokyros I, et al. The TNBS-induced colitis animal model: An overview. Annals of Medicine and Surgery. 2016, 2012;**11**:9-15

[87] Grimm MC, Elsbury SK, Pavli P, Doe WF. Enhanced expression and production of monocyte chemoattractant protein-1 in inflammatory bowel disease mucosa. Journal of Leukocyte Biology. 1996;**59**(6):804-812

[88] Chen W, Lu C, Hirota C, Iacucci M, Ghosh S, Gui X. Smooth muscle hyperplasia/hypertrophy is the most prominent histological change in Crohn's fibrostenosing bowel strictures: A semiquantitative analysis by using a novel histological grading scheme. Journal of Crohn's & Colitis. 2017;**11**(1):92-104

[89] Komuro T, Seki K, Horiguchi K. Ultrastructural characterization of the interstitial cells of Cajal. Archives of Histology and Cytology. 1999;**62**(4):295-316

[90] Kurahashi M, Zheng H, Dwyer L, Ward SM, Koh SD, Sanders KM. A functional role for the 'fibroblast-like cells' in gastrointestinal smooth muscles. The Journal of Physiology. 2011;**589** (Pt 3):697-710

[91] Bassotti G, Villanacci V, Antonelli E, Morelli A, Salerni B. Enteric glial cells: New players in gastrointestinal motility? Laboratory Investigation. 2007;**87**(7):628-632

[92] Seguella L, Gulbransen BD. Enteric glial biology, intercellular signalling and roles in gastrointestinal disease. Nature Reviews Gastroenterology & Hepatology. Aug 2021;**18**(8):571-587. DOI: 10.1038/s41575-021-00423-7. Epub 2021 Mar 17. PMID: 33731961; PMCID: PMC8324524

[93] von Boyen GB, Steinkamp M, Reinshagen M, Schäfer KH, Adler G, Kirsch J. Proinflammatory cytokines increase glial fibrillary acidic protein expression in enteric glia. Gut. 2004;**53**(2):222-228

[94] Rosenbaum C, Schick MA, Wollborn J, Heider A, Scholz CJ, Cecil A, et al. Activation of myenteric glia during acute inflammation in vitro and in vivo. PLoS One. 2016;**11**(3):-e0151335

[95] Grubišić V, McClain JL, Fried DE, Grants I, Rajasekhar P, Csizmadia E, et al. Enteric glia modulate macrophage

phenotype and visceral sensitivity following inflammation. Cell Reports. 2020;**32**(10):108100

[96] Stoffels B, Hupa KJ, Snoek SA, van Bree S, Stein K, Schwandt T, et al. Postoperative ileus involves interleukin-1 receptor signaling in enteric glia. Gastroenterology. 2014;**146**(1):176-87.e1

[97] Brown IA, McClain JL, Watson RE, Patel BA, Gulbransen BD. Enteric glia mediate neuron death in colitis through purinergic pathways that require connexin-43 and nitric oxide. Cellular and Molecular Gastroenterology and Hepatology. 2016;**2**(1):77-91

[98] McClain J, Grubišić V, Fried D, Gomez-Suarez RA, Leinninger GM, Sévigny J, et al. Ca^{2+} responses in enteric glia are mediated by connexin-43 hemichannels and modulate colonic transit in mice. Gastroenterology. 2014;**146**(2):497-507.e1

[99] Stakenborg M, Abdurahiman S, De Simone V, Goverse G, Stakenborg N, van Baarle L, et al. Enteric glial cells favour accumulation of anti-inflammatory macrophages during the resolution of muscularis inflammation. bioRxiv. DOI: 10.1101/ 2021.06.10.447700

[100] Progatzky F, Shapiro M, Chng SH, et al. Regulation of intestinal immunity and tissue repair by enteric glia. Nature. 2021;**599**:125-130

[101] Liu M, Guo S, Stiles JK. The emerging role of CXCL10 in cancer (review). Oncology Letters. 2011;**2**(4):583-589. DOI: 10.3892/ ol.2011.300

[102] Krapp C, Hotter D, Gawanbacht A, McLaren PJ, Kluge SF, Stürzel CM, et al. Guanylate binding protein (GBP) 5 is an interferon-inducible inhibitor of HIV-1 infectivity. Cell Host & Microbe. 2016;**19**:504-514. DOI: 10.1016/j. chom.2016.02.019

[103] Challis C, Hori A, Sampson TR, et al. Gut-seeded α-synuclein fibrils promote gut dysfunction and brain pathology specifically in aged mice. Nature Neuroscience. 2020;**23**:327-336

[104] Esposito G, Capoccia E, Turco F, Palumbo I, Lu J, Steardo A, et al. Palmitoylethanolamide improves colon inflammation through an enteric glia/ toll like receptor 4-dependent PPAR-α activation. Gut. 2014;**63**(8):1300-1312

Chapter 6

The Tale of Mastering Macrophage Environment through the Control of Inflammasome-Mediated Macrophage Activation and cAMP Homeostasis by the Protozoan Parasite *Leishmania*

Anindita Bhattacharjee, Arunima Biswas and Pijush K. Das

Abstract

Leishmania, being an intelligent protozoan parasite, modulates the defensive arsenals of the host to create a favorable niche for their survival. When the intracellular parasite is encountered by the host, multimeric complexes of inflammasomes get assembled and activated, thereby leading to genesis of inflammatory response. In order to subvert host defensive strategies, *Leishmania* utilizes their cyclic adenosine monophosphate (cAMP) and cAMP-induced response to neutralize macrophage oxidative damage. In this chapter, we summarize our current understanding of the mechanisms of inflammasome activation in macrophages and cAMP homeostasis of the parasite, leading to parasite viability within the macrophages and establishment of infection. Furthermore, we took into account, recent progresses in translating these research areas into therapeutic strategies, aimed at combating macrophage associated diseases.

Keywords: inflammasome, NLRP3, cAMP homeostasis, phagosome, *Leishmania*, macrophage

1. Introduction

Leishmaniases involve a broad spectrum of neglected tropical diseases that are caused by kinetoplastid parasites belonging to the genus *Leishmania*, that is transmitted by female sandflies belonging to the genus *Phlebotomus* [1]. From the clinical manifestations and symptoms occurring in hosts harboring various species of *Leishmania,* three major forms of *Leishmania* can be delineated: visceral, cutaneous and mucocutaneous leishmaniasis. Visceral leishmaniasis is the chronic and often fatal, if left untreated, form of the disease primarily caused by *Leishmania donovani* and *Leishmania infantum,* infecting visceral organs including bone marrow, liver and spleen. Cutaneous leishmaniasis, generally caused by *Leishmania major*, produces self-healing ulcerative lesions on the skin. Another variant of cutaneous leishmaniasis is mucocutaneous leishmaniasis that is characterized by damaged oro-naso-pharyngeal tissues. The infective stage, i.e., the metacyclic promastigotes, are found to be embedded in a proteophosphoglycan-rich gel derived from the parasite itself in the anterior mid-gut of the sandfly, which plays important role in parasite regurgitation during blood meal feeding of the sandfly [1]. The moment the parasites enter the host system, they are rapidly phagocytosed by the macrophages where they differentiate into aflagellar, nonmotile amastigotes that multiply within the acidic phagolysosomal compartment of the macrophages [2]. In order to survive within the unfriendly environment of the macrophage, *Leishmania* evolved several approaches to counter the microbicidal power of the macrophage and to mount an effective immune response against the parasite. After the primary encounter of the parasites with neutrophils during early stages of host infection, the monocytes and macrophages in the blood stream participate in the act of engulfing *Leishmania* parasites by phagocytosis. Monocytes that express CD11-c on their surface have recently been identified as the major cellular micro-environment for *Leishmania* to proliferate and also acts as a reservoir of *Leishmania*, providing ample number of parasites required for infecting neighboring cells [2]. On the other hand, recruitment and activation of the inflammatory monocytes protect the host system by limiting proliferation of the parasites by reactive oxygen species (ROS) and inducible nitric oxide synthase (iNOS) generation. However, tissue macrophages become the primary host cells responsible for parasite elimination after infection has been established in the tissues. The macrophages are activated by two components of the immune system like interferon gamma (IFN-γ) and tumor necrosis factor alpha (TNF- α), that synergistically induce iNOS expression, the enzyme responsible for production of free radical NO which actively kills *Leishmania* parasites through oxidative stress induction. Apart from the induction of oxidative stress by the macrophage, monocyte-derived macrophages were found to be responsible for activation of inflammasomes and secretion of cytokines like Interleukin-1 β (IL-1β) upon parasitic infection [3]. Inflammasomes are cytosolic complexes that gather upon sensing microbial molecules or cellular stress, leading to cytokine processing and an inflammatory programmed cell death called pyroptosis, activated by caspase-1. Different species of *Leishmania*, when subjected to analysis against inflammasome activation, were found to be capable of inducing the macrophages to release IL-β by activation of NLRP3 (Nod-like receptor), CASP1 (Caspase-1) and ASC (Apoptosis-associated speck-like protein containing CARD) [4]. IL-1β production by activated NLRP3 inflammasome induces specific signaling pathways triggering NO synthesis leading to parasite killing and disease resistance. In a recent study, it is documented that *Leishmania* lipophosphoglycan (LPG) activates Caspase-11 which in turn activates the non-canonical NLRP3 inflammasomes. Strikingly, the amastigote form of the parasite causes lesser activation of inflammasomes owing to the fact that they display fewer LPG on their surface as compared to the promastigote forms. Moreover, the amastigotes destruct the NLRP3 inflammasome activation pathway in the macrophages by targeting histone H3 [5]. Therefore, it can be considered as an excellent strategy adapted by the parasites to combat the hostility offered by the macrophages against them.

Another major modulator of cytological events in *Leishmania* and other related kinetoplastids is cAMP (cyclic adenosine monophosphate), which is one of the primary factors responsible for parasite transformation and parasite survival. cAMP plays a major role in differentiation-induced cell cycle arrest in G_0/G_1 phase in both *Leishmania* and *Trypanosoma* [6]. It has significant role in modulating promastigote proliferation, flagellar length and motility and regulation of mitochondrial membrane potential [7]. Moreover, the oxidative burst that the parasites encounter as the first line of defense in mammalian macrophage is associated with elevation of cAMP in the parasite triggering cell cycle arrest and stage differentiation [8]. Thus, it is quite evident that there is a delicate interconnection between the immune response offered by the macrophage upon *Leishmania* infection and the cAMP homeostasis inside the parasite that prevents their killing withing the host. This chapter will discuss the host–parasite interaction, inflammasome activation by the infected macrophages and cAMP homeostasis within the parasite leading to parasite survival.

2. Epidemiology of leishmaniasis

Visceral leishmaniasis, also known as kala-azar, is a deadly disease and in over 95% of instances it is found to be direful when left untreated. Approximately 50,000–90,000 new incidents of visceral leishmaniasis seem to occur globally each year in countries like Bangladesh, Brazil, China, Ethiopia, India, Kenya, Nepal, Somalia, South Sudan and Sudan. Cutaneous and mucocutaneous leishmaniasis occur in South American countries, Mediterranean river basin, the Central Asia and Middle East. Over 90% of mucocutaneous leishmaniasis cases occur in Bolivia, Brazil, Ethiopia and Peru [9]. The diseases collectively affect more than 1 million people every year, visceral leishmaniasis being the main reason for the death of a vast population of about 20,000–40,000 people annually [10]. Apart from humans, the primary host of the diseases, dogs, rodents, other mammals and few reptilian species act as the reservoir hosts of leishmaniases [11].

3. Parasite infection and activation of parasite-dependent host biology modulation

3.1 Initial events of parasite infection and macrophage activation

The disease manifestation of VL strictly relies on host immunocompetency ranging from asymptomatic forms to severe disease conditions, which if left untreated, can be fatal. Clinical conditions such as HIV infection or immunosuppression due to any drug treatment leading to immunodepression in host weaken the efficiency of the host immune system to deal with the infection and permit recurrence of the disease. The contrast in host–parasite interactions between cutaneous and visceral leishmaniasis is quite noteworthy, suggesting the role of infecting species of *Leishmania* in diversification of complexity of immune responses to the pathogen [12]. Resistance and susceptibility of the host to the infection is associated with various genetic factors impacting both severity of the disease and its diagnosis in case of visceral leishmaniasis. One of the most crucial factors that determine the clinical outcome of the disease is host immune response upon parasite entry. One of the components of innate immunity, the complement system, is activated immediately after penetration of the dermis by the promastigotes, resulting in effective clearance of about 90% of all injected parasites within a moment or two [13, 14]. Cells of the innate immune system including dendritic cells, NK (natural killer) cells, T cells and the cytokines they release, altogether participate to mount immune response against *Leishmania*. IL-12 released by the dendritic cells activates NK cells that produce IFN-γ that enhance killing mechanisms in macrophages, the main target of *Leishmania* [15]. Apart from interleukins and interferons, tumor necrosis factors (TNFs) play a pivotal role in both parasite clearance and tissue damage in liver and spleen, respectively. *Leishmania* parasites modify the chemokine profiles of the host–parasite persistence is promoted. IFN-γ release triggered by Th1 response correlates with infection resistance by induction of some leishmanicidal mechanism in the phagocytes. However, Th2 response results in infection susceptibility and disease manifestation due to replication of intracellular parasite as macrophage activation is inhibited [16]. Thus, symptoms and extent of disease manifestation largely depends on immunocompetency of the host and the fine interplay between the pathogen and the immunological and genetic characteristics of the infected host.

3.1.1 Recognition and uptake

During the parasite's transfer from its vector to the vertebrate host, neutrophils and macrophages are quickly recruited to the sand fly bite site [17]. The parasites secret proteophosphoglycans inside sandfly midgut which acts as a potent stimulator for recruiting macrophages at the site of infection as found in both *L. mexicana* and *L. infantum* [18, 19]. Parasites initially infect the neutrophils but since neutrophils are unsuitable for parasitic differentiation into the amastigote forms, they start infecting the macrophages, their actual site of transformation [20–22]. As a result, the macrophage is a crucial host cell for parasite infection and persistence. The parasite flagellum initiates the contact between the promastigote and the macrophage. This may induce the parasite to release intrinsic survival factors, hence modulating phagocytic activity of the macrophages [20]. The complexity of *Leishmania*-macrophage interaction largely depends on the type of macrophage receptors involved with parasite recognition. Complement receptor-mediated uptake of the parasite results in parasite survival within the macrophage phagosomes because of inhibition of oxidative burst and inflammation, and lysosomal markers like Cathepsin D and LAMP1 accumulation. On the other hand, increased inflammatory conditions developed by fibronectin receptor-mediated uptake leads to parasite clearance. Other receptors including mannose receptors and FCγ receptors trigger inflammatory responses and NADPH oxidase activation in the phagosomes, respectively [23].

After the event of parasite recognition by macrophage cell surface, promastigotes are internalized by cholesterol-rich caveolae for both *L. chagasi* and *L. donovani* uptake [24–26]. However, lipid microdomains is found to have no effect on amastigote phagocytosis, highlighting the importance of membrane lipid-microdomains in the phagocytosis of *Leishmania* by the mammalian macrophages [24]. It is demonstrated in recent studies that lipid microdomain synthesis is promoted by *Leishmania* promastigotes by conversion of sphingomyelin into ceramide, the main constituent of lipid microdomain, by the activation of host acid sphingomyelinase [27]. *De novo* ceramide production is induced by the parasite at late stage of infection leading to disruption of lipid microdomain and impaired antigen presentation [27]. Moreover, *L. donovani* targets a macrophage transcription factor, SREBP2, which promotes parasite internalization and persistence through regulation of macrophage membrane cholesterol and mitochondrial ROS generation [28]. As a result, precise modulation of lipid microdomains is likely to be one of the important actors in host–parasite interactions in *Leishmania* infection.

3.1.2 Phagosome maturation and parasite differentiation

Following phagocytosis of the promastigotes by the macrophages and their internalization into the phagosome, the parasites fuse with lysosomes and adapt to the hostile environment where they must survive for disease manifestations. Despite the fact that this is one of the most difficult habitats for most infectious pathogens, *Leishmania* is one of the few protozoan parasites that can survive and reproduce in such conditions. Phagosomes that contain *L. donovani* promastigotes showed reduced fusogenicity towards lysosomes and late endosomes [29, 30]. LAMP1, a lysosome marker, was employed to the parasitophorous vacuoles leading to reorientation of the parasites with their cell body facing the macrophage nucleus and the flagellum in the direction of the periphery of the cell. This orientation of the parasites endorsed the parasitophorous vacuole to move outwards causing cell injury, accelerated lysosome docking followed by exocytosis. Some of the parasite containing lysosomes might fuse with the parasitophorous vacuoles promoting transformation of promastigote into amastigote, whereas cell injury might disrupt the integrity of the plasma membrane and the capacity of the host to fight infection [31].

Differentiation from promastigote to amastigote is triggered by an increase in temperature from 22–37°C and a decrease in pH from 7.2 to 5.5 in mammalian phagolysosomes. Furthermore, iron uptake followed by hydrogen peroxide generation has been found to be a significant trigger for parasitic differentiation in *L. amanzonensis* [32, 33]. *Leishmania* iron transporter (LIT1) triggers the conversion of ROS into hydrogen peroxide by the enzyme iron superoxide dismutase; hydrogen peroxide being the major trigger for promastigote-to-amastigote differentiation to occur [34]. From previous studies, it was well documented that there is a close association between this transformation and the elevated levels of cAMP and cAMP-dependent Protein Kinase A (PKA) within the parasite [35]. cAMP plays a very crucial role in the transformation and regulation of the cell cycle of the parasites. cAMP acts as a cyto-protector which increase peroxide neutralizing capacity of the parasite increasing their chance of survival and is also known to trigger G_1 arrest [8]. Several isoforms of leishmanial phosphodiesterases (LdPDEA and LdPDED) also showed roles in controlling the cAMP levels during transformation along with the leishmanial receptor adenylate cyclases (LdracA and LdracB) and pyrophosphatases (V-H^+PPase) proving beyond doubt the importance of cAMP signaling cascade in the parasite [35, 36].

3.1.3 Macrophage activation: host: parasite interaction

Macrophages, apart from acting as a phagocytic cell, respond to and regulate different signaling molecules [37]. Circulating monocytes are the precursors of tissue macrophages that secrete various antimicrobial and immunoregulatory molecules capable of inactivating pathogens through ROS and NO generation [38–40]. Monocyte–macrophage lineage show notable plasticity and can modify their physiology according to the environmental stimuli giving rise to diversified cell population with different functions [41, 42]. The state of activation of macrophages can be changed in response to different cytokines, growth factors and microbial molecules. When stimulated by TNF-α or IFN-γ or lipopolysaccharide, macrophages undergo classical activation that is characterized by surface marker CD80 expression [43, 44]. On the other hand, macrophages undergoing alternative activation is induced by IL-4 and IL-13 by the activation of a common receptor, IL-4R [45]. Production of high levels IL-13, CCL14, CCL17, CCL18, CCL22, IL-10, TGF-β, urea, and ornithine which is an essential substrate for both polyamine and collagen synthesis, are observed in alternatively activated macrophages [44, 46, 47]. One of the mechanisms for the establishment of intra-macrophage parasite infection is the inhibition of host defense mechanism which is achieved by inhibiting inflammatory cytokine secretion and apoptosis. One such target of *L. donovani* promastigotes is AKT signaling and its downstream components, β-catenin and FOXO-1, modulation of which inhibits both cytokine production and apoptosis [48]. Thus, the initial interaction of *Leishmania* with macrophages leads to their activation and polarization that is essential for the survival of the parasite inside the macrophage and establishment of disease manifestation.

3.2 Inflammasome activation by *Leishmania*: mastering the macrophage environment exploiting macrophage biology

Upon detection of pathogenic organisms, the cytoplasm of the cells of innate immunity assembles multiprotein complexes called inflammasomes that cause an inflammatory programmed cell death called pyroptosis. The nucleotide-binding domain leucine-rich repeat protein (NLR) family is the widely studied inflammasome that is activated by cell membrane damage-inducing pathogens and molecules (**Figure 1**) [49]. Caspase-1 activation is promoted upon NLRP3 activation and oligomerization which leads to ASC polymerization exposing the CARD domains of the ASC, leading to recruitment of Caspase-1 through CARD/CARD interaction. The NLRP3 inflammasome undergoes both canonical and non-canonical activation. Initially, TLR (toll-like receptors) or TNFRs are stimulated by microbial components or TNF-α leading to numerous inflammatory gene transcription, Nlrp3, Casp11 and Il1b for instance. But inspite of the presence of a first signal, a second signal is required for canonical NLRP3 activation that occurs via pore formation by the microbial toxins, and subsequent rupture of the host cell membrane, resulting in K^+ efflux

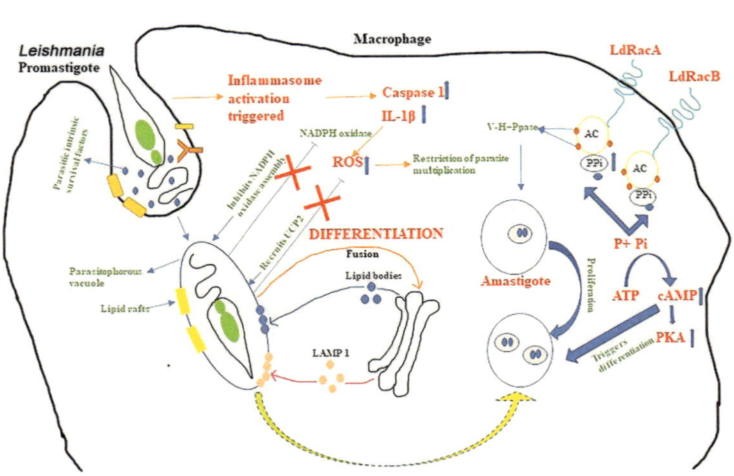

Figure 1.
Interaction of Leishmania *promastigotes with macrophage receptors triggers phagocytosis of the parasite and release of intrinsic survival factors by the pathogen that modify phagosome synthesis and results in inhibition of proinflammatory pathways. The schematic diagram is the summary of the fine interplay between inflammasome-induced and cAMP-mediated differentiation of the parasite through modulation of ROS and activation by Ld receptor adenylate cyclases (LdRacs) by acidocalcisomal pyrophosphatase (V-H$^+$PPase) resulting in upregulation of cAMP, respectively. PPi = inorganic pyrophosphate pool, AC = acidocalcisome.*

and decrease in K^+ concentration the cytoplasm [50]. Apart from potassium efflux, lysosomal cathepsin and ROS production is also essential for canonical activation of NLRP3. In contrast, non-canonical activation of NLRP3 inflammasomes is promoted by Caspase-11 which is activated by bacterial LPS. Different species of *Leishmania* use different strategies of limiting or inhibiting inflammasome activation in the macrophages. *L. mexicana* and *L. major*, as demonstrated by Shio et al., use GP63, a virulence factor that inhibit IL1b production in THP-1 cells, either by ROS inhibition or by inflammasome components cleavage [51]. Inhibition of NLRP3 inflammasome by *L. donovani* is achieved by A20, a negative regulator of NF-κβ and UCP2, mitochondrial uncoupling protein 2 manipulation by inhibiting ROS generation [52]. Leishmania infection induces the expression of UCP2 leading to downregulation of ROS generation by the macrophage, thus probably averting ROS-mediated inactivation of protein tyrosine phosphatases which in turn suppresses defense mechanism of the infected macrophages [53]. In two recent findings, *L. donovani* and *L. amazonensis* was shown to transcriptionally inhibit the components of inflammasome in infected macrophages [52, 54]. Though inflammation activation might not be fully blocked by the pathogens, but the magnitude or extent of inflammasome activation is surely noticeably limited by *Leishmania* as compared to other infectious pathogens like bacteria or protozoan parasites like *Trypanosoma cruzi* and *Toxoplasma gondii* [4].

3.3 The NLRP3 inflammasome and its activation during *Leishmania* sp. infection

Initial stage of macrophage infection by *Leishmania* triggers inflammasome activation in the infected macrophages prompting Caspase-1 activation and production of IL-1b. The role of NLRP3 inflammasome in Caspase-1 activation was established by the absence of the process in NLRP3 or ASC deficient cells [55]. Macrophage inflammasome activation restricted parasite multiplication by Caspase-1 and IL-1b production and stimulation of ROS generation via p47phox and arachidonic acid-NADPH oxidase signaling pathway in *L. infantum* [56]. In conjunction with these findings, it was revealed that *L. amazonensis* triggered Dectin-1 activation, which resulted in Syk kinase activation and ROS production by NADPH oxidase, a step required for NLRP3 activation in macrophages [57]. Furthermore, inhibiting ROS and NADPH oxidase during the primary infection was sufficient to prevent inflammasome activation, demonstrating that the earliest signals for inflammasome activation occur during parasite phagocytosis [57]. These findings highlight the role of ROS in the activation of NLRP3 during *Leishmania* infection. Lipophosphoglycan (LPG) from several *Leishmania* species has recently been demonstrated to activate caspase-11 in macrophages, suggesting non-canonical NLRP3 inflammasome activation [58]. It was also observed that mitochondrial phosphatase phosphoglycerate mutase family member five, a protein involved in restricting *Leishmania* multiplication in macrophages, is required for the production of IL-1b in response to *Leishmania* infection, implying that this protein is involved in the NLRP3 inflammasome activation [59]. Compounds that activate inflammasomes and promote IL-1b production, such as polyester poly (lactide-co-glycolide acid) nanoparticles infused with an 11 kDa *Leishmania* antigen, the antiprotozoal drug diterpene kaurenoic acid, and the conventional anti-leishmanial drug Amphotericin B, have also been shown to limit parasite replication in macrophages [60, 61]. In a visceral Leishmaniasis model, anti-IL-1b treatment inhibited parasite clearance by Amphotericin B. These investigations show indisputably that the inflammasome is activated as a result of *Leishmania* infection and plays a key role in limiting proliferation of *Leishmania* in macrophages.

4. *Leishmania* evades host defense

4.1 Curbing inflammation

To counter host defenses, *Leishmania* exploits a multitude of intervention mechanisms by targeting various signaling pathways in macrophages. Even before the parasites are inoculated by the sand fly vector, the proteophosphoglycan rich secretory gel produced by the parasites promotes *L. mexicana* viability by increasing alternative activation and arginase activity in the macrophages [18]. Interestingly, *Leishmania* amplified the production of the proinflammatory cytokines IL-1, TNF, MIP-1, and MCP-1 as well as the anti-inflammatory cytokine IL-10 induced by leishmanial LPS [62]. Murine peritoneal macrophages infected with *L. donovani* promastigotes has recently been observed to stimulate expression of PPARγ of the host, which is believed to suppress inflammation and guard the host from irreparable damage. The parasite was easier to remove when PPAR was inhibited [63]. *Leishmania* also activated host PTPs (protein tyrosine phosphatases) such as PTP1B, TC-PTP, PTP-PEST, and SHP-1. PTP activation causes a wide range of beneficial events for the parasite, including a decrease in proinflammatory processes, a decrease in IL-12, NO, TNF, phagolysosomal maturation, and antigen presentation by class II MHC molecules [64, 65]. TRAF3 is another newly discovered target of *L. donovani* promastigotes. In RAW 264.7 cells and bone marrow-derived macrophages, the parasite blocked TRAF3 (TNF receptor-associated factor) degradation to impede TLR4-mediated inflammatory response in the host. TLR4 activation requires TRAF3 degradative ubiquitination. TRAF3 knockdown by shRNA reduced parasite load [66]. The preceding investigations demonstrate the wide range of host targets that *Leishmania* uses to avoid macrophage activation and the consequent proinflammatory response. As *Leishmania* develops infection and multiplies within the macrophage, the macrophage may ultimately undergo apoptosis. The parasite postpones apoptosis of macrophage but eventually uses the apoptotic cell to propagate to nearby non - infected macrophages with limited access to extracellular immune recognition systems. Hence, when it is at its most susceptible phases, *Leishmania* skillfully manipulates its host to escape immune detection and associated inflammation.

4.2 Interfering with host cell signaling

Leishmania-infected macrophages lack events associated with activation and are insensitive to IFN-γ [51]. It has also been found that IFN-γ receptors are downregulated by *L. donovani* promastigotes and promote the expression of the cytokine signaling suppressor SOCS3 [67]. As a result, *L. donovani* promastigotes may effectively turn off the main signaling cascade of one of the most essential macrophage activators. *L. donovani* amastigotes, like promastigotes, suppressed IFN-induced MHC class II and iNOS expression. Infection with *L. donovani* amastigotes, on the other hand, reduced IFN-induced gene expression without changing STAT1 activation. Rather, amastigotes decreased IFN-induced nuclear translocation of STAT1 through interfering with STAT1's interaction with karyopherin importin-α5 [68]. The fundamental mechanics are yet unknown.

4.3 Avoiding oxidative damage

The reactions of *Leishmania* to oxidative stress is different for different *Leishmania* species and host cell they infect [69]. For instance, peritoneal macrophages infected with *L. major*, when elicited by thioglycolate, triggered ROS generation by stationary phase promastigotes whereas the same was inhibited in macrophages infected with *L. amazonensis* [70]. To combat oxidative stress, various Leishmania species employ a variety of strategies. *L. donovani* axenic amastigotes, for example, were able to reduce both intracellular and mitochondrial ROS by inducing mitochondrial uncoupling protein 2 (UCP2) upregulation, hence ROS inhibition [53]. *Leishmania* can also escape oxidative damage by inhibiting the assembly of phagolysosomal membrane NADPH oxidase and the formation of ROS within the parasitophorous vacuoles [71]. The parasite's insertion of the surface glycolipid lipophosphoglycan (LPG) in the phagosomal membrane may further hinder recruitment of the NADPH oxidase components to the parasitophorous vacuoles [30]. In addition to directly damaging the parasite's oxidative damage caused by ROS promotes macrophage apoptosis, destroying the parasite's replicative niche.

4.4 Countering antigen presentation

Antigen cross-presentation is a significant aspect in pathogen immunity. It entails presenting phagocytosed cargo-derived foreign proteins on class I MHC for cytotoxic CD8+ T cells recognition and a systemic immune response coordination. The macrophage, as a specialized antigen presenting cell (APC), contributes in the cross-presentation of proteins generated from *Leishmania*. In macrophages infected with *L. donovani* or *L. major*, the parasite strategically escapes immune responses offered by the host by inducing SNARE VAMPS cleavage, thus preventing antigen cross-presentation [34]. No such inhibition is observed in *L. donovani* amastigote infected macrophages. VAMP8 disruption inhibited assembly of NADPH oxidase, resulting in more effective phagosomal acidification and proteolysis, and thereby reducing presentation by MJHC class I and activation of T cells [71–73]. The parasite also inhibited antigen cross-presentation by disrupting membrane lipid microdomains [74]. Indeed, infected cells had lower membrane cholesterol levels, and the defect in antigen presentation could be repaired with liposomal administration of exogenous cholesterol. Liposomal cholesterol was also found to be enhancing ROS and RNI degeneration, as well as expression of proinflammatory cytokine and intracellular parasite death, and was linked to cellular stress and ROS-induced apoptosis in peritoneal cells infected with *L. donovani* promastigotes [75].

4.5 Inducing autophagy

L. amazonensis amastigotes and stationary phase promastigotes increased intracellular parasite survival by autophagy induction in peritoneal exudate cells or macrophages derived from bone marrow. Autophagy inhibitors like 3-methyladenine (3MA) or wortmannin lowered parasite burden, but autophagy inducers like rapamycin or starvation had little effect or increased parasite load [76, 77]. Autophagy induction was related with a decrease in NO, emphasizing the importance of this mechanism in infection establishment.

4.6 Exploiting macrophage environment to activate its antioxidant defense mechanism through cyclic nucleotide signaling pathway

Following phagocytosis by macrophages in the early stages of infection, the parasites are subjected to severe oxidative stress as a result of a respiratory burst offered by the macrophages releasing ROS and RNS [78, 79]. Superoxide dismutase, peroxidoxin, and trypanothione reductase are three *Leishmania* components involved in antioxidant defense against ROS and RNIs. The parasites are rendered susceptible to death in the ROS producing macrophages upon the disruption of the above-mentioned genes [80–83]. Furthermore, resistance against oxidative damage is induced when the organism is pre-exposed to environmental stress [78, 84]. In many unicellular eukaryotes, the cAMP response has been linked as one of the key environmental sensing machineries related with environmental stress response. Despite the fact that *Leishmania* parasites are subjected to extreme stress, which is a trigger for differentiation, and the relevance of cAMP in parasite differentiation has been documented, knowledge about the function of cAMP in *Leishmania* pathogenicity and resistance against oxidative stress is still obscure. A high temperature of 37°C, a low pH of 5.5 and nutritional starvation, all these collectively trigger cell cycle arrest in promastigote resulting in differentiation into aflagellar amastigote forms inside the macrophage. Occurrence of the major antioxidant gene upregulation was confirmed by analyzing the mRNA expression of these genes under stressed condition and maximum elevation of Ldpxn1 level was found indicating the activity of antioxidant genes in *Leishmania* during stress [8]. Not only that, antioxidant gene protein upregulation was also observed in *Leishmania* treated with cAMP analogues, suggesting a crucial role of cAMP in promoting antioxidant defense in *Leishmania*. Chemical or genetic inhibition of intracellular cAMP resulted in a decrease in the mRNA and protein levels of these anti-oxidant genes. The role of cAMP in parasite infectivity was reinforced by the discovery that promastigotes with a steadily overexpressed pde gene had a lower ability to infect IFN-γ activated macrophages than normal cells. The cAMP response is most likely one of several environmental sensing tools connected with *Leishmania* differentiation, and many other biochemical reactions may collaborate with cAMP in the process of differentiation resulting in parasite transformation.

5. Role of cAMP in survival and infectivity of the parasites

In eukaryotes, cAMP, a second messenger which is formed from ATP by the membrane- bound enzyme, receptor adenylate cyclases (RAC), is a key component that controls a wide range of cellular activities such as cytoskeletal modeling, cell proliferation, virulence, cellular differentiation, and death [85]. There have been reports of various isoforms of both membrane-bound receptor adenylate cyclases and soluble adenylate cyclases in *Leishmania* [86]. cAMP has been found to be involved in signal transduction processes that occur during transformations not only in *Leishmania*, but also in other similar kinetoplastid protozoa. In *Trypanosoma brucei* [87] and *Trypanosoma cruzi* [88], various life cycle phases have variable intracellular cAMP concentrations. Owing to the importance of cAMP and the role it plays in the transformation of kinetoplastid parasites, receptor adenylate cyclases in *L. donovani* have further been investigated. In *L. donovani*, the occurrence of receptor adenylate cyclase (RAC) has also been revealed, and a membrane associated RAC-A has been established to be functional when exposed to phagolysosome conditions (PC) actively catalyzing cAMP production [89]. In addition to the direct action of LdRAC-A in stress-induced intra-cellular cAMP generation, intracellular PPi and pyrophosphatases also perform a significant role in modulating cAMP concentration in the cell. A higher PPi concentration might be modulating adenylate cyclase reactions and thus, inhibits cAMP generation in the parasites (**Figure 1**) [90]. Aside from pyrophosphatases, which control intracellular cAMP synthesis by receptor adenylate cyclases, other aspects of cAMP regulation must be investigated. Intramacrophage cAMP concentration is increased upon infection-induced Prostaglandin E2 production in the *Leishmania*-infected macrophage [91]. Intracellular cAMP level is maintained by phosphodiesterases (PDEs) which are universal enzymes that hydrolyze cAMP to 5′-AMP or cGMP to 5′-GMP to terminate the cyclic nucleotide signaling pathway, are the only mechanism for the cell to get rid of the cAMP generated for managing various cellular activities [92]. Cytosolic PDE activities decrease throughout stage differentiation, although the activity of membrane bound PDEs remains constant. This data suggests that PDEs have a crucial function as a regulating factor during stage differentiation of *Leishmania* [93]. Not only membrane-bound phosphodiesterases, but cytosolic phosphodiesterase, PDED, is also important in the regulation of cAMP homeostasis by enhanced hydrolytic property through PKA-mediated activation of PDED [94]. PDED plays a role in the regulation of PKA activity and in turn maintains cAMP homeostasis in the parasite when initially exposed to stress conditions.

Despite the fact that cAMP-dependent protein kinase (PKA) exists and functions in eukaryotes, the role of PKA in cAMP signaling in this specific parasite is still ambiguous. PKA, being the first downstream effector of cAMP in the RAC pathway, facilitate γ-P transfer to particular ser/thr residue from ATP [95]. Upon exposure of *Leishmania* to environmental stress, a significant upregulation of PKA activity, concomitantly with cAMP level increase, is observed, suggesting a connection between cAMP and PKA during parasite differentiation. PKA activity of five distinct *Leishmania* species was shown to be relatively high in logarithmic, as well as stationary phase promastigotes, with *L. amazonensis* being the most active and *L. donovani* being the least active [96]. A regulatory subunit of cAMP-dependent PKA, LdPKAR1, have been identified in *L. donovani* which plays significant role in metacyclogenesis, intra-macrophage survival and enhanced infectivity of the parasite [97]. Thus, cAMP is emerging as a key regulator of cytological processes in kinetoplastida parasites [98]. Despite the discovery of multiple cyclic nucleotide binding effector molecules, there is still lack of complete understanding on cAMP signaling from receptor to effector.

6. Conclusion

Being an intracellular parasite, *Leishmania* has adopted various ways to enter the host cells efficiently and then subsequently try to neutralize the hostile environment of macrophages. Although various strategies have been adopted by this parasite to establish successful infection, we are mainly concerned about stressing the role of inflammasome activation in host cells and cAMP homeostasis of the parasite in this chapter. To summarize, it can be stated that recent advances in research have increased our understanding of the role of cAMP signaling in kinetoplastid parasites such as *Leishmania* and its relationship to parasite infectivity. These findings shed light on the activity of many enzymes involved in cAMP metabolism. It can be suggested that modulating cAMP levels in the parasite might be one of the methods for controlling leishmaniasis, and that the molecules involved could be explored as powerful therapeutic targets against the leishmaniases.

Acknowledgements

We would like to thank Personal Research Grant (PRG), University of Kalyani, DST-PURSE, University of Kalyani and INSA Senior Scientist Fellowship for contingent costs associated with the drafting of this chapter.

Conflict of interest

The authors declare no conflict of interest.

Author details

Anindita Bhattacharjee[1], Arunima Biswas[1*] and Pijush K. Das[2*]

1 Molecular Cell Biology Laboratory, Department of Zoology, University of Kalyani, Kalyani, India

2 Department of Infectious Diseases and Immunology, CSIR-Indian Institute of Chemical Biology, Kolkata, India

*Address all correspondence to: arunima10@klyuniv.ac.in and pijushdas@iicb.res.in

References

[1] Rogers ME. The role of Leishmania Proteophosphoglycans in sand Fly transmission and infection of the mammalian host. Frontiers in Microbiology. 2012;**3**:223

[2] Heyde S, Philipsen L, Formaglio P, Fu Y, Baars I, Höbbel G, et al. CD11c-expressing Ly6C+CCR2+ monocytes constitute a reservoir for efficient Leishmania proliferation and cell-to-cell transmission. PLoS Pathogens. 2018;**14**(10):e1007374

[3] Kelley N, Jeltema D, Duan Y, He Y. The NLRP3 Inflammasome: An overview of mechanisms of activation and regulation. International Journal of Molecular Sciences. 2019;**20**(13):3328

[4] de Carvalho RVH, Zamboni DS. Inflammasome activation in response to intracellular protozoan parasites. Trends in Parasitology. 2020;**36**(5): 459-472

[5] Lecoeur H, Prina E, Rosazza T, Kokou K, N'Diaye P, Aulner N, et al. Targeting macrophage histone H3 modification as a Leishmania strategy to dampen the NF-κB/NLRP3-mediated inflammatory response. Cell Reports. 2020;**30**(6):1870-1882.e4

[6] Biswas A, Bhattacharya A, Das PK. Role of cAMP Signaling in the survival and infectivity of the protozoan parasite, Leishmania donovani. Molecular Biology International. 2011;**2011**:e782971

[7] Saha A, Bhattacharjee A, Vij A, Das PK, Bhattacharya A, Biswas A. Evaluation of modulators of cAMP-response in terms of their impact on cell cycle and mitochondrial activity of Leishmania donovani. Frontiers in Pharmacology. 2020;**11**:782

[8] Bhattacharya A, Biswas A, Das PK. Role of intracellular cAMP in differentiation-coupled induction of resistance against oxidative damage in Leishmania donovani. Free Radical Biology & Medicine. 2008;**44**(5):779-794

[9] Casalle N, de Barros Pinto Grifoni L, Bosco Mendes AC, Delort S, Massucato EMS. Mucocutaneous Leishmaniasis with rare manifestation in the nasal mucosa and cartilage bone septal. Case Reports in Infectious Diseases. 2020;**2020**:8876020

[10] Alvar J, Vélez ID, Bern C, Herrero M, Desjeux P, Cano J, et al. Leishmaniasis worldwide and global estimates of its incidence. PLoS One. 2012;**7**(5):e35671

[11] Ready PD. Epidemiology of visceral leishmaniasis. Clinical Epidemiology. 2014;**6**:147-154

[12] McMahon-Pratt D, Alexander J. Does the Leishmania major paradigm of pathogenesis and protection hold for New World cutaneous leishmaniases or the visceral disease? Immunological Reviews. 2004;**201**:206-224

[13] Domínguez M, Moreno I, Aizpurua C, Toraño A. Early mechanisms of Leishmania infection in human blood. Microbes and Infection. 2003;**5**(6):507-513

[14] Maurer M, Dondji B, von Stebut E. What determines the success or failure of intracellular cutaneous parasites? Lessons learned from leishmaniasis. Medical Microbiology and Immunology. 2009;**198**(3):137-146

[15] Scharton TM, Scott P. Natural killer cells are a source of interferon gamma that drives differentiation of

CD4+ T cell subsets and induces early resistance to Leishmania major in mice. The Journal of Experimental Medicine. 1993;**178**(2):567-577

[16] Sundar S, Reed SG, Sharma S, Mehrotra A, Murray HW. Circulating T helper 1 (Th1) cell- and Th2 cell-associated cytokines in Indian patients with visceral leishmaniasis. The American Journal of Tropical Medicine and Hygiene. 1997;**56**(5):522-525

[17] Peters NC, Egen JG, Secundino N, Debrabant A, Kimblin N, Kamhawi S, et al. In vivo imaging reveals an essential role for neutrophils in leishmaniasis transmitted by sand flies. Science. 2008;**321**(5891):970-974

[18] Rogers M, Kropf P, Choi B-S, Dillon R, Podinovskaia M, Bates P, et al. Proteophosophoglycans regurgitated by Leishmania-infected sand flies target the L-arginine metabolism of host macrophages to promote parasite survival. PLoS Pathogens. 2009;**5**(8):e1000555

[19] Rogers ME, Corware K, Müller I, Bates PA. Leishmania infantum proteophosphoglycans regurgitated by the bite of its natural sand fly vector, Lutzomyia longipalpis, promote parasite establishment in mouse skin and skin-distant tissues. Microbes and Infection. 2010;**12**(11):875-879

[20] Rotureau B, Morales MA, Bastin P, Späth GF. The flagellum-mitogen-activated protein kinase connection in Trypanosomatids: A key sensory role in parasite signalling and development? Cellular Microbiology. 2009;**11**(5):710-718

[21] Peters NC, Sacks DL. The impact of vector-mediated neutrophil recruitment on cutaneous leishmaniasis. Cellular Microbiology. 2009;**11**(9):1290-1296

[22] Mollinedo F, Janssen H, de la Iglesia-Vicente J, Villa-Pulgarin JA, Calafat J. Selective fusion of azurophilic granules with Leishmania-containing phagosomes in human neutrophils. The Journal of Biological Chemistry. 2010;**285**(45):34528-34536

[23] Ueno N, Wilson ME. Receptor-mediated phagocytosis of Leishmania: Implications for intracellular survival. Trends in Parasitology. 2012;**28**(8):335-344

[24] Rodríguez NE, Gaur Dixit U, Allen L-AH, Wilson ME. Stage-specific pathways of Leishmania infantum chagasi entry and phagosome maturation in macrophages. PLoS One. 2011;**6**(4):e19000

[25] Chattopadhyay A, Jafurulla M. Role of membrane cholesterol in leishmanial infection. Advances in Experimental Medicine and Biology. 2012;**749**:201-213

[26] Roy S, Kumar GA, Jafurulla M, Mandal C, Chattopadhyay A. Integrity of the actin cytoskeleton of host macrophages is essential for Leishmania donovani infection. Biochimica et Biophysica Acta. 2014;**1838**(8):2011-2018

[27] Majumder S, Dey R, Bhattacharjee S, RubA, GuptaG, BhattacharyyaMajumdarS, et al. Leishmania-induced biphasic ceramide generation in macrophages is crucial for uptake and survival of the parasite. The Journal of Infectious Diseases. 2012;**205**(10):1607-1616

[28] Mukherjee M, Basu Ball W, Das PK. Leishmania donovani activates SREBP2 to modulate macrophage membrane cholesterol and mitochondrial oxidants for establishment of infection. The International Journal of Biochemistry & Cell Biology. 2014;**55**:196-208

[29] Vinet AF, Fukuda M, Turco SJ, Descoteaux A. The Leishmania donovani

lipophosphoglycan excludes the vesicular proton-ATPase from phagosomes by impairing the recruitment of synaptotagmin V. PLoS Pathogens. 2009;**5**(10):e1000628

[30] Moradin N, Descoteaux A. Leishmania promastigotes: Building a safe niche within macrophages. Frontiers in Cellular and Infection Microbiology. 2012;**2**:121

[31] Forestier C-L, Machu C, Loussert C, Pescher P, Späth GF. Imaging host cell-Leishmania interaction dynamics implicates parasite motility, lysosome recruitment, and host cell wounding in the infection process. Cell Host & Microbe. 2011;**9**(4):319-330

[32] Mittra B, Cortez M, Haydock A, Ramasamy G, Myler PJ, Andrews NW. Iron uptake controls the generation of Leishmania infective forms through regulation of ROS levels. The Journal of Experimental Medicine. 2013;**210**(2):401-416

[33] Mittra B, Andrews NW. IRONy OF FATE: Role of iron-mediated ROS in Leishmania differentiation. Trends in Parasitology. 2013;**29**(10):489-496

[34] Podinovskaia M, Descoteaux A. Leishmania and the macrophage: A multifaceted interaction. Future Microbiology. 2015;**10**(1):111-129

[35] Vij A, Biswas A, Bhattacharya A, Das PK. A soluble phosphodiesterase in Leishmania donovani negatively regulates cAMP signaling by inhibiting protein kinase a through a two way process involving catalytic as well as non-catalytic sites. The International Journal of Biochemistry & Cell Biology. 2014;**57**:197-206

[36] Biswas A, Bhattacharya A, Vij A, Das PK. Role of leishmanial acidocalcisomal pyrophosphatase in the cAMP homeostasis in phagolysosome conditions required for intra-macrophage survival. The International Journal of Biochemistry & Cell Biology. 2017;**86**:1-13

[37] Wynn TA, Chawla A, Pollard JW. Macrophage biology in development, homeostasis and disease. Nature. 2013;**496**(7446):445-455

[38] Nathan CF, Hibbs JB. Role of nitric oxide synthesis in macrophage antimicrobial activity. Current Opinion in Immunology. 1991;**3**(1):65-70

[39] Forman HJ, Torres M. Reactive oxygen species and cell signaling: Respiratory burst in macrophage signaling. American Journal of Respiratory and Critical Care Medicine. 2002;**166**(12 Pt 2):S4-S8

[40] Franken L, Schiwon M, Kurts C. Macrophages: Sentinels and regulators of the immune system. Cellular Microbiology. 2016;**18**(4):475-487

[41] Gordon S, Taylor PR. Monocyte and macrophage heterogeneity. Nature Reviews. Immunology. 2005;**5**(12):953-964

[42] Mosser DM, Edwards JP. Exploring the full spectrum of macrophage activation. Nature Reviews. Immunology. 2008;**8**(12):958-969

[43] Sica A, Mantovani A. Macrophage plasticity and polarization: in vivo veritas. The Journal of Clinical Investigation. 2012;**122**(3):787-795

[44] Jaguin M, Houlbert N, Fardel O, Lecureur V. Polarization profiles of human M-CSF-generated macrophages and comparison of M1-markers in classically activated macrophages from GM-CSF and M-CSF origin. Cellular Immunology. 2013;**281**(1):51-61

[45] Gordon S, Martinez FO. Alternative activation of macrophages: Mechanism and functions. Immunity. 2010;**32**(5):593-604

[46] Mills CD. Macrophage arginine metabolism to ornithine/urea or nitric oxide/citrulline: A life or death issue. Critical Reviews in Immunology. 2001;**21**(5):399-425

[47] Tarique AA, Logan J, Thomas E, Holt PG, Sly PD, Fantino E. Phenotypic, functional, and plasticity features of classical and alternatively activated human macrophages. American Journal of Respiratory Cell and Molecular Biology. 2015;**53**(5):676-688

[48] Gupta P, Srivastav S, Saha S, Das PK, Ukil A. Leishmania donovani inhibits macrophage apoptosis and pro-inflammatory response through AKT-mediated regulation of β-catenin and FOXO-1. Cell Death and Differentiation. 2016;**23**(11):1815-1826

[49] Broz P, Dixit VM. Inflammasomes: Mechanism of assembly, regulation and signalling. Nature Reviews. Immunology. 2016;**16**(7):407-420

[50] Di A, Xiong S, Ye Z, Malireddi RKS, Kometani S, Zhong M, et al. The TWIK2 potassium Efflux Channel in macrophages mediates NLRP3 Inflammasome-induced inflammation. Immunity. 2018;**49**(1):56-65.e4

[51] Shio MT, Christian JG, Jung JY, Chang K-P, Olivier M. PKC/ROS-mediated NLRP3 Inflammasome activation is attenuated by Leishmania zinc-metalloprotease during infection. PLoS Neglected Tropical Diseases. 2015;**9**(6):e0003868

[52] Gupta AK, Ghosh K, Palit S, Barua J, Das PK, Ukil A. Leishmania donovani inhibits inflammasome-dependent macrophage activation by exploiting the negative regulatory proteins A20 and UCP2. The FASEB Journal. 2017;**31**(11):5087-5101

[53] Ball WB, Mukherjee M, Srivastav S, Das PK. Leishmania donovani activates uncoupling protein 2 transcription to suppress mitochondrial oxidative burst through differential modulation of SREBP2, Sp1 and USF1 transcription factors. The International Journal of Biochemistry & Cell Biology. 2014;**48**:66-76

[54] Saha G, Khamar BM, Singh OP, Sundar S, Dubey VK. Leishmania donovani evades caspase 1 dependent host defense mechanism during infection. International Journal of Biological Macromolecules. 2019;**126**:392-401

[55] Lima-Junior DS, Costa DL, Carregaro V, Cunha LD, Silva ALN, Mineo TWP, et al. Inflammasome-derived IL-1β production induces nitric oxide-mediated resistance to Leishmania. Nature Medicine. 2013;**19**(7):909-915

[56] Lefèvre L, Lugo-Villarino G, Meunier E, Valentin A, Olagnier D, Authier H, et al. The C-type lectin receptors dectin-1, MR, and SIGNR3 contribute both positively and negatively to the macrophage response to Leishmania infantum. Immunity. 2013;**38**(5):1038-1049

[57] Lima-Junior DS, Mineo TWP, Calich VLG, Zamboni DS. Dectin-1 activation during Leishmania amazonensis phagocytosis prompts Syk-dependent reactive oxygen species production to trigger Inflammasome assembly and restriction of parasite replication. Journal of Immunology. 2017;**199**(6):2055-2068

[58] de Carvalho RVH, Andrade WA, Lima-Junior DS, Dilucca M, de

Oliveira CV, Wang K, et al. Leishmania Lipophosphoglycan triggers Caspase-11 and the non-canonical activation of the NLRP3 Inflammasome. Cell Reports. 2019;**26**(2):429-437.e5

[59] Farias Luz N, Balaji S, Okuda K, Barreto AS, Bertin J, Gough PJ, et al. RIPK1 and PGAM5 control Leishmania replication through distinct mechanisms. Journal of Immunology. 2016;**196**(12):5056-5063

[60] Santos DM, Carneiro MW, de Moura TR, Soto M, Luz NF, Prates DB, et al. PLGA nanoparticles loaded with KMP-11 stimulate innate immunity and induce the killing of Leishmania. Nanomedicine. 2013;**9**(7):985-995

[61] Miranda MM, Panis C, da Silva SS, Macri JA, Kawakami NY, Hayashida TH, et al. Kaurenoic acid possesses leishmanicidal activity by triggering a NLRP12/IL-1β/cNOS/NO pathway. Mediators of Inflammation. 2015;**2015**:392918

[62] Lapara NJ, Kelly BL. Suppression of LPS-induced inflammatory responses in macrophages infected with Leishmania. Journal of Inflammation. 2010;**7**(1):8

[63] Chan MM, Adapala N, Chen C. Peroxisome proliferator-activated receptor-γ-mediated polarization of macrophages in Leishmania infection. PPAR Research. 2012;**2012**:796235

[64] Gómez MA, Olivier M. Proteases and phosphatases during Leishmania-macrophage interaction: Paving the road for pathogenesis. Virulence. 2010;**1**(4):314-318

[65] Liu D, Uzonna JE. The early interaction of Leishmania with macrophages and dendritic cells and its influence on the host immune response. Frontiers in Cellular and Infection Microbiology. 2012;**2**:83

[66] Gupta P, Giri J, Srivastav S, Chande AG, Mukhopadhyaya R, Das PK, et al. Leishmania donovani targets tumor necrosis factor receptor-associated factor (TRAF) 3 for impairing TLR4-mediated host response. The FASEB Journal. 2014;**28**(4):1756-1768

[67] Bhattacharya P, Gupta G, Majumder S, Adhikari A, Banerjee S, Halder K, et al. Arabinosylated lipoarabinomannan skews Th2 phenotype towards Th1 during Leishmania infection by chromatin modification: Involvement of MAPK signaling. PLoS One. 2011;**6**(9):e24141

[68] Matte C, Descoteaux A. Leishmania donovani amastigotes impair gamma interferon-induced STAT1alpha nuclear translocation by blocking the interaction between STAT1alpha and importin-alpha5. Infection and Immunity. 2010;**78**(9):3736-3743

[69] Olivier M, Atayde VD, Isnard A, Hassani K, Shio MT. Leishmania virulence factors: Focus on the metalloprotease GP63. Microbes and Infection. 2012;**14**(15):1377-1389

[70] Almeida TF, Palma LC, Mendez LC, Noronha-Dutra AA, Veras PST. Leishmania amazonensis fails to induce the release of reactive oxygen intermediates by CBA macrophages. Parasite Immunology. 2012;**34**(10):492-498

[71] Matheoud D, Moradin N, Bellemare-Pelletier A, Shio MT, Hong WJ, Olivier M, et al. Leishmania evades host immunity by inhibiting antigen cross-presentation through direct cleavage of the SNARE VAMP8. Cell Host & Microbe. 2013;**14**(1):15-25

[72] Savina A, Jancic C, Hugues S, Guermonprez P, Vargas P, Moura IC,

et al. NOX2 controls phagosomal pH to regulate antigen processing during crosspresentation by dendritic cells. Cell. 2006;**126**(1):205-218

[73] Rybicka JM, Balce DR, Chaudhuri S, Allan ERO, Yates RM. Phagosomal proteolysis in dendritic cells is modulated by NADPH oxidase in a pH-independent manner. The EMBO Journal. 2012;**31**(4):932-944

[74] Chakraborty D, Banerjee S, Sen A, Banerjee KK, Das P, Roy S. Leishmania donovani affects antigen presentation of macrophage by disrupting lipid rafts. Journal of Immunology. 2005;**175**(5):3214-3224

[75] Ghosh J, Guha R, Das S, Roy S. Liposomal cholesterol delivery activates the macrophage innate immune arm to facilitate intracellular Leishmania donovani killing. Infection and Immunity. 2014;**82**(2):607-617

[76] Pinheiro RO, Nunes MP, Pinheiro CS, D'Avila H, Bozza PT, Takiya CM, et al. Induction of autophagy correlates with increased parasite load of Leishmania amazonensis in BALB/c but not C57BL/6 macrophages. Microbes and Infection. 2009;**11**(2):181-190

[77] Cyrino LT, Araújo AP, Joazeiro PP, Vicente CP, Giorgio S. In vivo and in vitro Leishmania amazonensis infection induces autophagy in macrophages. Tissue & Cell. 2012;**44**(6):401-408

[78] Zarley JH, Britigan BE, Wilson ME. Hydrogen peroxide-mediated toxicity for Leishmania donovani chagasi promastigotes. Role of hydroxyl radical and protection by heat shock. The Journal of Clinical Investigation. 1991;**88**(5):1511-1521

[79] Gantt KR, Goldman TL, McCormick ML, Miller MA, Jeronimo SM, Nascimento ET, et al. Oxidative responses of human and murine macrophages during phagocytosis of Leishmania chagasi. Journal of Immunology. 2001;**167**(2):893-901

[80] Tovar J, Wilkinson S, Mottram JC, Fairlamb AH. Evidence that trypanothione reductase is an essential enzyme in Leishmania by targeted replacement of the tryA gene locus. Molecular Microbiology. 1998;**29**(2):653-660

[81] Barr SD, Gedamu L. Cloning and characterization of three differentially expressed peroxidoxin genes from Leishmania chagasi. Evidence for an enzymatic detoxification of hydroxyl radicals. The Journal of Biological Chemistry. 2001;**276**(36):34279-34287

[82] Ghosh S, Goswami S, Adhya S. Role of superoxide dismutase in survival of Leishmania within the macrophage. The Biochemical Journal. 2003;**369** (Pt 3):447-452

[83] Plewes KA, Barr SD, Gedamu L. Iron superoxide dismutases targeted to the glycosomes of Leishmania chagasi are important for survival. Infection and Immunity. 2003;**71**(10):5910-5920

[84] Miller MA, McGowan SE, Gantt KR, Champion M, Novick SL, Andersen KA, et al. Inducible resistance to oxidant stress in the protozoan Leishmania chagasi. The Journal of Biological Chemistry. 2000;**275**(43):33883-33889

[85] Dremier S, Kopperud R, Doskeland SO, Dumont JE, Maenhaut C. Search for new cyclic AMP-binding proteins. FEBS Letters. 2003;**546**(1):103-107

[86] Hansen BD, Chiang PK, Perez-Arbelo J. Evidence for a membrane

adenosine receptor in Leishmania mexicana mexicana (WR 227). Advances in Experimental Medicine and Biology. 1986;**195**(Pt B):547-551

[87] Mancini PE, Patton CL. Cyclic 3′,5′-adenosine monophosphate levels during the developmental cycle of Trypanosoma brucei brucei in the rat. Molecular and Biochemical Parasitology. 1981;**3**(1):19-31

[88] Rangel-Aldao R, Allende O, Triana F, Piras R, Henriquez D, Piras M. Possible role of cAMP in the differentiation of Trypanosoma cruzi. Molecular and Biochemical Parasitology. 1987; **22**(1):39-43

[89] Sanchez MA, Zeoli D, Klamo EM, Kavanaugh MP, Landfear SM. A family of putative receptor-adenylate cyclases from Leishmania donovani. The Journal of Biological Chemistry. 1995;**270**(29):17551-17558

[90] Seebeck T, Schaub R, Johner A. cAMP signalling in the kinetoplastid protozoa. Current Molecular Medicine. 2004;**4**(6):585-599

[91] Saha A, Biswas A, Srivastav S, Mukherjee M, Das PK, Ukil A. Prostaglandin E2 negatively regulates the production of inflammatory cytokines/ chemokines and IL-17 in visceral leishmaniasis. Journal of Immunology. 2014;**193**(5):2330-2339

[92] Conti M, Beavo J. Biochemistry and physiology of cyclic nucleotide phosphodiesterases: Essential components in cyclic nucleotide signaling. Annual Review of Biochemistry. 2007;**76**:481-511

[93] Bhattacharya A, Biswas A, Das PK. Role of a differentially expressed cAMP phosphodiesterase in regulating the induction of resistance against oxidative damage in Leishmania donovani. Free Radical Biology & Medicine. 2009;**47**(10):1494-1506

[94] Gettys TW, Vine AJ, Simonds MF, Corbin JD. Activation of the particulate low km phosphodiesterase of adipocytes by addition of cAMP-dependent protein kinase. The Journal of Biological Chemistry. 1988;**263**(21):10359-10363

[95] Mochly-Rosen D. Localization of protein kinases by anchoring proteins: A theme in signal transduction. Science. 1995;**268**(5208):247-251

[96] Mukhopadhyay NK, Saha AK, Lovelace JK, Da Silva R, Sacks DL, Glew RH. Comparison of the protein kinase and acid phosphatase activities of five species of Leishmania. The Journal of Protozoology. 1988;**35**(4):601-607

[97] Bhattacharya A, Biswas A, Das PK. Identification of a protein kinase a regulatory subunit from Leishmania having importance in metacyclogenesis through induction of autophagy. Molecular Microbiology. 2012;**83**(3): 548-564

[98] Tagoe DNA, Kalejaiye TD, de Koning HP. The ever unfolding story of cAMP signaling in trypanosomatids: Vive la difference! Frontiers in Pharmacology. 2015;**6**:185

Chapter 7

Inflammation-Associated Wound Healing through a Monocytic Lens

Avi Petroff

Abstract

The development of macrophages from monocytes during wound healing is a complicated and convoluted process. Classically or alternatively activated macrophages result from a complex network of cytokine signaling between circulating monocytes entering tissue, resident macrophages, and stromal fibroblasts. This network of signaling constitutes a continuous communication between these cell types, influencing factors such as inflammatory duration, healthy or fibrotic tissue repair, and downstream macrophage functionality. "Forward talk" from monocytes to fibroblasts, as well as "back talk" from fibroblasts to monocytes, can greatly influence the behavior of each cell type. This cell-cell communication, though difficult to fully encapsulate *in vitro*, can be facilitated through implementation of specific cell culture techniques. 3D cell culture systems enable a more representative assessment of myofibroblast phenotypes that would likely be seen during wound repair. Co-culture systems further enable cell-cell interactions in the inflammatory and wound repair cascades to be assessed in coordination with each other. Looking ahead, these cell culture techniques, alongside novel concepts such as organ-on-a-chip models, can provide deeper insight into the myriad molecular mechanisms we claim to understand currently. Our improved understanding of these cellular interactions can lead to improved clinical outcomes for pathologies associated with these complex cell types.

Keywords: monocyte, macrophage, fibroblast, inflammation, communication, cell culture, wound repair, fibrosis, cytokine, cellular development

1. Introduction

To truly appreciate the history of our understanding of macrophages, we must first understand how macrophages manifest from earlier cellular lineages. Just as humans have common ancestors and lineages with other primates, so too do macrophages with other cells derived from myeloid progenitor cells. All this is to say, just as humans are complex organisms, macrophages have fantastic intricacies and potential fates. The whole world is its oyster, or petri dish, if you will.

So, how do macrophages come to be? We'll go over some key points here, and some will be expanded upon in subsequent sections within this chapter. Discussion in this chapter will pertain to macrophages, monocytes, and fibroblasts in a broad cellular sense but will also have a focus on human physiology. Briefly, macrophages comprise a heterogenous and highly variable group of myeloid cells that function within the innate immune system [1]. The functions of macrophages are largely attributed to inflammation, which will be discussed further below.

2. Mention of macrophage manifestation

What makes macrophages particularly fascinating is the plasticity of their manifestation. In other words, macrophages have the innate ability to alter their phenotype during development in response to, and in conjunction with, myriad environmental signals [1]. This plasticity in "activation" of macrophages is a growing area of research in fields such as immunology, disease progression, tissue and extracellular matrix homeostasis, and resolution of inflammation [2].

More specifically, the activation of macrophages can come about by stimuli such as cytokines—special cellular signaling proteins—that influence levels of gene and protein expression [2]. The unique composition of cell surface receptors, intracellular enzymes, and cytokines allows us to create distinctions that organize our understanding of macrophage activation.

The exact categories of macrophage activation go beyond the scope of this chapter, and such distinctions are still a point of ongoing scientific discussion. However, for the purpose of our understanding, there are two primary routes of macrophage activation. The first is commonly known as "classically activated" or "type 1" macrophages (M1), and the second is known as "alternatively activated" or "type 2" (M2) [2]. These states of activation have been described as polarized extremes within a continuum of macrophage functionality [3]. Indeed, various subsets of nomenclature have been established, such as M2a and M2b, that expand upon the basic M1 and M2 classifications, accounting for the possibility of activation within a spectrum of phenotypes [2]. For the purpose of this chapter, we'll delve deeper into M1 and M2, bearing in mind the continuum within which we are exploring.

Classically activated macrophages are purported to be involved in the canonical response to tissue injury and/or infection. As expected, this pathway of activation is characterized by macrophage expression of many pro-inflammatory cytokines, such as TNF-α, and interleukins such as IL-1β, IL-6, and IL-12 [1]. These M1 macrophages are heavily involved in the inflammatory cascade discussed in subsequent sections within this chapter, primarily through the production of reactive oxygen and nitrogen species [1].

Alternatively activated macrophages, in contrast to M1 macrophages, secrete minimal pro-inflammatory cytokines [1]. Instead, M2 macrophages secrete numerous anti-inflammatory cytokines such as IL-10, CCL18, and CCL22 [1]. Further, alternatively activated macrophages play a crucial role in counteracting pro-inflammatory and cellular immune mechanisms, with inhibitory and regulatory functions in such pathways [4]. In this respect, M1 macrophages are broadly categorized as the pro-inflammatory side of the spectrum, whereas M2 macrophages pertain mostly to the anti-inflammatory side of the spectrum [1].

Though more complicated than necessary for the purpose of discussion in this chapter, there are various *in vitro* protocols employed to induce M1 and M2 phenotypes [5]. Because M1 and M2 phenotypes represent such polarized and opposite activation states within the macrophage continuum, these basic classifications provide an opportunity to study and assess macrophages in a wound healing context. However, we must remember that *in vivo* macrophage phenotypes in tissue wounds would likely demonstrate a much more complex and variable phenotype.

To conclude our introduction to the manifestation of macrophages, it should additionally be noted that IL-10 is a much more complex cytokine than previously thought. Difficult to describe and fully encapsulate in experimental data or scientific publications, IL-10 can behave as both a pro-inflammatory and anti-inflammatory cytokine in various environmental conditions [6, 7]. With the presence of IL-10 during the developmental process of macrophages, it is exciting to consider that there is potentially still much to learn about macrophages, and that our history of understanding these cells continues into our future.

3. Inflammation during wound healing

Now that we understand a bit more about the manifestation of macrophages, let us now turn our attention to the myeloid cells from which macrophages are themselves derived—monocytes. Monocytes are another complex and intriguing cell type and will be one of our focuses for the bulk of this chapter. However, it would be inappropriate to discuss the functions and fates of monocytes without also discussing the role of another cell type involved in would healing—fibroblasts. Fibroblasts are largely involved in the structuring and maintenance of the extracellular matrix (ECM) of tissue and play a vital role in the wound healing process.

In most human tissues, healthy wound healing is predicted to occur following hemostasis (blood clotting) via orderly and efficient progression through various stages of a signaling cascade (**Figure 1**). These stages include local inflammation, inflammatory resolution, tissue cell proliferation, and tissue remodeling [8]. Fibrosis—the formation of dysfunctional and often distorted scar tissue—occurs when these sequential events are dysregulated by dynamic signaling pathways [9, 10].

The inflammatory phase of wound healing is when circulating monocytes, as well as neutrophils, infiltrate tissue at the site of injury via cytokine recruitment [8]. Upon arrival, these circulating monocytes, in addition to local tissue monocytes, may differentiate into tissue macrophages (**Figure 2**) [8]. Classically or alternatively activated macrophages then play a role in tissue debridement, phagocytosis of foreign particles, and interaction with other cell types at the wound site such as fibroblasts and lymphocytes. This communication is in the form of secreted cytokines and growth factors, such as platelet-derived growth factor (PDGF), fibroblast growth factor

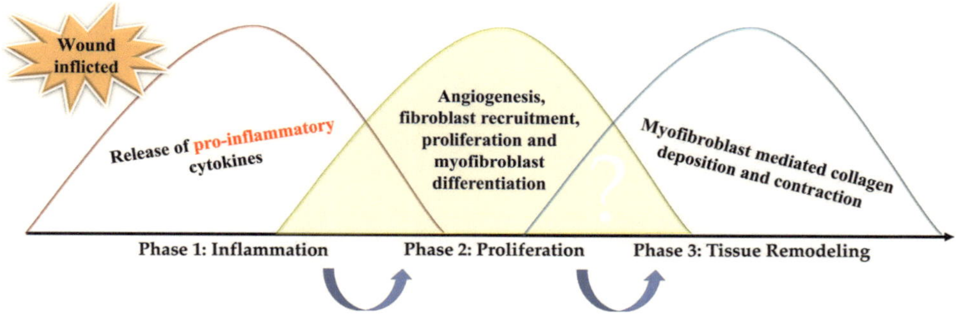

Figure 1.
Signaling cascade following hemostasis during wound healing. Progression through these stages, either subsequently or in an overlapping fashion, leads to the healthy remodeling of tissue. Dysregulation at various points within this cascade can result in aberrant wound repair, as is seen in fibrosis.

(FGF), and transforming growth factor β (TGFβ) [8]. Macrophages also play a role in antigen presentation for T-lymphocytes for development of downstream memory immune responses [8]. Without the vital role of macrophages, there would be slowed growth of damaged tissue, persistence of cellular and particulate debris, and slowed progression through the subsequent stages of wound healing (**Figure 1**).

The plasticity of activated macrophages is quite impressive. The elegant balance between classically and alternatively activated macrophages is crucial for preventing pathologies or acute reactions within wounded tissue [11]. This balance is made possible by the macrophage phenotypic plasticity; classically activated macrophages within the wound site can kill pathogens, neutralize toxins, and debride the wound [11]. In turn, alternatively activated macrophages are recruited via cytokines to repair tissue and heal the wound [11]. To prevent recruitment of circulating monocytes beyond this point, classically activated macrophages can switch their apparent phenotype to alternatively activated macrophages, based on signals from the local stromal tissue (**Figure 2**) [11]. This interesting signaling between stromal tissue, macrophages, and circulating monocytes will be discussed further later in this chapter.

In many human tissues, wound healing initiates the TGFβ signaling pathway, distinct from macrophage-secreted TGFβ [10]. Exposure of tissue fibroblasts to TGFβ induces another type of cellular activation. In this situation, tissue fibroblasts can become activated into myofibroblasts, characterized by expression of α-smooth muscle actin (α-SMA) [8]. Myofibroblasts play a prominent role in wound healing by synthesizing and secreting large quantities of ECM material, and additionally obtain a phenotype of increased contractility. The ECM secretions and increased contractility of these cell types facilitate wound healing, though excessive levels are characteristic of tissue fibrosis [8].

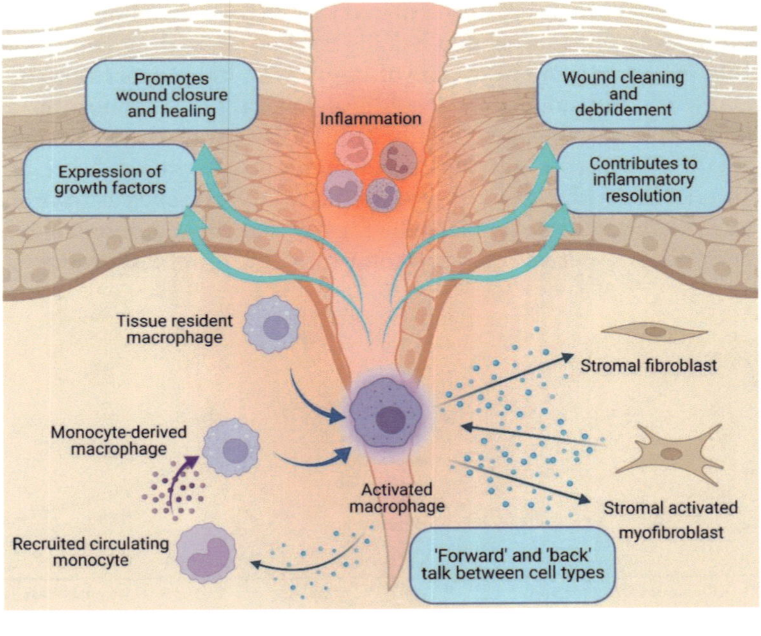

Figure 2.
Schematic of the central role of macrophages in wound healing. Circulating monocytes that differentiate into macrophages, in addition to tissue resident macrophages, can be classically or alternatively activated. Activated macrophages then contribute to various processes associated with wound healing. Cellular crosstalk between monocytes, macrophages, and stromal myofibroblasts further contributes to the complexity of the wound repair process.

The magnitude and duration of the proliferative stage of wound healing is correlated to the duration of the inflammatory phase [12]. Indeed, the amount of collagen deposited by myofibroblasts can be reduced by attenuating the inflammatory response [13]. During remodeling, fibrovascular tissue formed during the proliferative stage matures into scar tissue [12]. Normal reduction in myofibroblast numbers through apoptosis is important during this ECM remodeling, and prolongation of myofibroblast survival leads to excessive scar tissue formation [12].

Before moving to the next section of this chapter, let us connect these concepts and ideas surrounding cell types to form a clearer picture for our understanding. It certainly wasn't an exaggeration on my part when I described monocytes, macrophages, and fibroblasts as complex cell types! In a vacuum, each of these cells can behave in unique ways, demonstrating variable phenotypes even when assessed individually as a mono-culture of cells. This is a focal point of many *in vitro* studies that aim to articulate the innate behavior of these cells. However, the world of possibilities becomes even larger when considering these cells in coordination with each other. The myriad interactions between just these three cell types *in vivo* presents a niche area of modern cellular research, quite literally.

4. Stromal influence on monocyte signaling: a game of broken telephone

The canonical understanding of wound healing involves the "forward talk" from circulating immune cells to stromal cells, such as fibroblasts, to induce paracrine signaling or activation of these fibroblasts into myofibroblasts [8]. Indeed, it has long been accepted that the processes of monocyte recruitment, differentiation into classically or alternatively activated macrophages, and signaling to fibroblasts follow an organized and stringent process [14]. However, our general understanding is somewhat lacking when considering the "back talk" from stromal cells to monocytes, and the effects of this communication on monocyte cytokine production and downstream macrophage differentiation (**Figure 2**).

As a brief aside, a commonly used cell line for assessing monocyte cellular processes is the THP-1 cell line. THP-1 cells are immortalized human monocytes derived from an acute monocytic leukemia patient [15]. These cells are invaluable because they potentiate a simplistic but widely available *in vitro* cell model of inflammatory infiltrate. These cells allow for meaningful immune modulation analyses because they demonstrate few changes during cell culture periods, maintain minimal genetic variation, and present few obstacles in terms of ethical issues or donor availability [15]. Lastly, these cells are very useful because they can be classically or alternatively activated into macrophages through various experimental techniques. We will not go into these specific laboratory protocols, but it must be understood that THP-1 monocytes provide an informative tool for exploring macrophage differentiation.

However, as is the case with many *in vitro* studies, it is difficult to fully recapitulate cell-cell interactions that would occur *in vivo*, and thus studies using THP-1 cells should be assessed with this in mind. In any experimental model that does not incorporate all physiological components, there are elements missing that can only be compensated to a certain degree. Even the most optimal *in vitro* models fails to include the plethora of microenvironmental and cellular niches that can contribute to cellular processes *in vivo*. Nevertheless, there is much to learn about the characteristics of monocytes using THP-1 cells, and so we'll include these cells in our discussion.

Previous studies have shown that gene expression in THP-1 monocytes encoding macrophage differentiation markers is influenced by co-culture with fibroblasts [16]. However, there are currently few studies of this type that assess the relative effects of co-culture on both cell types, particularly in the context of wound healing. Could it be the case that multiple cell types influence each other's behavior in cell culture? Let us explore this for a moment.

As outlined earlier, fibroblast activation into myofibroblasts is largely induced by mechanical properties of the ECM through various mechanotransduction pathways [14]. Strain caused by fibroblast focal adhesions within the collagen meshwork of the ECM enables efficient mechanical activation of latent TGFβ1 through integrin-mediated cell-pulling [14]. Increased TGFβ1 signaling can then induce further fibroblast activation into myofibroblasts in a positive feedback loop. As well, myofibroblast activation facilitates active ECM remodeling during wound healing, producing mechanical cues for other cell types such as circulating blood monocytes [14]. Such signaling characterizes the "back talk" from ECM myofibroblasts to monocytes. Erroneous and persistent communication from ECM signals to monocytes can promote further myofibroblast activation and fibrosis [14], characterizing a feedback loop of "forward talk". Thus, a 3D cell culture model that closely resembles physiological ECM would likely be most appropriate for the assessment of myofibroblast activation via TGFβ1 signaling pathways.

That there have been relatively few studies assessing the relative effects of co-culture on circulating monocytes and fibroblasts is unfortunate. It is troubling because of a phenomenon previously demonstrated via *in vitro* fibrosis models in which immunologically-activated myofibroblasts promoted monocyte migration into tissue through cellular "back talk" [17]. This "back talk" could have been the result of pro-inflammatory stimuli of myofibroblasts inducing subsequent changes in monocytic gene expression and physiological chemotactic recruitment [18]. In other words, the importance of co-culturing these cell types together is emphasized by the role of myofibroblasts as immunoregulatory "sentinel cells" [18].

All this is to say, there are complex cell-cell interactions between stromal fibroblasts in a 3D ECM and circulating blood monocytes. Indeed, stromal cells, specifically fibroblasts, are becoming increasingly prominent in research regarding pathogenesis of tissue inflammation, immunomodulation of tissue microenvironments, transition from acute to chronic inflammation, and inflammation persistence associated with rheumatoid arthritis [19]. In this context, fibroblasts play a functional role in the progression of chronic inflammation, in addition to their role in tissue fibrosis highlighted earlier.

Beyond involvement in chronic inflammation and tissue fibrosis, fibroblasts and stroma in a broad sense play a functional role in another chronic pathology: malignant disease. In this instance, stromal cells lay down the components of the non-tumor ECM that potentiates growth of solid tumors [19]. However, stromal cells can also be a key driver of tumor progression through the inhibition of apoptosis in malignant cells in breast carcinoma [20]. Further, stromal cells and cancer-associated fibroblasts are purported to facilitate tumorigenesis and eventual metastasis through production of oncogenic signals and promotion of angiogenesis [19].

While reading this, you may notice that we have veered onto tangential thinking. Our main discussion involves monocytes, fibroblasts, and macrophages in the context of wound healing following acute inflammation. How, then, does chronic inflammation and malignant disease progression relate to this? The answer lies within the interactions between the cell types involved in these processes. The "forward talk" and "back talk" in each of these situations is critical for the progression of cell migration, development, signaling, and proliferation. Just as communication is vital for a healthy relationship between humans, so too is it vital for these cellular processes—even if pathological!

To realign our thinking regarding fibroblasts, it is purported that even in the absence of external stimuli, fibroblasts are capable of promoting monocyte migration through the production of similar protein signals to cytokines, called chemokines [17]. Further, this behavior is not limited to one cell type, but instead is an intrinsic property of fibroblasts [17]. This alludes to the concept of immunologically-activated myofibroblast "back talk" inducing monocytic migration, which then ties into our understanding of downstream fates of monocytes into classically or alternatively activated macrophages, for example.

With this in mind, lets tie a few more strings together. At a site of wound injury, circulating blood monocytes are recruited to the site of injury via the process of inflammation [21]. Through a multitude of cytokine signals between monocytes, tissue macrophages, and stromal cells, monocytes quickly acquire certain macrophage phenotypic characteristics once at the wound site [21]. The coordination between blood-derived and tissue macrophages allows for the synthesis and release of many different types of regulatory cytokines and chemokines that are crucial for the wound healing process [21]. This "forward talk" from monocytes and macrophages allows for stromal fibroblasts to acquire a myofibroblast phenotype in many cases, and facilitates processes such as matrix deposition, tissue contraction, and cellular reorganization. The last point of discussion for the purpose of this chapter will thus be how the "forward talk" and "back talk" demonstrate an elegant interplay, influencing the quality and quantity of wound repair.

5. Implications toward our understanding of macrophages

Up to this point, we have discussed the key players of the inflammatory cascade, some cell types involved in wound repair, and the significance of the "forward talk" and "back talk" between some of these cellular driving forces. What implications, then, does all of this have with regards to our understanding of macrophages?

The answer to this question, as is the case with many scientific inquiries, lies in how we observe and assess the communicatory phenomena surrounding monocytes and macrophages. We've already alluded to how each cell type can innately behave one way when assessed in mono-culture, and how this behavior can be altered when assessed in co-culture. However, the extent to which we can improve our experimentation on these cell types is dependent on how accurately we can recapitulate some of the physiological processes that occur *in vivo* using mimetic cell culture models.

Two potential ways through which the scientific community can better understand the complex interplay of monocytes, macrophages, and fibroblasts is through the use of co-culture systems, but also through the use of 3D cell culture systems. Such 3D systems could more intimately mimic the biological interactions that occur in living tissues and can provide novel perspectives beyond those attainable through 2D cell cultures [16, 22]. Current cell culture models that lack 3D and co-culture techniques are likely to underestimate potential immunomodulatory effects of stromal fibroblasts on monocytes and macrophage development due to the omission of complex bi-directional signaling that can occur between these cell types in living tissue [22].

For example, a novel macrophage and fibroblast co-culture model was designed and employed to assess the effect of material surface properties on inflammatory response regulation *in vitro* [23]. This co-culture system was used because it more closely mimicked autocrine, paracrine, and juxtacrine signaling between these two cell types [23]. As well, the comparison between macrophage behavior in mono-culture vs. co-culture was made possible [23]. Together, this exemplifies the usefulness of co-culture models when understanding the inflammatory processes that occur physiologically, particularly in the context of biomaterial assessment.

A similar model designed by many of the same authors was also used to assess physiological host responses of biomaterials *in vitro* [24]. This model maintained the advantage of spatially-controlled interactions between macrophages and fibroblasts in a co-culture system [24]. Further, data showed that macrophages could induce wound healing and even fibrotic responses via upregulation of fibroblast outgrowth, cytokine production, and myofibroblast activation [24]. Use of this model was also advantageous because additional factors, such as cytokines, could also be assessed *in vitro* for their effects on cell-cell communication in a co-culture system [24].

A step in the right direction toward a more comprehensive experimental system for monocytes, macrophages, and fibroblasts is the recent development of organ-on-a-chip (OOC) models. These models employ microfluidic *in vitro* systems that markedly improve our ability to assess how immune cells interact with parenchymal cells to mediate immune responses to inflammation [25, 26]. These models are powerful and flexible, but they can be difficult to manufacture. In addition, they are not usually designed to accommodate cell-type specific nor sensitive analyses of cellular responses to co-culture conditions, such as changes in gene expression of cytokine markers [22].

6. Conclusion

Our understanding of macrophages has immensely improved over the past 140 years. So too has our understanding of myriad cellular interactions, such as inflammation, wound healing, and tissue homeostasis. This has, in part, been made possible by our simultaneous understanding of other crucial cell types, such as monocytes and stromal fibroblasts, and the role these cells have in our greater understanding of macrophages.

The importance of experimental models that employ both 3D and co-culture techniques for assessing cellular responses to inflammatory cytokine stimuli thus cannot be understated. To that end, we must appreciate the potential to accumulate incomplete or perhaps even fallacious data from mono-culture or 2D systems that do not incorporate various physiological factors that are at play during the "forward talk" and "back talk" of these cellular processes.

Looking ahead, our understanding of macrophages can and should be expanded upon. By designing cell culture systems that better enable assessment of the many cell-cell communications during inflammation, wound healing, and tissue homeostasis, we can continue to explore these incredible feats of nature. Advancements in these areas could improve clinical outcomes for patients suffering from numerous pathologies discussed in this chapter, such as chronic inflammation, tissue fibrosis, and even cancer formation. I look forward to the "forward talk" that we have yet to discover.

Conflict of interest

The authors declare no conflict of interest.

Notes/thanks/other declarations

I would like to personally thank my undergraduate research thesis advisors, Dr. Cindy Hutnik and Dr. David O'Gorman, for their role in shaping my fascination for this area of scientific discovery. You both challenged me to learn and explore topics surrounding wound healing, inflammation, and fibrosis and enabled me to branch into fields of research that I had never thought to consider prior.

I would also like to personally thank Jelena Vrdoljak, the Author Service Manager for IntechOpen, for her role in supporting the production of this chapter. Her patience, guidance, and communication made submission to this book seamless and organized.

Author details

Avi Petroff
Sackler School of Medicine, New York State/American Program, Tel Aviv University, Tel Aviv, Israel

*Address all correspondence to: avipetroff@mail.tau.ac.il

References

[1] Genin M, Clement F, Fattaccioli A, Raes M, Michiels C. M1 and M2 macrophages derived from THP-1 cells differentially modulate the response of cancer cells to etoposide. BMC Cancer. 2015;**15**:577

[2] Murray PJ, Allen JE, Biswas SK, Fisher EA, Gilroy DW, Goerdt S, et al. Macrophage activation and polarization: Nomenclature and experimental guidelines. Immunity. 2014;**41**(1):14-20

[3] Mantovani A, Sozzani S, Locati M, Allavena P, Sica A. Macrophage polarization: Tumor-associated macrophages as a paradigm for polarized M2 mononuclear phagocytes. Trends in Immunology. 2002;**23**(11):549-555

[4] Gordon S, Martinez FO. Alternative activation of macrophages: Mechanism and functions. Immunity. 2010;**32**(5):593-604

[5] Ploeger DT, Hosper NA, Schipper M, Koerts JA, de Rond S, Bank RA. Cell plasticity in wound healing: Paracrine factors of M1/M2 polarized macrophages influence the phenotypical state of dermal fibroblasts. Cell Communication and Signaling: CCS. 2013;**11**(1):29

[6] Cavaillon JM. Pro- versus anti-inflammatory cytokines: Myth or reality. Cellular and Molecular Biology (Noisy-le-Grand, France). 2001;**47**(4):695-702

[7] Fernandes JC, Martel-Pelletier J, Pelletier J-P. The role of cytokines in osteoarthritis pathophysiology. Biorheology. 2002;**39**(1-2):237-246

[8] Seibold LK, Sherwood MB, Kahook MY. Wound modulation after filtration surgery. Survey of Ophthalmology. 2012;**57**(6):530-550

[9] Gabbiani G. The myofibroblast in wound healing and fibrocontractive diseases. The Journal of Pathology. 2003;**200**(4):500-503

[10] Schlunck G, Meyer-ter-Vehn T, Klink T, Grehn F. Conjunctival fibrosis following filtering glaucoma surgery. Experimental Eye Research. 2016;**142**:76-82

[11] Chistiakov DA, Myasoedova VA, Revin VV, Orekhov AN, Bobryshev YV. The impact of interferon-regulatory factors to macrophage differentiation and polarization into M1 and M2. Immunobiology. 2018;**223**(1):101-111

[12] Zada M, Pattamatta U, White A. Modulation of fibroblasts in conjunctival wound healing. Ophthalmology. 2018;**125**(2):179-192

[13] Serhan CN, Savill J. Resolution of inflammation: The beginning programs the end. Nature Immunology. 2005;**6**(12):1191-1197

[14] Pakshir P, Hinz B. The big five in fibrosis: Macrophages, myofibroblasts, matrix, mechanics, and miscommunication. Matrix Biology. 2018;**68-69**:81-93

[15] Chanput W, Mes JJ, Wichers HJ. THP-1 cell line: An in vitro cell model for immune modulation approach. International Immunopharmacology. 2014;**23**(1):37-45

[16] Kuen J, Darowski D, Kluge T, Majety M. Pancreatic cancer cell/fibroblast co-culture induces M2 like macrophages that influence therapeutic response in a 3D model. PLoS One. 2017;**12**(7):e0182039

[17] Enzerink A, Salmenpera P, Kankuri E, Vaheri A. Clustering of

fibroblasts induces proinflammatory chemokine secretion promoting leukocyte migration. Molecular Immunology. 2009;**46**(8-9):1787-1795

[18] Kaufman J, Graf BA, Leung EC, Pollock SJ, Koumas L, Reddy SY, et al. Fibroblasts as sentinel cells: Role of the CDcd40-CDcd40 ligand system in fibroblast activation and lung inflammation and fibrosis. Chest. 2001;**120**(Suppl. 1):53S-55S

[19] Patel R, Filer A, Barone F, Buckley CD. Stroma: Fertile soil for inflammation. Best Practice & Research. Clinical Rheumatology. 2014;**28**(4):565-576

[20] Wiseman BS, Werb Z. Stromal effects on mammary gland development and breast cancer. Science. 2002;**296**(5570):1046-1049

[21] Brancato SK, Albina JE. Wound macrophages as key regulators of repair: Origin, phenotype, and function. The American Journal of Pathology. 2011;**178**(1):19-25

[22] Petroff A, Pena Diaz A, Armstrong JJ, Gonga-Cavé BC, Hutnik C, O'Gorman DB. Understanding inflammation-associated ophthalmic pathologies: A novel 3D co-culture model of monocyte-myofibroblast immunomodulation. Ocular Immunology and Inflammation. 2021:1-12. DOI: 10.1080/09273948.2021.1980816. PMID: 34648419

[23] Zhou G, Loppnow H, Groth T. A macrophage/fibroblast co-culture system using a cell migration chamber to study inflammatory effects of biomaterials. Acta Biomaterialia. 2015;**26**:54-63

[24] Zhou G, Liedmann A, Chatterjee C, Groth T. In vitro study of the host responses to model biomaterials via a fibroblast/macrophage co-culture system. Biomaterials Science. 2016;**5**(1):141-152

[25] Polini A, Del Mercato LL, Barra A, Zhang YS, Calabi F, Gigli G. Towards the development of human immune-system-on-a-chip platforms. Drug Discovery Today. 2019;**24**(2):517-525

[26] Sasserath T, Rumsey JW, McAleer CW, Bridges LR, Long CJ, Elbrecht D, et al. Differential monocyte actuation in a three-organ functional innate immune system-on-a-chip. Advancement of Science. 2020; 7(13):2000323

Chapter 8

The Role of Macrophages in Controlling the Adaptive Response to Injury: Regeneration Vs. Scarring

Dale Feldman

Abstract

This chapter will cover the apparent role macrophages play in orchestrating the adaptive response to injury. The chapter will first explore the differences in adaptive response to injury for fetal vs. adult wound healing. In addition, the differences in adaptive response between animals that regenerate vs. ones that heal more by scarring. This information will be used to propose a theory of how to control the adaptive response by controlling the macrophages response. Part of this theory will be what is the evolutionary change in macrophages that tips the scale between regeneration and scarring as well as what is different about the response of macrophages in fetal vs. adult wound healing. The body responds to changes (stimuli) with an adaptive response. Additional stimuli can be added to an injury to alter the response of macrophages to effect the overall adaptive response. The theory developed helped to explain why specific strategies to control the adaptive response are successful.

Keywords: macrophage, wound healing, adaptive response control, burn treatment, pressure ulcer treatment

1. Introduction

This chapter will cover the apparent role macrophages play in orchestrating the adaptive response to injury. Although macrophages are potent innate immune cells injury triggers an inflammatory response and a non-specific foreign body response virtually independent of an immune response (unless antigens such as bacteria are introduced into the wound).

As with any stimuli, there is a normal adaptive response to injury. Macrophages play an important role in controlling this adaptive response as well as why there are differences between species or as we age. The goal of this chapter is to explore the role of macrophages in this adaptive response to develop a theory on how macrophages control the response.

The chapter will first explore the differences in adaptive response to injury for fetal vs. adult wound healing. In addition, the differences in adaptive response between animals that regenerate vs. ones that heal more by scarring. This information will be used to propose a theory of how to control the adaptive response by controlling the response of macrophages. Part of this theory will be what is the evolutionary change in macrophages that tips the scale between regeneration and scarring as well as what is different about the response of macrophages in fetal vs. adult wound healing. This theory will be used to explain why specific strategies to control the adaptive response are successful.

2. Adaptive response to injury

The body responds to changes (stimuli) with an adaptive response. The goal of this review is to understand how macrophages control the normal adaptive response, in this case for a skin injury, as well as how additional stimuli can be added to alter the macrophage response to control the overall adaptive response.

This section will look at the normal adaptive response to a skin injury as well as differences between animals that regenerate and those that do not. In addition, the difference in adult wound healing vs. fetal wound healing will be explored. Based on these observations a theory will be presented on how the macrophage causes these differences in adaptive response to injury.

2.1 Adaptive responses to injury

The adaptive response to injury can be regeneration, grow larger to fill the space (hypertrophy), or use scar tissue to fill the space [1–4]. In many cases, it can be a combination of these responses. Although the adaptive response is seen at the tissue/organ level [3] it is first triggered at the cellular level [4], which coordinates the ultimate response [5].

2.1.1 Regeneration

Regeneration in this case is to recapitulate structure and function of tissue after an injury. An important issue is how good are humans at regeneration? Of the four tissue types (epithelium, muscle, nerve, and connective tissue) only epithelium is totally regenerative [2, 3]. The regenerative ability, however, is limited and requires assistance in some cases.

For each tissue type, we have had successes in small amounts, but not large areas. The biggest reason is the inability to get blood supply fast enough for a large area. Even in skin grafts, they do not get blood supply fast enough (a few weeks in many cases), but it is able to recover sufficiently to take (heal in) [6]. This inability to form blood vessels in graft substitutes has hampered the ability to create actual graft substitutes that heal in [2, 6–16]. It also hampers the ability to seed scaffolds to use *in vivo* [2, 6–9, 14]. The cells in the middle do not get blood supply fast enough to survive [1, 2, 6].

2.1.2 Loss of regeneration

Limits on regenerative healing is driven by evolution [8, 17, 18]. Certain species still have the ability to regenerate large structures (epimorphic regeneration) [8]. In humans, the loss of regenerative ability is seen as we age [8]. In utero, healing is regenerative and scarless. Even newborns can regenerative digits that are accidently cut off [19]. The length that can regenerate, however, decreases over time [19].

The question is how much of this ability can we get back? Understanding why we probably lost this ability and what changes occur between fetal and adult wound healing can shed some light on how we may be able to better control the healing response. It is likely that the normal adaptive response is genetic (evolutionary). However, adding additional stimuli will create additional adaptive responses that can alter the overall adaptive response. It is also likely that the differences that occur due to age are not genetic, since the genes do not change over time.

Through evolution and natural selection, the scale has tipped toward scarring over regeneration in humans [20]. Not entirely, however, since we can regenerate blood as well as other tissues and organs to a limited degree (e.g. bone, smooth muscle, liver, and epithelial tissue) [21]. It is not that we really lost it, since virtually all tissue is turned over at some rate (days to years depending on the tissue); most tissue has at least limited regenerative ability [1–3, 5, 8, 22, 23]; and we can increase the rate of regeneration with things like growth factors, stem cells, and electrical stimulation [1, 2]. Typically tissue that heals quickly (higher mitotic rate) has the fastest turnover rate [3, 4]. For example, epithelium is the fastest growing tissue and has the quickest turnover rate [21]. Even in thick layers of epithelium like epidermis, it only takes about 30 days for a basal cell to move upward to form all the layers of stratified squamous epithelium [1, 3, 21].

Further, babies up until about 6 months can regenerate an amputated finger and in utero surgery is essentially scarless [8, 19, 22, 23]. So we have the machinery to regenerate, but scarring normally dominates; and even more so when healing time increases as in larger wounds, more inflammation, or less stem cells (as we get older or with certain diseases) [1, 2, 8]. So many strategies geared toward speeding up healing have the added benefit of reducing scarring [1, 2].

So what has tipped the scales from regeneration to repair or scarring? From an evolutionary standpoint it is probably related to speed of recovery [4, 18, 23]; possibly why scarring increases as healing rate decreases. It may be as simple as if a wound does not heal within a specified time frame, the wound contracts and scars. Also from an epimorphic regeneration standpoint it could be how quickly the skin can cover the wound. The only thing that seems to shift is the maximum length of healing time before scarring starts to replace regenerative healing. There also are individuals that have a more robust scarring than the average, which can lead to hypertrophic scarring for even small wounds.

Why is scarring an evolutionary advantage? In part, "survival of the fittest" (natural selection) is more about those who can reproduce vs. that only the strongest survive [18, 19, 22, 23]. Many animals can regenerate large parts of their body [18]. As the species and/or part gets larger (and more complicated) it takes longer to regenerate and in most higher animals it serves more as a defense mechanism than for healing [18]. For example, a lizard's tail comes off easily and will distract the prey, but requires nine months to regenerate [18, 23]. The African Spiny Mouse (skin comes off) and the axolotl salamander are other good examples of larger animals regenerating [18, 23].

Although evolution and natural selection may have kept regeneration as a defense mechanism to help in survival, for many larger species, the length of time for regeneration and the metabolic demand probably made it an evolutionary disadvantage [3, 4, 18]. It could make an animal easier prey, reduce their ability to reproduce, and increase the risk of infection [18, 22]. To that end, many mammals will kill their young if they are injured or deformed and zoos often have to rescue babies who might be killed by their parents [24].

Some claim it is partly due to mammals being warm blooded and becoming terrestrial [18, 22]. Warm blooded, makes infection easier [23]. Terrestrial means that legs would need to be weight bearing during regeneration and could be easily damaged [18]. Also as animals got larger and warm blooded the length of survival time without food has diminished [18]. It has been shown that the shorter the time an animal can survive without food the less likely it can have regenerative healing [18].

This is all also consistent with the theory that the only evolutionary change is how quickly scarring starts replacing regenerative healing. This means that the normal adaptive response tips more toward scarring. In many cases, in today's world, with better infection control and the reduction in the need for fast healing, it is probably beneficial to tip the scales more toward regenerative healing. Since waiting for an evolutionary change could take at least 50 generations, once the mutation starts showing up [18, 22], strategies to control the response are a better option.

It appears, therefore that the bioprocess to control is time to complete healing. There are two bioprocesses that affect the time to heal: the delay in healing due to inflammation (since healing is limited during inflammation) and the rate of healing in the repair phase.

2.1.3 Mammalian regenerative healing

To explore this concept of shortening the inflammation part of healing more it would be helpful to look at examples of regenerative healing in mammals (including fetal wound healing). There are very few cases in adult mammals that undergo true (epimorphic) regeneration [8]. These include deer antlers and the ear of a rabbit [8]. These require blastema formation and require the epidermis to seal the growing blastema [8]. A hole punched in the rabbit ear can undergo epimorphic regeneration where ears of dogs will scar vs. regenerate [8].

Most injured tissue in adult mammals heal by repair and scarring (going through the inflammation, repair, remodeling phases) [8, 17, 18]. In the case of small defects the tissue can expand (hypertrophy) without mitosis to fill the gap—skeletal muscle is one example [8]. Also part of repair and scarring is wound contraction to reduce the amount of hypertrophy necessary [1, 2].

Regeneration of the finger of an infant is like epimorphic regeneration, but is more outgrowth of the bone [9, 19]. Fetal wound healing is essentially scarless, but does not require a blastema [23]. Without a skin wound, some internal structures can heal scarlessly and do not have a blastema formed [8].

Although we have learned much about epimorphic regeneration, it is unlikely to be a useful strategy in adults [8]. Besides the examples of deer antlers and rabbit ears, the process has not been able to be recreated in mammals, even with similar tissue to those found in other animals [21]. This is because there are a few requirements that are difficult to recreate at the same time including: skin injury, epidermal tissue quickly covering the injury, enervation, low or no inflammation, and the ability to start repair quickly (local cells or recruited cells) [4, 8].

It is also probably both a size and complexity issue, which is why it is only found in small animals less complex than mammals [8]. This would be consistent with the theory that it is about time to heal (including the time with little healing due to inflammation) as the trigger for scarring. Even, if we could get it to work for large structures like digits or limbs, however, it is unlikely that the size would be an adult size; since it takes almost two decades for human digits and limbs to grow to adult size [23].

Without a blastema, regeneration of structures such as digits and limbs has a number of hurdles we have not solved yet including: shutting down the natural scarring response, revascularization, re-innervation, acceleration of healing, and duplicating the 3D architecture macroscopically and microscopically [6, 23]. These would be both growing *in vitro* as a graft substitute or *in vivo* with a degradable regenerative scaffold [2, 6, 7]. A graft substitute has the additional problem of attachment to and integrating with the host [2, 6, 7].

2.1.4 Fetal wound healing

To further explore the theory that it is the time to heal that is the trigger for scarring, it is helpful to look at fetal wound healing vs. adult wound healing. Again since wound healing in utero is scarless and the regenerative ability decreases over time, understanding the differences between adult and fetal wound healing can offer some potential control strategies [23]. Although there are many specific differences, between the two, it is possible they are mostly related to two phenomena that change over time: the ability for cells to do multiple things (due to stem cells) at the same time and the size of the injury [4, 8, 25]. Both affect the time to start healing and the length of time for healing to occur [2, 4, 25]. In fetal wounds there are more local stem cells and therefore do not require as much homing of stem cells from the circulation (primary source in adult wounds) [2, 4, 25]. It also is possible that there is no true scarless healing without epimorphic regeneration and scarless healing is just no detectable scar [2, 23]. Then the amount of scarring increases as we age [17, 23].

Again, time to heal is both the length of the inflammatory phase and the length of the repair phase. The ability to heal during the inflammatory phase (due to stem cells) reduces the normal delay in healing due to the inflammatory response. The size difference between the fetus and the adult leads to a shorter repair phase for the same type of injury. Both of these advantages in fetal wound healing decrease as we age, helping to explain the decrease in regeneration as we age.

2.1.5 Developing strategies to reduce scarring and increase regeneration

Based on the differences between fetal wound healing and adult wound healing as well as potential reasons some animals have more regenerative ability than others, some control strategies can be developed. Again, the theory is that the length of time to heal is the trigger to start the scarring process. This is both the delay in healing due to inflammation as well as the amount of tissue to be healed determining the length of the repair phase. For example, incision wounds can heal without visible scarring even in adults, if clean and protected from forces that will break newly formed tissue [2, 25]. The amount of cleaning up (foreign material, necrotic tissue, bleeding, etc.) determines both the amount of inflammation and the length of the inflammatory phase [2, 25].

Although there are many biochemical differences between animals that regenerate (or fetal wound healing) and adults, the main evolution change could be just the length of healing time required to trigger scarring. This can be the total time to heal and/or the time required before healing is complete. Therefore, shortening the inflammatory phase or the repair phase should reduce scarring. In addition, increasing the relative amount of regenerative healing vs. scarring during the inflammatory phase, which appears to occur in fetal wound healing, or repair phase should also reduce scarring.

Looking at the typical adaptive response to injury can shed some light on what the specific evolutionary change might be as well as ways to control the adaptive response. This means, which bioprocesses control the time to heal and how they do it.

2.2 The usual adaptive response

2.2.1 Healing response

Since regenerative epimorphic healing is not an option in adults and hypertrophy only occurs to a limited extent, then healing occurs mostly through a repair process. Healing of an injury normally has four phases: hemostasis, inflammation, repair, and remodeling. The first step (hemostasis) is essentially stopping the bleeding. This normally occurs via the blood clotting cascade and ends up with fibrinogen, a blood protein, being cleaved by thrombin to allow polymerization into a fibrin clot [2, 21, 25]. The next step is the inflammatory response, which is to clean up the wound [25]. This can be removal of foreign material, dead tissue, and or products of hemostasis including: red blood cells, edema, and fibrin clot [25]. Neutrophils and macrophages are responsible for this phase [2, 25].

In adults, typically, little healing occurs during the inflammatory phase. If any it is predominantly granulation tissue (repair tissue with inflammatory cells and well vascularized) and/or scarring to wall off the granulation tissue [2, 8].

Once the inflammation subsides it turns into the repair phase. In some cases, the inflammation never goes away and becomes chronic inflammation (common with non-degradable implants particularly ones that are fibrous scaffolds) [2, 8]. Therefore, there is not always a clear demarcation between the inflammation and repair phases. In the repair phase, new tissue is formed to fill the defect. It is a mix of granulation tissue and regenerated tissue (similar to the tissue being repaired). This requires a number of interrelated events. To form the extracellular matrix (ECM) repair, cells need to migrate into the wound space once cleaned up by inflammation. The cells need to produce the ECM scaffold in front of them to allow them to grow into the wound [2, 5]. The cells need enough oxygen to produce the ECM, which requires blood vessels to grow into the wound as well [2, 25]. The cells, usually fibroblasts, need the blood supply to be within 100 μm to provide enough oxygen via diffusion to produce the scaffold [2, 6]. This works in a centripetal fashion from the wound edges until the defect is repaired; shutting down probably due to contact inhibition [2, 5]. In most cases, the repair tissue gets remodeled (fourth phase) over time to be closer in structure and function to the normal tissue [2, 5, 6]. The closer the repair tissue is to the surrounding tissue the less remodeling needs to be done.

Due to underlying pathology, the defect may not completely heal. The most common problem, however, is the production of scar tissue, which reduces function [2, 21, 25]. Although not fully understood, it appears that the extent and time frame of the inflammatory phase is one of the most important factors to determine the extent of the scarring [2, 8, 23]. Also typically the more the repair tissue is granulation tissue vs. regenerated tissue, the more scarring will occur [2, 8].

There are a number of interrelated bioprocesses that determine the extent of scarring [5]. These include: the amount of inflammation, the length of the inflammatory phase, the length of the repair phase, and the activity of both macrophages and fibroblasts [2, 26]. Although, it is unclear, which bioprocesses are triggers for the other bioprocesses, the end result is less regenerative healing until wound closure (end of the repair phase), which leads to a higher percent of granulation tissue and increased wound contraction (producing scar tissue) to reduce the size of the wound and thus shorten the healing time [2–5, 7, 25]. Many diseases are due to inflammation leading to scar tissue including: arteriosclerosis and cirrhosis of the liver [2, 5, 21].

Figure 1a shows granulation vs. regeneration tissue percentages (in the repair phase) as the amount or time of inflammation increases due to cleaning up the wound. It is likely that in some cases, particularly in small wounds, inflammation does not trigger granulation immediately.

2.2.2 Evolutionary control of the adaptive response

Although it is not known what the evolutionary change is to push toward scarring, it is unlikely to be a biological clock. The difference is probably the amount of wound contraction due to the fibroblast/myofibroblast transformation, but the actual genetic difference has not been identified [1, 2, 26]. It is likely that macrophages control this transformation as well as any mechanical stress present. Many claim that macrophages orchestrate all the healing responses [2, 26]. The adaptive response of macrophages can be to help in the healing process or create a chronic inflammatory response. In addition, macrophages present antigens to lymphocytes to start the immune response [2, 26].

Although there has been work on identifying different phenotypes of macrophages (what they do and produce) and what are the triggers to change phenotype, there still is much to learn about how to control the phenotype of macrophages as well as if there are evolutionary differences in activation of macrophages between animals that heal more by regeneration vs. those that heal more by scarring. One change is the ability to form a blastema, for complete regeneration. The change between animals that heal without a blastema would be different. It is possible that the evolutionary change is the amount of stimulus to increase the ratio of pro-inflammatory macrophages to pro-healing macrophages as shown in **Figure 1b**. This could be a conversion of phenotype of resident macrophages or a recruitment of different types of macrophages from the blood. Macrophages, even in adults, can clean up some debris, like red blood cells and dead tissue without triggering an inflammatory response [26]. **Figure 1b** shows how the percentage of each type of macrophage could change based on the sensitivity of macrophages to cleanup/inflammation.

It is also possible that a given macrophage can be on the continuum from pro-healing to pro-inflammatory in addition to the relative amount of macrophages that are pro-healing vs. pro-inflammatory. It is also possible that different types of macrophages recruit different types and or numbers of macrophages from the blood or that they can change phenotype after they get to the wound. All of these are still consistent with the theory. It is also likely that the more pro-inflammatory macrophages in the wound the longer the inflammatory process, since resolving the inflammation involves removal of the pro-inflammatory macrophages.

Lengthening the inflammation phase will increase the overall healing time, since little healing besides scarring occurs in the inflammatory phase. Much of the regenerative healing, during inflammation, could be due to recruited stem cells from the blood, which again is why fetal wounds heal more by regenerative healing due to the presence of more local stem cells.

In adult wounds, the type of tissue formed is mostly due to the fibroblast to myofibroblast transition (**Figure 1c**), which is most likely controlled by the pro-healing to pro-inflammatory ratio. Myofibroblasts are responsible for the granulation tissue that contracts and leads to scarring (**Figure 1a** and **d**) [2, 23].

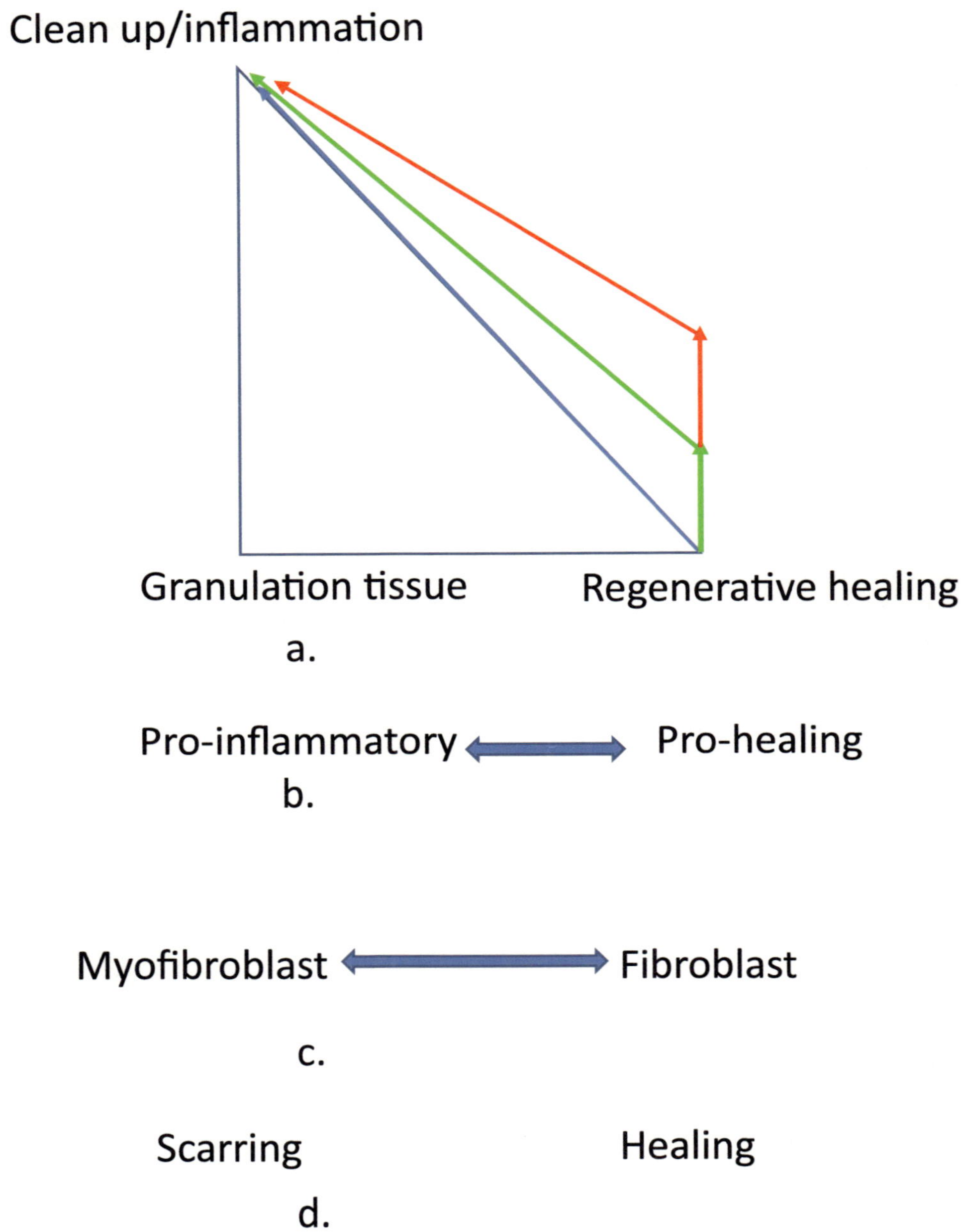

Figure 1.
Cell and tissue changes during the repair phase of wound healing. a. As the amount and time of inflammation increases (mostly due to cleaning up of the wound), the higher percentage of healing is granulation tissue. Part of the theory proposed is that animals that are more regenerative would require more clean-up/inflammation before increasing the percentage of granulation tissue formed (green and red lines). b. As the amount and time of inflammation increases (mostly due to cleaning up of the wound), a higher and higher percent of macrophages are pro-inflammatory vs. pro-healing. Again, animals that are more regenerative would probably require more clean-up/inflammation before increasing the percentage of pro-inflammatory macrophages (green and red lines). c. The ratio of pro-inflammatory macrophages to pro-healing macrophages should control the ratio of myofibroblasts to fibroblasts, which in turn will control the ratio of granulation tissue to regenerative healing (a), which will control the ratio of scarring to healing (d).

So, the evolutionary change could be the amount of clean up macrophages can do in a wound without shifting to a pro-inflammatory phenotype where only scarring can occur until the inflammation is resolved. There also is a trigger based on the length of time to close the wound (dependent on the application). This probably is a big factor in why adult wound healing scars relative to fetal wound healing.

Part of the theory is that the fibroblast to myofibroblast ratio set by the phenotype ratio of macrophages lasts through most of the repair phase, although a macrophages phenotype will revert back to pro-healing (unless there is a chronic inflammation). This ratio does set the granulation tissue/regenerative healing (G/R) ratio, however, it is likely that the granulation tissue healing rate is faster than the regenerative healing rate; leading to an increase in the G/R ratio over time. Therefore the longer the wound is in the repair phase the more there is tissue that contracts and scars relative to tissue that has regenerative healing.

Understanding the evolutionary changes as well as the fetal to adult wound healing differences can help in selecting designs to control the adaptive response. It can be by controlling the triggers for the transitions for macrophages and/or fibroblasts as well as controlling the biological responses to these transitions.

Although the theory presented is most likely a simplistic view of the actual mechanisms, it will be used to justify the selection of control strategies. The goal is not to prove the validity of the theory, but to see whether control strategies selected based on the theory do lead to meeting the desired outcomes in animal and clinical studies.

3. Control strategies

Although the desired adaptive response can be different for different clinical presentations, the mechanisms for control are the same. The control strategies can be used in different ways to achieve the desired adaptive response. There are essentially two types of control strategies for wound healing, ones that control the inflammation phase and ones that control the repair phase.

3.1 Inflammation control

3.1.1 Causes of inflammation

Both the level of inflammation and the time to resolution can alter the adaptive response. Inflammation is the normal adaptive response to injury. In adults, it functions to prepare the wound for the repair phase. In the beginning, (acute inflammation) neutrophils and macrophages are recruited to clean up the wound from foreign debris, necrotic tissue and cells, and byproducts of hemostasis such as fibrin and free red blood cells.

The recruited cells produce cytokines to recruit cells and blood vessels for the repair phase [2–4, 21, 25]. The pathological response normally results when the inflammation becomes chronic and slows or delays the repair phase, resulting in scarring [1, 3–5, 7–9]. In addition, the cytokines and enzymes produced by the inflammatory cells can damage local healthy tissue (leading to more inflammation to clean it up) as well as produce systemic effects [1, 4, 21, 25–27]. Histamine and other substances produced by inflammatory cells can increase inflammation in other parts of the body [5, 25]. Although not well understood many inflammatory diseases such as autoimmune (including arthritis) or colitis are made worse (exacerbated) by increases in histamine levels from injury or foods that are eaten [1, 4, 5].

3.1.2 Inflammation control strategies

These are mostly centered around reducing the amount of material that has to be cleaned up. In many cases, skin wounds are debrided to remove foreign material and necrotic tissue. This helps to reduce the inflammatory response that would have been necessary to remove the foreign material and necrotic tissue as well as reduces the likelihood of an infection, which stimulates both an immune and inflammatory response [1, 2, 21, 25, 26]. Similarly, limiting the bleeding and swelling reduces the inflammatory response by reducing the amount of clean up required [1, 5, 25]. Also in some cases, once repair has begun too much movement at the healing site can lead to microtears and a new cycle of inflammation [1, 2, 25]. In soft tissue, stabilizing the healing parts of the wound with sutures, staples, glue, etc. can limit this [1, 2, 25].

In many cases, foreign materials are used to stabilize the wound or help in the repair phase [1, 21, 25]. Reducing inflammation in these cases is tied to reducing macrophage activation [1, 5, 21, 23, 25, 26, 28–30]. As long as the materials chosen do not leach out chemicals that directly or indirectly activate macrophages, then size of the foreign material is the most important determination of inflammation [1, 2, 21, 28]. Macrophages are most activated in the size range where the foreign material can be phagocytized, but either cannot be or it is not easily done [1, 21, 28–32]. This is normally in the 1–50 μm range [1, 2]. Below 1 μm the foreign material is easily removed and above 50 μm individual macrophages do not try to phagocytize or surround it [28–32]. **Figure 2** shows the change in activation of macrophages when fiber diameter is below 60 μm [1, 2].

The immune response can also occur in the inflammatory phase by using antigenic materials as the foreign material (proteins typically) as well as increased by increasing the response of macrophages, since macrophages typically present the antigens to the lymphocytes [1, 21, 25]. So, control of both the immune response and foreign body response is tied to the activation of macrophages.

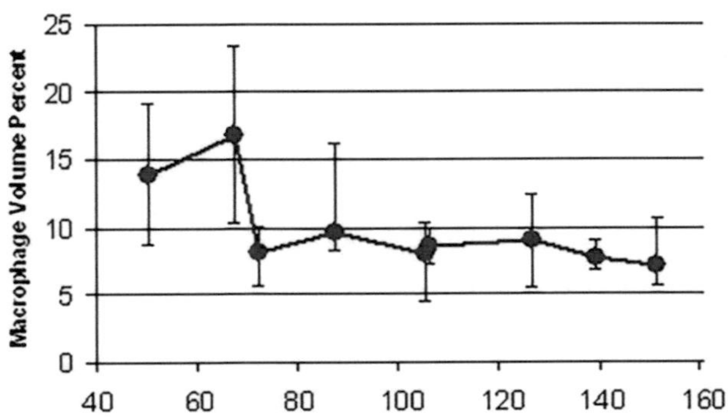

Figure 2.
Shows how size can affect the adaptive response of macrophages. As size of the fibers goes below 60 μm the response of macrophages increase in vivo. This suggests that the inflammatory response significantly increases for diameters (fibers and probably particles) below a certain threshold.

There can also be chemical and environmental changes to reduce the inflammatory response or enhance its efficiency. There are a number of anti-inflammatory drugs that work to either reduce the cellular response or the effect of what the cells produce. Environmental changes can also have an effect. Temperature can be used to slow bleeding or increase the efficiency of the clean-up. Oxygen can directly affect the activity of macrophages, with low oxygen (seen in the beginning of an injury) activating macrophages [1, 4, 5, 33–37].

3.2 Repair phase control

Assuming there is a defect, the speed in which new tissue fills the space determines the length of time it takes to repair the defect. In the case of skin, there is the connective tissue layer (dermis) and the epithelial layer (epidermis). The epidermis requires a vascularized layer to grow across, so the speed of dermal tissue formation controls it [2, 9, 38]. The dermal repair requires fibroblasts to grow into the defect [2, 9, 36, 38]. The fibroblasts require a scaffold to migrate into the wound [2, 9, 20]. The fibroblasts produce the collagen, but need oxygen from blood vessels to produce the collagen scaffold [2, 9, 16]. Therefore, fibroblasts, collagen, and the blood supply grow into the wound together [2]. The rate-limiting step is the blood vessel ingrowth (angiogenesis) [1, 37]. Speeding up fibroblast proliferation, migration, or ECM production is only effective if the angiogenic response is also enhanced. So controlling the angiogenic response controls the rate of dermal and epidermal repair [1, 25, 37]. If healing rate is distance the epidermal cells migrate inward toward the center of the wound, then it is both an epidermal healing rate plus a contraction rate [1, 2, 39].

To increase the rate of angiogenesis a scaffold can be used, to reduce the need for fibroblasts to produce ECM in order for blood vessels to grow in. [2, 25]. Fibroblasts still need to be within about 100 μm of a blood vessel to survive [2, 37]. There are different types of scaffolds that are used: different materials, different degradation profiles, different additives (cells, growth factors, etc.).

There are a number of strategies to increase the angiogenesis ingrowth rate into the defect. These include adding angiogenic growth factors or cell seeding with endothelial cells or endothelial progenitor cells [27, 35, 36]. Electrical stimulation and hyperbaric oxygen have also been used [1, 2].

4. Design selection

Previous sections have shown typical adaptive responses, why you want to control them, and general strategies of how to control the adaptive response. An important part of controlling the adaptive response is deciding the “best” strategy to do that. As it turns out there is hardly ever a best choice in design or for most things in life. In general, all you can do is select an option that has a reasonable probability of doing what you want it to do. In research, using the Scientific Method, we tend to think statistically better is good enough. It is critical to use the engineering design process vs. the Scientific Method to design a treatment.

In reality, the engineering design process uses the Scientific Method, but studies are design driven vs. hypothesis driven. In addition, there are other steps in the engineering design process, which do not have to be included when using the Scientific Method. Too often, based on previous studies, a treatment that is shown to be better than current treatments is tried clinically and although it proves the hypothesis, fails to meet the desired clinical outcome. Researchers try to come up with reasons why it did not work; besides that it was not designed to meet the desired clinical outcome.

The engineering design process is typically taught as a linear process (**Figure 3**). Normally, however, in order to design a clinical treatment there are many feedback loops. This is typically because clinical performance design constraints (desired outcomes) may change over time as well as the performance requirements of the

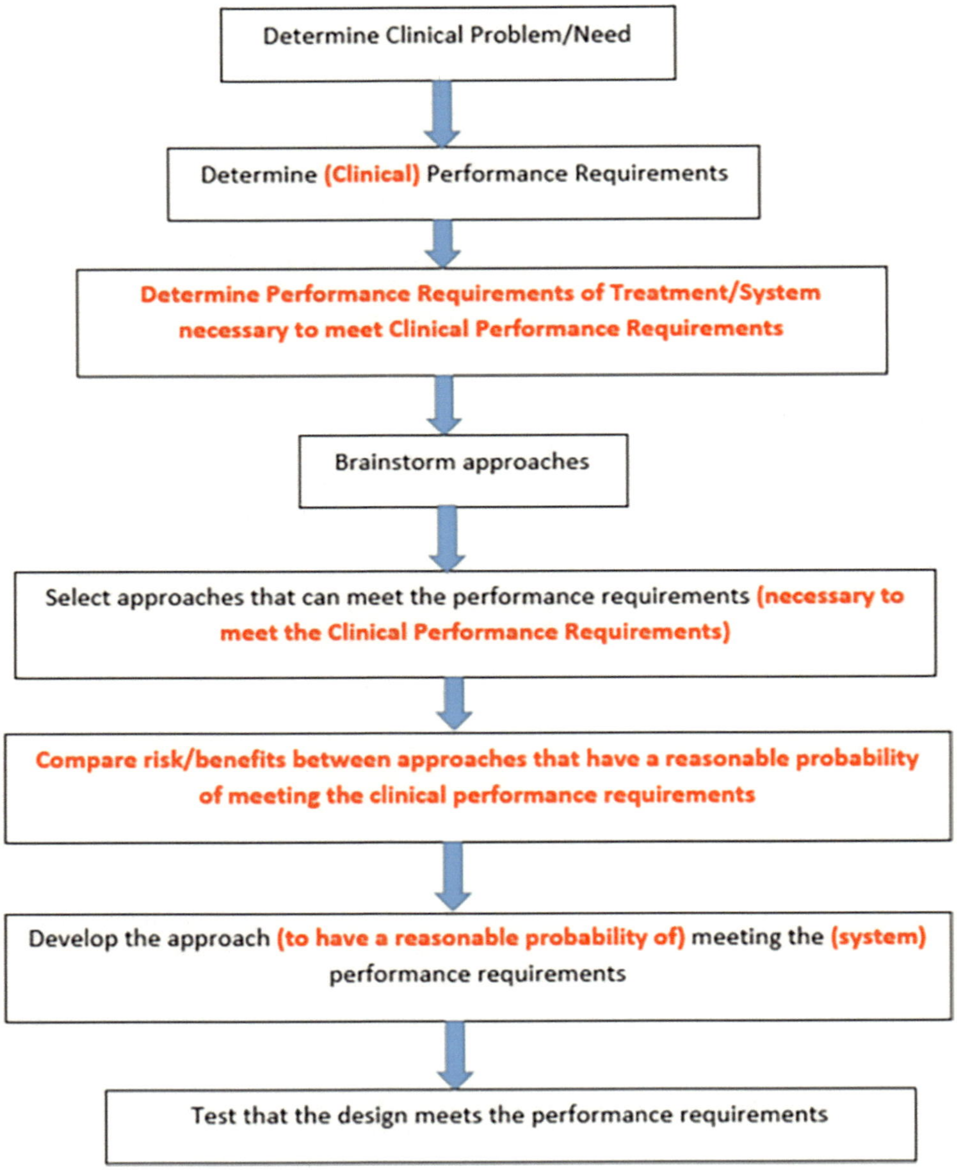

Figure 3.
The engineering design process.

treatment to meet the clinical performance design constraints are not always known. Also, most of the commercializability concerns require iterative processes as the design evolves.

This section (4) will describe the linear design process and then how some of the feedback loops could work. The specific design will depend on the desired clinical outcome (which is one of the steps left out by the Scientific Method) for a given clinical presentation.

4.1 Engineering design process

The linear steps of the design process are shown in **Figure 3** (without the parts in red). The Scientific Method part of the process does not occur until the testing phase (the last step), where studies are done to prove that the system meets the design constraints (design based experiments vs. hypotheses based). The other preceding steps are not required for the Scientific Method, but are essential to design a clinical treatment.

These steps also can be used to justify a research study that is suggesting a better design than current treatments. Without them, it is difficult to justify why a different treatment option should be looked at. First, there needs to be a clinical problem that is not being met by current treatment, otherwise why do we need other options. Then what success looks like (performance requirements) have to be the listed and quantified. It is usually helpful to have a minimum level of acceptable benefits and a maximum level of acceptable harms. Also, additional design constraints can be listed as "would like to" design constraints that can be additional desires or higher levels of benefits as well as lower levels of harms.

Then there is brainstorming to come up with potential approaches. With the "best" one selected to develop further based on meeting all of the performance requirements and a desirable mix of the "would like to" constraints. Then the selected approach is fully developed and tested to assure it meets the performance requirements.

4.2 The real world engineering design process for skin wounds

4.2.1 Modified design process

In practice, however, this process is not linear and needs to be implemented with more detail. The more detailed approach is outlined in **Figure 3** (with the text in red added) and the non-linear elements are described in the next section (4.2.2). The main difference is to make sure the right level of design constraints are used for selection. First, the clinical performance design constraints must be selected. This is again generally functional recovery rate (on the business side they are called "value propositions" if they are better than current treatments). Then the requirements of the system/treatment needed to meet the clinical performance requirements need to be specified. Then brainstorming is done for approaches and the "best" approach is selected.

4.2.2 Iterative nature of the design process

Again, there are two main reasons that this is not a linear process in practice: (1) performance requirements may change over time particularly after testing to see if performance design constraints are actually predictive of the next level up design constraint (e.g., does meeting the system performance requirements assure meeting the clinical performance design constraints) and (2) many of the commercializability concerns require iterative processes as the design evolves.

In most cases, the feedback loop would be after testing to determine, if the design requirements can be met and are predictive of meeting the clinical performance requirements. This iterative process more closely approximates the Design Controls required for FDA regulatory approval.

Again many of the commercializability issues have to be determined in an iterative fashion and can be written as design constraints. Although they should be used to select approaches and specific designs, the commercializability is not really known until the design is complete. In general, they can be looked at as either value added (benefit) to each stakeholder or additional costs to each stakeholder. This risk/benefit analysis is also something typically left out of Scientific Method based studies.

5. Conclusion

The goal of this Chapter was to explain how macrophages can orchestrate the adaptive response to various stimuli, in order to understand the specific role of macrophages in controlling the adaptive response to injury as well as to suggest the introduction of additional stimuli to modify the response of macrophages in an attempt to get a more desired overall adaptive response. In many cases, the normal adaptive response to injury leads to a clinical outcome that falls short of the desired clinical outcome.

Although there has been much work on the different phenotypes of macrophages *in vitro* and *in vivo* [26, 40]. There does not seem to be an on and off switch between pro-inflammatory (M1) and pro-healing (M2a) macrophages [26, 40]. There probably is a continuum and likely that not all macrophages in a wound are in the same place [26, 40]. There is general consensus on what cytokine changes occur during healing of an injury (**Table 1**), however it has been suggested that instead of sorting out phenotypes and cytokine production it would be better to just look at functions (as was done in this review) [26, 40].

A theory was developed to help understand why the normal macrophage orchestrated adaptive response was different in different situations. This theory was also used to suggest why specific clinical strategies could have a significant effect on activation of macrophages and therefore clinical outcome.

Cytokine	Production during repair from onset to the end	
	Increasing	Decreasing
TNFα		X
IL-1β. IL-6		X
YM1		X
TGFβ	X	
CD206	X	

Table 1.
Changes in macrophage cytokine production during injury repair.

To actually design a system based on this theory a specific application would have to be used. This is because different applications would have different desired clinical outcomes. Many of the references cited in this chapter go into more detail (including clinical studies): e.g. [1, 2, 41–44].

Another important aspect of design for injury is that the desired clinical outcome is almost always the rate of return of function to a certain percent of what it was pre-injury. Although it was important to understand how sensitivity of macrophages to stimuli is probably the difference between animals that regenerate and those that do not, regeneration is hardly ever the actual clinical goal. This is mostly because, based on current technology, there are very few cases that we have the ability to regenerate the native structure.

A recent panel discussion at the Society for Biomaterials [45], asked the question "Is it better to regenerate *in vitro* (graft substitute) or *in vivo* (degradable regenerative scaffold)." Both sides gave some very good arguments to justify their approach to a particular wound/injury. Someone from the audience made a good point that it is application dependent and our abilities are different in each area.

However, the panel discussion question missed the point. Again, it is not about regeneration but functional recovery. In particular, with skin wounds, we are not able to make graft substitutes that work like skin grafts nor are we able to make degradable/regenerative scaffolds that completely regenerate skin. Although it may be possible someday, until we are able to, the design goal should not be to move closer to regeneration either *in vitro* or *in vivo*, but to achieve the desired functional recovery.

An important corollary to this is the importance of determining the minimum desired clinical benefits (functional recovery). This requires identifying the problem to solve and describing quantitatively what the minimum clinical outcome requirements are for solving the problem. Too often a researcher proves that a specific design is significantly (statistically at a high confidence level) better than current treatment in one or more desired clinical outcomes, but does not get the desired results clinically (even though it was statistically better than current treatments); and is uncertain why this happened. This is because, in design, it is only important if it allows a better than the minimum desired clinical outcome; better than current treatment is meaningless in design.

Acknowledgements

The concepts and research examples came from research and book chapters written with graduate students and collaborators (who were cited with the applicable references). Funding for this research has come from the CDC, NIH, NSF, and Biofisica.

Conflicts of interest

The author declares no conflict of interest.

Author details

Dale Feldman
Department of Biomedical Engineering, University of Alabama at Birmingham, Birmingham, Alabama, USA

*Address all correspondence to: dfeldman@uab.edu

References

[1] Feldman D. Quantification and modeling of biological processes for tissue engineering and regenerative medicine. Biomedical Journal of Scientific & Technical Research. 2019;**12**(5):1

[2] Feldman DS. Biomaterial enhanced regeneration design research for skin and load bearing applications. Journal of Functional Biomaterials. 2019;**10**(1):10

[3] Palsson B, Bhatia SN. Tissue Dynamics: In Tissue Engineering. Upper Saddle River, NJ: Pearson Education; 2004. pp. 34-45

[4] Palsson B, Bhatia SN. Cellular-Fate Processes: In Tissue Engineering. Upper Saddle River, NJ: Pearson Education; 2004. pp. 74-104

[5] Palsson B, Bhatia SN. Coordination of Cellular-Fate Processes: In Tissue Engineering. Upper Saddle River, NJ: Pearson Education; 2004. pp. 105-131

[6] Wax MK. Split-thickness skin grafts. Medscapes Online. 2019

[7] Boyce ST, Supp DM. Biologic skin substitutes. In: Albanna MZ, Holmes JH, editors. Skin Tissue Engineering and Regenerative Medicine. New York, NY, USA: Academic Press; 2016. pp. 211-238

[8] Goss R. In: Cohen I, Diegelmann R, Lindblad W, editors. Regeneration Versus Repair: In Wound Healing: Biochemical and Clinical Aspects. Philadelphia PA: W.B. Saunders, Co.; 1992. pp. 20-29

[9] Vig K, Chaudhari A, Tripathi S, Dixit S, Sahu R, Pillai S, et al. Advances in skin regeneration using tissue engineering. International Journal of Molecular Sciences. 2017;**18**:789

[10] Duranceau L, Genest H, Bortoluzzi P, Moulin V, Auger FA, Germain L. Successful grafting of a novel autologous tissue-engineered skin substitutes (dermis and epidermis) on twelve burn patients. Journal of Burn Care & Research. 2014;**35**:S121

[11] Boyce ST, Simpson PS, Rieman MT, Warner PM, Yakuboff KP, Bailey JK, et al. Randomized, paired-site comparison of autologous engineered skin substitutes and split-thickness skin graft for closure of extensive, full-thickness burns. Journal of Burn Care & Research. 2017;**38**:61-70

[12] Varkey M, Ding J, Tredget EE. Advances in skin substitutes—Potential of tissue engineered skin for facilitating anti-fibrotic healing. Journal of Functional Biomaterials. 2015;**6**:547-563

[13] Thomas-Virnig CL, Allen-Hoffmann BL. A bioengineered human skin tissue for the treatment of infected wounds. Advances in Wound Care. 2012;**1**:88-94

[14] Boyce ST, Kagan RJ, Greenhalgh DG, Warner P, Yakuboff KP, Palmieri T, et al. Cultured skin substitutes reduce requirements for harvesting of skin autograft for closure of excised, full-thickness burns. Journal of Trauma and Acute Care Surgery. 2006;**60**:821-829

[15] Kagan RJ, Peck MD, Ahrenholz DH, Hickerson WL, Holmes IVJ, Korentager R, et al. Surgical management of the burn wound and use of skin substitutes: An expert panel white paper. Journal of Burn Care & Research. 2013;**34**:e60-e79

[16] Heimbach DM, Warden GD, Luterman A, Jordan MH, Ozobia N,

Ryan CM, et al. Multicenter postapproval clinical trial of Integra dermal regeneration template for burn treatment. The Journal of Burn Care & Rehabilitation. 2003;**24**:42-48

[17] Atala A, Irvine DJ, Moses M, Shaunak S. Wound healing vs. regeneration. Role of the tissue environment in regenerative medicine. MRS Bulletin. 2010;**35**(8):597-606

[18] Bely AE, Nyberg KG. Evolution of animal regeneration: Re-emergence of a field. Trends in Ecology & Evolution. 2009;**25**(3):131-198

[19] Shieh SJ, Cheng TC. Regeneration and repair of human digits and limbs: Fact and fiction. Regeneration. 2015;**2**(4):149-168

[20] Yannas IV, Burke JF, Gordon PL, Huang C, Rubenstein R. Design of an artificial skin. II. Control of chemical composition. Journal of Biomedical Materials Research. 1981;**14**:107-131

[21] Black J. Biological Performance of Materials: Fundamentals of Biocompatibility. New York, NY, USA: Marcel Dekker, Inc; 1981

[22] Feldman D. Regeneration vs. scarring: Did evolution get it right? Current Trends in Biomedical Engineering & Biosciences. 2018;**12**(4):55

[23] Goss R. In: Cohen I, Diegelmann R, Lindblad W, editors. Tissue Repair in the Mammalian Fetus: In Wound Healing: Biochemical and Clinical Aspects. Philadelphia PA: W.B. Saunders, Co.; 1992. pp. 326-343

[24] Morrell V. Why Do Animals Sometimes Kill their Babies? March 28. 2014. National.Geographic.com.

[25] Dee KC, Puleo DA, Bizios R, editors. Wound Healing: In an Introduction to Tissue Biomaterials Interactions. Hoboken, NJ: Wiley-Liss, Inc.; 2002. pp. 127-147

[26] Mosser DM, Edwards JP. Exploring the full spectrum of macrophage activation. Nature Reviews Immunology. 2008;**8**(12):958-969

[27] Barrientos S, Stojadinovic O, Golinko MS, Brem H, Tomic-Canic M. Growth factors and cytokines in wound healing. Wound Repair and Regeneration. 2008;**16**:585-601

[28] Williams DF. On the mechanism of biocompatibility. Biomaterials. 2008;**29**:2941-2953

[29] Shanbhag A, Jacobs J, Black J, Galante J, Glant T. Macrophage/particle interaction: Effect of size, composition, and surface area. Journal of Biomedical Materials Research. 1994;**28**(1):81-90

[30] Gonzalez O, Smith R, Goodman S. Effect of size, concentration, surface area, and volume of polymethylmethacrylate particles on human macrophages *in vitro*. Journal of Biomedical Materials Research. 1996;**30**:463-473

[31] Nagse M. Host reactions to particulate biomaterials. In: Wise D, editor. Encyclopedic Handbook of Biomaterials and Bioengineering. New York: Marcel Dekker; 1995. pp. 269-303

[32] Mooney D, Langer S. Engineering biomaterials for tissue engineering: The 10-100 micron size scale. In: Bronzino J, editor. The Biomedical Engineering Handbook. Hartford, CT: CRC Press; 1995. pp. 1609-1617

[33] Tenenhaus M, Rennekamoff HO. Current concepts in tissue engineering:

Skin wound healing. Plastic and Reconstructive Surgery. 2016;**138**(Suppl. 3):42S-50S

[34] Whitneey JA. Physiologic effects of tissue oxygenation on wound healing. Heart & Lung. 1989;**18**(5):466-467

[35] Knighton DR, Fiegel V. Macrophage-derived growth factors in wound healing: Regulation of growth factor production by the oxygen microenvironment. The American Review of Respiratory Disease. 1989;**140**:1109-1110

[36] Hunt TK, Pai MP. The effect of varying ambient oxygen tensions on wound metabolism and collagen synthesis. Surgery, Gynecology & Obstetrics. 1972;**135**:561

[37] Winter G. Oxygen and epidermal wound healing. Advances in Experimental Medicine and Biology. 1977;**94**:673-674

[38] Gibran NS, Boyce S, Greenhalgh DG. Cutaneous wound healing. Journal of Burn Care & Research. 2007;**28**:577-579

[39] Feldman D, Jennings A. Healing equations. Wounds. 2003;**15**(11):385

[40] Novak ML, Koh TJ. Macrophag2 phenotype during tissue repair. Journal of Leukocyte Biology. 2013;**93**(6):875-881

[41] Feldman DS, McCauley JF. Mesenchymal stem cells and transforming growth factor-β_3 (tgf-β_3) to enhance the regenerative ability of an albumin scaffold in full thickness wound healing. Journal of Functional Biomaterials. 2018;**9**(4):65

[42] Feldman DS, Osborne D. Fibrin as a tissue adhesive and scaffold with an angiogenic agent (FGF-1) to enhance burn graft healing in vivo and clinically. Journal of Functional Biomaterials. 2018;**9**(4):68

[43] Feldman DS. The feasibility of using pulsatile electromagnetic fields (PEMFs) to enhance the regenerative ability of dermal biomaterial scaffolds. Journal of Functional Biomaterials. 2018;**9**(4):66

[44] Jennings A, Andino R, Feldman D. Clinical evaluation of an electrical stimulation bandage (Posifect dressing). Wound Repair and Regeneration. 2005;**13**(2):A13

[45] Regeneration: Better *In Vitro* or *In Vivo*, Panel Discussion SFB. 2019

Section 3

Macrophages in Parasitic Infections

Chapter 9

Elucidating the Complex Interrelationship on Early Interactions between *Leishmania* and Macrophages

Patrícia Sampaio Tavares Veras, Thiago Castro-Gomes and Juliana Perrone Bezerra de Menezes

Abstract

The host's ability to eradicate or control infection caused by intracellular pathogens depends on early interactions between these microorganisms and host cells. These events are related to the organism's nature and stage of development and host immune status. Pathogens are recognized by host cells, which respond to infection by either mounting an efficient response or becoming a replication niche. Early interactions between the protozoan *Leishmania* parasite and host cell receptors activate different signaling pathways that can result in microbe elimination or, alternatively, infection establishment and the migration of *Leishmania* infected cells to other host tissues. This chapter focuses on *Leishmania*-macrophage interaction via phagocytosis, which involves a range of parasite ligands characteristic of Leishmania species and parasite stage of development and diverse host cell receptors. We also discuss alternative *Leishmania* entry by cell invasion and review how *Leishmania* spp. survive and replicate within the phagocytic compartment they induce.

Keywords: *Leishmania* spp., early interactions, parasite survival, macrophage, phagocytosis

1. Introduction

Leishmaniasis is a wide-ranging group of diseases caused by different species of *Leishmania* parasites that result in a broad spectrum of clinical manifestations. Cutaneous leishmaniasis (CL) is characterized by skin and mucosal lesions. At the same time, Visceral leishmaniasis (VL) affects internal organs, such as the liver, spleen, and bone marrow, which can be fatal if left untreated [1]. The WHO has estimated that 30,000 new cases of VL and more than 1 million new cases of CL occur annually, with more than one billion people at risk of infection worldwide [2].

Clinical manifestations of Leishmaniasis are dependent on the infecting parasite species and host immune response [3]. The host's ability to eradicate or control infection caused by intracellular pathogens depends on early interactions between these microorganisms and host cells. Firstly, pathogens are recognized by host cells, which either respond to infection by mounting an efficient response or becoming a replication niche. Early interactions between the protozoan *Leishmania* parasite and host cell receptors result in microbe elimination or infection establishment and the migration of *Leishmania* infected cells to other host tissues. The dissemination of infected cells containing *Leishmania* is crucial to parasite survival and infection in the vertebrate host [4].

Macrophages are crucial in the host response to *Leishmania* infection since these cells are considered the primary host cell for *Leishmania* parasites [5]. This chapter focuses on *Leishmania*–macrophage interaction via phagocytosis, which involves a range of parasite ligands characteristic of *Leishmania* species and parasite stage of development and diverse host cell receptors. We also discuss alternative *Leishmania* entry by cell invasion and how *Leishmania* parasites survive and replicate within the phagocytic compartment they induce and macrophage's effector mechanisms and parasite killing.

2. General aspects of phagocytosis

Phagocytosis is a metabolism-dependent process involving the internalization of particulate material (>0.5 mm) by professional and non-professional phagocytes that can differentiate self from non-self, modified or damaged self-particles. It occurs in a series of distinct and complementary steps [6, 7]. Initially, when the phagocyte recognizes ligands of the particulate material by receptors on cellular membranes, occurs an increase in phosphatidyl bisphosphate (PIP2) levels, followed by a reduction in PIP2 mediated by the conversion of PIP2 to phosphatidyl triphosphate (PIP3) [8]. Next, PLCγ hydrolyzes PIP3 into diacylglycerol and inositol triphosphate (IP3) [9]. After the phagosome formation, maturation of this compartment by the acquisition of different proteins begins [10]. The parasite can promote changes in the kinetics of recruitment to the membrane and activation of these molecules, interfering with phagosome maturation and the microbicidal activity of macrophages [11].

The best-known receptors that induce the attachment and ingestion of different particles, opsonized or not, are those for the complement fractions (CR1 and CR3), those for the Fc region of antibodies (Fc RI, RII, and RIII), as well as the mannose and beta-glycan receptors involved in the recognition and phagocytosis of particles derived from yeast [12] or by circulating collectins and pentraxins [13]. In addition, microbial products defined by Medzhitov and Janeway in 1997 [14] as "pathogen-associated molecular patterns" (PAMPs) are recognized by pattern recognition receptors (PRRs), mainly the toll-like receptors (TLRs) [15] nod-like receptors [16] and dendritic cell receptors such as C-type lectins [17, 18]. The PRRs interplay between innate and adaptive immune responses by directly activating effector mechanisms and alerting the host organism to the presence of infectious agents, including the expression of a group of endogenous signals, such as inflammatory cytokines and chemokines [14, 19].

Like professional phagocytes, nonprofessional phagocytic cells have the machinery, cytoskeleton, and components for signal transduction necessary for phagocytosis [20]. Although intestinal epithelial cells and many nonprofessional cell lines phagocytose bacteria such as *Shigella*, *Yersinia*, and *E. coli*, the mechanisms involved in pathogen recognition by these nonprofessional phagocytes are less well-known than those by professional cells [21, 22]. The significant difference between the two types of phagocytes may be the presence of a broader spectrum and a more substantial number of receptors capable of performing phagocytosis on the membrane of professional cells [20, 23–25].

The molecular processes involved in the uptake of particulate material have been well studied using particles opsonized by immunoglobulins (Ig) class G (IgG) and cells expressing a receptor for the Fc region of IgGs. This interaction results in the clustering of ligand-associated receptors on the phagocytic cell surface. The signaling steps leading to IgG engulfment of opsonized particles are also well studied. These steps comprise the recruitment and activation of kinases, phosphorylation of the cytosolic portion of the receptor, and stimulation of GTPases of the Rac and Cdc42 families, which cooperate with phosphatidyl bisphosphate promoting the stabilization of WASP family proteins. In turn, the WASP protein activates the Arp2/3 complex, promoting actin filaments polymerization, followed by the emission of pseudopodia around the particle [26]. The phagocytosed agent will be internalized in a vesicle called a phagosome. The phagosome will then fuse with lysosomes, forming the phagolysosome. Phagocytosis depends on a complex network of vesicle trafficking pathways that interconnect most intracellular compartments linked to the membrane and actin cytoskeleton and requires the use of a large amount of plasma membrane for pseudopod extension around the target particle [27].

3. Phagosome biogenesis

By analogy with the flow of substances through the endocytic pathway, it is most likely that the ligands present on the surface of particles or microorganisms contribute to the determination of particle destiny within the cell [28, 29]. In addition, the particles and microorganisms' composition present in vacuoles determines both the nature of the vacuolar contents [30, 31] and the ability of the organelles to fuse with other vesicles of the endocytic pathway [32, 33].

Newly formed phagosomes undergo a maturation process from the plasma membrane, which comprises a series of modifications, usually leading to the internalized particle's degradation [6]. In the past, biochemical analyses have been performed on phagosomes isolated and purified at different time points after uptake by antibody-fixed and antibody-coated staphylococcus aureus present in J774 macrophages. These studies revealed that changes in the protein composition of phagosomes are similar to those already identified during endosome maturation or for compartments successively formed during the internalization of soluble components. Identical to the maturation process of endosome compartments, the protein content within phagosomes is partly recycled and sorted. These organelles, probably by fusion with prelysosomes, produce a final compartment that presents at the membrane lysosomal glycoproteins, mannose-6 phosphate receptors, and the ATP-dependent proton pump [29]. The maturation of phagosomes containing IgG-opsonized particles has already been well described for the recognition process. This process involves the remodeling of membranes, gaining and losing proteins, and lipid markers during their biogenesis. These steps comprise acquisition of Rab5 with the participation of Rab20 [34]; acquisition of proton pump V-ATPases, with the release of protons in the phagosomes and acidification of the intracellular medium [35]; conversion of the membrane of the initial phagosome into a late one, due to the recruitment of some proteins such as

Mon1-Ccz1 by Rab5, which by the action of guanine exchange factor (GEF) recruit and activate Rab7. The formation of phagolysosomes culminates in the fusion between late phagosomes with lysosomes [36, 37].

4. Host cell and *Leishmania* interactions during phagocytosis - binding molecules and internalization process

The contact of promastigote forms of *Leishmania* spp. with different cell types, such as neutrophils, dendritic cells, and mainly macrophages, when entering the vertebrate host organism and some cells of the immune system will play an essential role in the development of the disease. The role of different cells, immune or not, at each stage of the infection remains controversial; however, it is possible to state that the parasites are mostly confined within macrophages in the chronic phase of Leishmaniasis. Regarding the cell invasion mechanism employed by the promastigote forms inoculated by the insect vector, it is believed that the main route of penetration into the host cell occurs by phagocytosis. Once phagocytosed, the parasite travels through the host cell endosomal pathway and not only survives but also replicates inside acidic parasitophorous vacuoles that fuse with host cell lysosomes [38–40].

The first studies showing the interaction of infective promastigotes with macrophages were carried out in the 70s [41] and focused on the observation of the interaction of the parasite with its host cell from the very first moments of interaction until its complete internalization, passing by all intermediate stages of parasite uptake. These studies carried out using scanning electron microscopy also showed, in a pioneering way, that the phagocytosis seems to start preferentially by the tip of the parasite's flagellum. Although parasites could be found being phagocytosed by the cell body, the flagellum appears to be the preferred portion to trigger the internalization process. The promastigote flagellum is an anterior structure, extremely active and motile, towards which the parasite moves its body. Interestingly, and due to these morphological characteristics, there is an increasing debate proposing that the promastigote flagellum is, in fact, a sensory structure and that it is probably the first portion of the parasite to interact with host cells. When macrophages were treated with cytochalasin-D, a potent phagocytosis inhibitor, about 75% of the infection was blocked [42].

Given that 25% of the cells continued to be infected even with the drug treatment, these data showed the importance of phagocytosis as a way of invasion. Furthermore, they pointed to alternative routes of infection yet to be explored. As discussed below, we now know that these parasites can penetrate cells also through non-phagocytic pathways.

The internalization process of the *Leishmania* parasite is partially orchestrated like Fc receptor-dependent phagocytosis, particularly those steps involving the recognition of molecules on parasite surface by classical phagocytosis receptors or PRRs on the host cell membrane. Promastigotes have a dense glycocalyx on their surface, mainly consisting of lipophosphoglycan (LPG) molecules, which have long carbohydrate chains with repeating phosphoglycan units that are attached to the membrane by glycophosphatidylinositol (GPI) and glycoinositol phospholipid (GIPL) anchors [43]. The 63 kDa glycoprotein (gp63) is also abundant on the surface of amastigotes and exhibits proteolytic activity. Studies show that gp63 degrades immunoglobulins, complement factors, and lysosomal proteins. Thus,

LPG and gp63 molecules protect the parasite from lysis by complement [44] and are involved in the interaction of the parasite with macrophages [45–47]. In addition to the direct interaction with parasite surface molecules such as LPG, gp63, and CR3 [48] the interaction of *Leishmania* with the macrophage can happen indirectly with receptors for complement fractions, such as CR1 and CR3, after opsonization of the parasite with C3b and C3bi, respectively [49–53]. Additionally, CR1 and CR3 act cooperatively with various receptors present on the macrophage surface, promoting phagocytosis of different *Leishmania* species [49, 52–54]. Complement receptors can interact with receptors for the Fc portion of Ig (FcR) when opsonized by IgGs [55–57]. Alternatively, the receptor for mannose and CR3 may act together to bind and internalize *L. donovani* [50, 58, 59].
In addition, the receptor for fibronectin [60, 61], as well as CR4 [48] and the receptor for C-reactive protein [62], may jointly participate in the phagocytosis of promastigotes of various *Leishmania* species, such as *L. donovani, L. mexicana,* and *L. infantum*.

In addition to classical phagocytosis receptors, PRRs also participate in the interaction of *Leishmania* with macrophages, being involved not in parasite internalization but rather in macrophage activation [63] and control of parasite proliferation [64] These *Leishmania*-macrophage interacting receptors have an influence on phagocytosis steps following ligand-receptor binding, such as actin polymerization [65] production of microbicidal molecules [66, 67], and the formation of the parasitophorous vacuole [68]. Scavenger Receptors (SRs) are PRRs that are part of a protein family with multiple transmembrane domains involved in receptor-mediated endocytosis of polyanionic ligands, including LDL (low-density lipoproteins) [69]. MARCO (Macrophage Receptor with Collagenous Structure), a specific scavenger receptor of the SR-A family, has a collagenous structure, and SRCR (Scavenger Receptor Cysteine-Rich) domain has also been implicated in infection of *L. major* by macrophages in vitro and in vivo [70] (**Figure 1**).

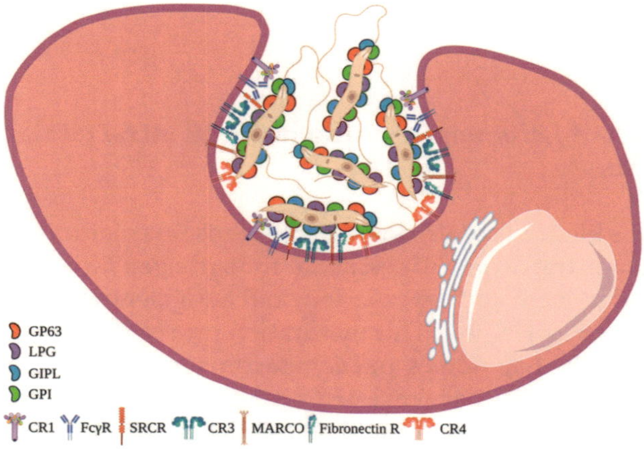

Figure 1.
Binding of Leishmania *during parasite phagocytosis by macrophages. This image depicts the recognition step of the* Leishmania *internalization process by phagocytes. Before being internalized, promastigotes presenting several surface molecules, such as LPG, GPI, GIPL, and GP63, are recognized by host cell surface molecules, including CR1, CR3, CR4, Fc gamma receptors (FcγRs), fibronectin receptor, and the scavenger receptors, SRCR and MARCO. Some of these receptors, such as FcgRs and fibronectin, only recognize opsonized parasites. Alternatively, CR3 can bind to opsonized and non-opsonized* Leishmania. *For clarity, the opsonization process is not illustrated in this image.*

5. A non-phagocytic route of invasion for *Leishmania* spp.

The fact that *Leishmania* spp. infect phagocytic cells created the perception that these parasites have a passive role in their internalization process, needing only to survive after being actively captured by the phagocyte. However, several groups have already described the infection of non-phagocytic cells in vivo and in vitro [71–74]. Thus, as mentioned before, treatment with phagocytosis blocking agents did not abolish infection since a considerable percentage of parasites end up internalized in macrophages even in the presence of such blockers [41]. Taken together, these data pointed to something that remained unexplored until very recently: parasites of the genus *Leishmania* are capable of penetrating host cells through mechanisms that are independent of the host cell cytoskeleton, thus by non-phagocytic means. Recently, this mechanism was elucidated using non-phagocytic cells as host cells and promastigote forms of the parasite. It was clearly demonstrated that *L. amazonensis* promastigotes actively induce cell invasion without any cytoskeleton activity, therefore, by a mechanism distinct from phagocytosis [75]. Similar to what was observed for *Trypanosoma cruzi* [76], the infection involves calcium signaling, recruitment, and exocytosis of lysosomes engaged in the process of plasma membrane repair and lysosome-triggered endocytosis. Briefly, when damaged, eukaryotic cells respond to repair the plasma membrane in a sequential process that involves calcium-dependent exocytosis of lysosomes and endocytosis of plasma membrane lesions [77]. *Leishmania* parasites use this endocytic process to invade host cells in a cytoskeleton-independent manner. In the presence of inhibitory drugs, for example, this is likely the pathway that allows promastigotes to penetrate macrophages even if they cannot phagocytose them. The study of non-phagocytic invasion by *Leishmania* spp. and the role of non-phagocytic host cells in maintaining the pathogen's life cycle is a neglected aspect of the biology of these organisms with great potential yet to be explored. It is possible, for example, that different routes of infection play different roles in the intracellular destination of parasites, impacting their replication rates and their abilities to evade the immune response and manipulate their host cells.

6. Establishment of *Leishmania* within host cell intracellular compartments

Phagolysosome biogenesis, also known as phagosome maturation, is a highly regulated membrane traffic process essential for pathogen intracellular fate, survival or intracellular death and degradation, and antigen processing presentation by professional phagocytes [78, 79]. This maturation process results from sequential fusion events between phagosomes and compartments of the endocytic pathway. Classical cell biology studies have revealed several aspects of the biogenesis of *Leishmania*-induced parasitophorous vacuoles [80–83]. To date, the mechanisms that explain the differences in morphological characteristics of parasitophorous vacuoles have not been fully elucidated. However, above all, the relationship between these morphological differences and the course of infection needs further investigation.

For pathogens that live in intracellular compartments, the process of phagosome maturation does not necessarily follow the steps described for other particles. Once internalized, several microorganisms, including protozoa and bacteria, are adapted to live at least one phase of their life cycle inside host cells. It has been described at least three strategies adopted by different pathogens to evade the defense mechanisms developed by the host following infection. Some microorganisms induce the formation of vacuoles that do not acidify [84]. Other pathogens are phagocytosed and settle in acidified compartments from which they then escape to live in the cytoplasm of the host cell. The last group is formed by organisms adapted to survive in the phagolysosomes of the host cell, which is the case of *Leishmania* parasites [84].

After being recognized by receptors in the host cell surface, *Leishmania* parasites are internalized by macrophages and settle inside structures known as parasitophorous vacuoles. Once inside the parasitophorous vacuoles, the parasites transform into amastigote forms with a rounded shape without apparent flagellum. Recently, Batista et al. (2021) [85] have comprehensively revised several aspects of the dependence of host cell machinery on the biogenesis of *Leishmania*- and *T. cruzi*-induced parasitophorous vacuoles. It is well known that *Leishmania*-induced parasitophorous vacuoles are acidic compartments containing lysosomal enzymes that have access to soluble markers of the endocytic pathway [5, 86, 87]. Indeed, these compartments are bounded by a membrane enriched by late endosome and lysosome markers, including Rab 7, macrosialin, LAMP-1, LAMP-2, vacuolar ATPase, and MHC class II molecules [88–90] (**Figure 2**). These data support the hypothesis that *Leishmania*-induced parasitophorous vacuoles exhibit characteristics of phagolysosomes [83, 90]. In addition, several other biomolecules, including lipids, proteins, and sialoglycoproteins, are exchanged by parasites and host cells following contact. One example is the identification of endoplasmic reticulum

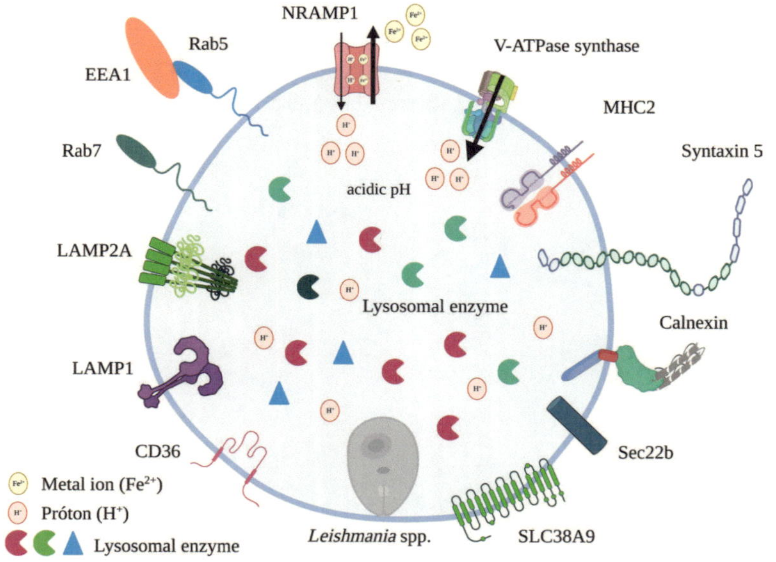

Figure 2.
Model of the parasitophorous vacuole composition induced by Leishmania*. This image illustrates a representative parasitophorous vacuole induced by* Leishmania *in macrophages. These compartments generated by* Leishmania *interact with the endocytic pathway and endoplasmic reticulum compartments. These compartments acquire by fusion markers from the late endosome and lysosome vesicles, such as Rab 7, macrosialin, LAMP-1, LAMP-2, vacuolar ATPase, Nramp1, SLC38A9, and MHC class II molecules. In addition, these compartments also acquire some molecules from host cell membrane, the integral membrane protein CD36, and the secretory pathway, including calnexin, SEC22b, and syntaxin 5.*

(ER) markers in the early steps of *Leishmania*-induced parasitophorous vacuole formation, indicating the participation of ER during phagosome membrane formation [91, 92].

Despite similar characteristics among *Leishmania*-induced vacuoles, the kinetics of their formation [89, 93] and the morphology of these parasite-containing compartments vary depending on the species and growth stage of *Leishmania*. It has been shown that, after phagocytosis of promastigotes of [90] *L. donovani* or *L. major*, the parasites localize in transient phagosomes with little ability to fuse with late endosomes [89]. This delay probably favors promastigote differentiation into amastigote forms if parasites settled within an acidic lysosomal enzyme-rich parasitophorous vacuole induced by *L. donovani*. Another possible mechanism involved in maturation delay by *L. donovani*-induced parasitophorous vacuole is the upregulation of Rab5a, an early endosome protein, along with the recruitment of its effector protein EEA1 [94]. In contrast, Rab5a and EEA1 are early recruited to *L. amazonensis* parasitophorous vacuole and then rapidly exchanged by late endosome and lysosome markers [95, 96]. On the other hand, after internalization, amastigotes of *L. donovani*, *L. amazonensis*, and *L. mexicana* are found in compartments that rapidly fuse with late compartments of the endocytic pathway, an environment in which parasites seem to be resistant [93, 97]. Another difference found to exist among parasite-induced parasitophorous vacuoles regards to their size. Despite *L. major, L. infantum,* and *L. braziliensis* living in tight vacuoles containing only one parasite inside [83], parasites from the Mexican complex are phagocytosed and settle in tight vacuoles that increase in size and become large parasitophorous vacuoles with a high number of parasites [80, 98, 99] (**Figure 3**). The usual large size of these parasitophorous vacuoles seems to be dependent on host cell factors, including lysosomal traffic regulator LYST/Beige [100] CD36 receptor [101] and V-ATPase subunit d isoform 2 (ATP6V0d2) [102] as recently revised by Bahia et al., 2021 [85]. Interestingly, the large size is shown to be related to infection success because in host cells lacking CD36 receptors, parasitophorous vacuoles are small in size, and parasite multiplication is impaired [101].

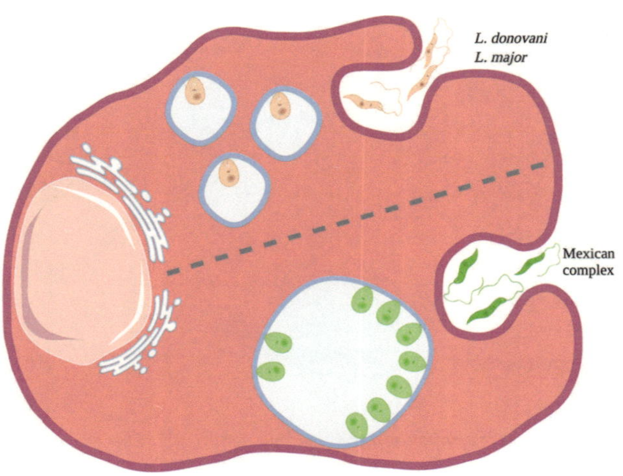

Figure 3.
Model of the parasitophorous vacuole induced by different Leishmania *species. Shown here a representative image of a tight parasitophorous vacuoles containing only one parasite inside induced by* L. major *and* L. donovani, *and a large parasitophorous vacuole with a high number of parasites induced by* L. amazonensis *and* L. mexicana.

7. Macrophage effector mechanisms, parasite replication and infection amplification

Once internalized within the parasitophorous vacuoles, the amastigotes multiply by binary fission, facilitating infection amplification, and persistence in the mammalian host (**Figure 4**). It is commonly assumed that amastigotes are released after host cell burst, which could be occasioned by the burden imposed by the unrestrained replication of the parasite. However, this is still an unproven hypothesis. Thus, the process of infection amplification during leishmaniasis is still a black box. Therefore, our knowledge about the mechanisms that lead to infection amplification during *Leishmania* infection is, in fact, quite limited. However, some crucial clues come from important observations made from in vivo experiments depicting the very first moments of the infectious process using mice and promastigotes of *Leishmania major* naturally transmitted to the mammalian model through the infective bite of the insect vector [38]. These experiments showed that just after promastigote inoculation, neutrophils are the first immune cells to reach the site of infection and phagocytose the parasite. It has been also demonstrated that the parasite could modulate neutrophil viability, which may delay or accelerate the host cell death through apoptosis [103, 104]. The modulation of neutrophil viability helps the survival of the parasites until their final targets and the macrophages. These cells reach the site of infection being attracted by different chemotactic factors such as MIP 1β, which stimulates the phagocytosis of infected apoptotic bodies [104]. Together with the macrophage recruitment, the inhibition of IL-12 secretion and the high secretion of IL-10 and TGF-β generate an anti-inflammatory environment, favoring the parasite's survival. This process of initial neutrophil invasion followed by phagocytosis of these infected and apoptotic cells by macrophages is known as the "Trojan horse" mechanism [105, 106]. From all this, at least one major conclusion can be made: macrophages do not need to be initially infected by the promastigotes inoculated by the vector. They can instead get infected by the ingestion of apoptotic cells or apoptotic cell bodies containing viable amastigotes previously internalized within another cell type. This

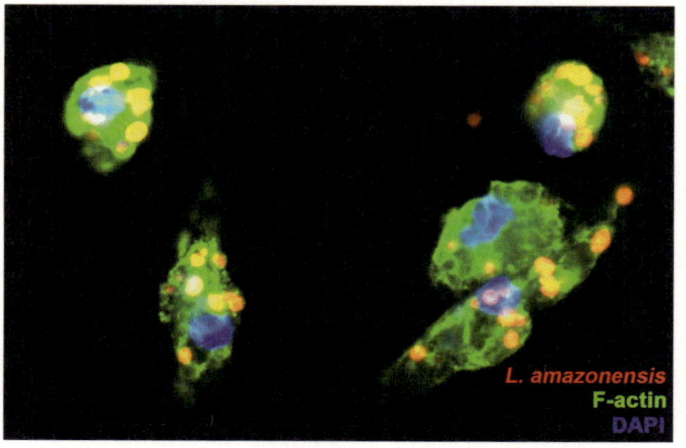

Figure 4.
Human macrophages infected by L. amazonensis. *Cells were infected* in vitro *using parasites expressing a red fluorescent protein, host cell cytoskeleton (F-actin - green) was labeled by Alexa 488-conjugated phalloidin (life technologies), and nuclei were labeled by DAPI (blue). The images show macrophages harboring* L. amazonensis *amastigote forms (red). Original images kindly provided by Prof. Jane Lima-Santos from Universidade Estadual de Santa Cruz, Bahia, Brazil.*

would be an interesting strategy for the parasite because apoptotic mechanisms do not trigger inflammation, as it would lead to a silent infection of macrophages, favoring parasite replication.

As mentioned earlier, cell disruption with the release of amastigotes into the extracellular environment has never been demonstrated despite being often assumed to be a mechanism of amastigote spread. On the other hand, it is entirely plausible to hypothesize that the amplification of infection in leishmaniasis occurs by the ingestion of apoptotic bodies of dead infected macrophages by new macrophages. This is even more logical if we consider that the clearance of dead cells is one of the leading roles these phagocytes play in tissue remodeling. This lack of knowledge about whether amastigotes are released extracellularly is also reflected in the few studies approaching cell invasion by free amastigotes [107–109].

Still, it is necessary to emphasize that other mechanisms have also been proposed regarding the infection amplification process. *Leishmania* amastigotes can be transferred cell to cell, from macrophage to macrophage, as already observed in in vitro studies [110]. Furthermore, other studies have shown that amastigotes can also be released by exocytosis of the parasite after the fusion of the parasitophorous vacuole membrane with host cell plasma membrane, thus without cell rupture [72]. Hence, several possibilities explain the spread of amastigotes and the amplification of infection during leishmaniasis, which do not involve the rupture of the parasitized cell. It is entirely plausible to hypothesize that these silent and non-necrotic pathways of infection amplification, without cell leakage or release of free amastigotes in the extracellular environment (which could be quickly cleared by immune effectors, such as the complement system) have been evolutionarily selected and are responsible for the susceptibility of macrophages to the infection and the amazing ability of *Leishmania* spp. to survive within the cell type that was supposed to kill them.

The dissemination of infected cells containing *Leishmania* is critical to parasite survival and the establishment of infection in the vertebrate host. Thus, the ability of *Leishmania*-infected host cells to migrate may be necessary for lesion distribution on the host and the dissemination of disease. As the main host cells for *Leishmania*, macrophages are crucial for the establishment of infection. However, the role played by these cells in parasite homing to specific tissues and how parasites modulate macrophage function is still poorly understood. Previously published work has shown that infection with *Leishmania* modulates phagocyte functions associated with cell migration [111–114]. Some of these studies have shown that infection with different *Leishmania* species reduces macrophage adhesion, which could facilitate parasite dissemination *in vivo* [113–115]. However, other authors have demonstrated that infection with *Leishmania* impairs the ability of macrophages to migrate [3, 111]. In contrast with previous work, it has been shown that the modulation induced by *Leishmania* could depend on parasite species [116]. Thus, the modulation of macrophage migration induced by *Leishmania*, as well as impacts on parasite dissemination, remains unelucidated.

In leishmaniasis, macrophages function as a replicative niche for *Leishmania* parasites and work as anti-leishmanial effector cells, as immunoregulators, and as permissive host cells for the long-term survival of persistent parasites [117]. Parasite recognition by macrophages and priming by cytokines, such as IFN-γ, lead to the activation of the macrophage's microbicide machinery and production of reactive species, especially superoxide by the multimeric enzyme NADPH oxidase and nitric oxide (NO) by inducible nitric oxide synthase (iNOS) [118]. These critical molecules are known to be involved in the macrophage-mediated innate host defense against

Leishmania parasites. Previously published studies have demonstrated that the killing of different *Leishmania* species (e.g., *L. major, L. donovani, L. braziliensis*) in vitro depended on ROS production. In addition, several studies in mouse models have provided convincing evidence for the crucial role of NO in *Leishmania* parasite killing [39, 117]. However, although IFN-γ has been recognized as the key activator of the leishmanicidal activity of human macrophages, the importance of both iNOS expression and NO production remains controversial in humans [119–121]. Thus, to survive within the hostile environment of macrophages, *Leishmania* parasites have evolved different strategies to circumvent the antimicrobial mechanisms developed by these cells.

8. Conclusions

Undoubtedly, *Leishmania* spp. parasites have evolved a series of adaptations to be captured by macrophages and, instead of succumbing after internalization, they not only survive in the endocytic pathway but also replicate within the intracellular compartment where several other parasites would meet death [122]. The mechanism involved in parasite survival within macrophages and their dissemination in the vertebrate host is still poorly understood. Thus, further studies to dissect the mechanisms involved in the early steps of *Leishmania*-macrophage interaction are critical for the full understanding of *Leishmania* pathogenesis.

Acknowledgements

This work was supported by grants from the Bahia State Research Support Foundation (FAPESB) and FAPEMIG; PSTV holds a grant (305235/2019-2) from National Council for Scientific and Technological Development (CNPq). PSTV and JPBMF are professors from PGPAT and PGBSMI financed by Higher Education Personnel Council–Brazil (CAPES)—Finance Code 001.

We thank Prof. Jane Lima-Santos for kindly providing the infected macrophage image.

Conflict of interest

The authors deny the existence of any conflict of interest.

Author details

Patrícia Sampaio Tavares Veras[1,2*], Thiago Castro-Gomes[3]
and Juliana Perrone Bezerra de Menezes[1]

1 Laboratory of Parasite-Host Interaction and Epidemiology, Gonçalo Moniz Institute–Fiocruz, Salvador, Brazil

2 National Council for Scientific Research and Development, National Institute of Science and Technology of Tropical Diseases, Salvador, Brazil

3 Department of Parasitology, Institute of Biological Sciences, Federal University of Minas Gerais, Belo Horizonte, Brazil

*Address all correspondence to: patricia.veras@fiocruz.br

References

[1] Podinovskaia M, Descoteaux A. Leishmania and the macrophage: A multifaceted interaction. Future Microbiology. 2015;**10**(1):111-129

[2] World Health O. Control of the leishmaniases. World Health Organization Technical Report Series. 2010;**949**:xii-xiii, 1-xii-xiii186. back cover

[3] de Menezes JP, Koushik A, Das S, Guven C, Siegel A, Laranjeira-Silva MF, et al. Leishmania infection inhibits macrophage motility by altering F-actin dynamics and the expression of adhesion complex proteins. Cellular Microbiology. 2017;**19**(3):e12668

[4] Bogdan C, Rollinghoff M. The immune response to Leishmania: Mechanisms of parasite control and evasion. International Journal for Parasitology. 1998;**28**(1):121-134

[5] Alexander J, Vickerman K. Fusion of host cell secondary lysosomes with the parasitophorous vacuoles of Leishmania mexicana-infected macrophages. The Journal of Protozoology. 1975;**22**(4):502-508

[6] Kumar V. Phagocytosis: Phenotypically simple yet a mechanistically complex process. International Reviews of Immunology. 2020;**118-150**:32141349

[7] Galli G, Saleh M. Immunometabolism of macrophages in bacterial infections. Frontiers in Cellular and Infection Microbiology. 2021;**10**:607650

[8] Jaumouille V, Farkash Y, Jaqaman K, Das R, Lowell CA, Grinstein S. Actin cytoskeleton reorganization by Syk regulates Fcgamma receptor responsiveness by increasing its lateral mobility and clustering. Developmental Cell. 2014;**29**(5):534-546

[9] Akashi K, Traver D, Miyamoto T, Weissman IL. A clonogenic common myeloid progenitor that gives rise to all myeloid lineages. Nature. 2000;**404**(6774):193-197

[10] Flannagan RS, Harrison RE, Yip CM, Jaqaman K, Grinstein S. Dynamic macrophage "probing" is required for the efficient capture of phagocytic targets. The Journal of Cell Biology. 2010;**191**(6):1205-1218

[11] Haas A. The phagosome: Compartment with a license to kill. Traffic. 2007;**8**(4):311-330

[12] Stahl PD, Ezekowitz RA. The mannose receptor is a pattern recognition receptor involved in host defense. Current Opinion in Immunology. 1998;**10**(1):50-55

[13] Deban L, Jaillon S, Garlanda C, Bottazzi B, Mantovani A. Pentraxins in innate immunity: Lessons from PTX3. Cell and Tissue Research. 2011;**343**(1):237-249

[14] Medzhitov R, Janeway CA Jr. Innate immunity: The virtues of a nonclonal system of recognition. Cell. 1997;**91**(3):295-298

[15] Beutler BA. TLRs and innate immunity. Blood. 2009;**113**(7):1399-1407

[16] Kersse K, Bertrand MJ, Lamkanfi M, Vandenabeele P. NOD-like receptors and the innate immune system: Coping with danger, damage and death. Cytokine & Growth Factor Reviews. 2011;**22**(5-6):257-276

[17] Geijtenbeek TB, van Vliet SJ, Engering A, BA TH, Van Kooyk Y. Self- and nonself-recognition by C-type lectins on dendritic cells. Annual Review of Immunology. 2004;**22**:33-54

[18] Underhill DM, Ozinsky A. Phagocytosis of microbes: Complexity in action. Annual Review of Immunology. 2002;**20**:825-852

[19] Bahia D, Satoskar AR, Dussurget O. Editorial: Cell Signaling in host-pathogen interactions: The host point of view. Frontiers in Immunology. 2018;**9**:221

[20] Rabinovitch M. Professional and non-professional phagocytes: An introduction. Trends in Cell Biology. 1995;**5**(3):85-87

[21] Isberg RR, Van Nhieu GT. The mechanism of phagocytic uptake promoted by invasin-integrin interaction. Trends in Cell Biology. 1995;**5**(3):120-124

[22] Galan JE. Salmonella interactions with host cells: Type III secretion at work. Annual Review of Cell and Developmental Biology. 2001;**17**:53-86

[23] Greenberg S, Chang P, Silverstein SC. Tyrosine phosphorylation is required for fc receptor-mediated phagocytosis in mouse macrophages. The Journal of Experimental Medicine. 1993;**177**(2):529-534

[24] Kruskal BA, Sastry K, Warner AB, Mathieu CE, Ezekowitz RA. Phagocytic chimeric receptors require both transmembrane and cytoplasmic domains from the mannose receptor. The Journal of Experimental Medicine. 1992;**176**(6):1673-1680

[25] Greenberg S, Burridge K, Silverstein SC. Colocalization of F-actin and Talin during fc receptor-mediated phagocytosis in mouse macrophages. The Journal of Experimental Medicine. 1990;**172**(6):1853-1856

[26] Gray M, Botelho RJ. Phagocytosis: Hungry, hungry cells. Methods in Molecular Biology. 2017;**1519**:1-16

[27] Huynh KK, Kay JG, Stow JL, Grinstein S. Fusion, fission, and secretion during phagocytosis. Physiology (Bethesda). 2007;**22**:366-372

[28] Desjardins M, Huber LA, Parton RG, Griffiths G. Biogenesis of phagolysosomes proceeds through a sequential series of interactions with the endocytic apparatus. The Journal of Cell Biology. 1994;**124**(5):677-688

[29] Pitt A, Mayorga LS, Stahl PD, Schwartz AL. Alterations in the protein composition of maturing phagosomes. The Journal of Clinical Investigation. 1992;**90**(5):1978-1983

[30] Joiner KA, Fuhrman SA, Miettinen HM, Kasper LH, Mellman I. Toxoplasma gondii: Fusion competence of parasitophorous vacuoles in fc receptor-transfected fibroblasts. Science. 1990;**249**(4969):641-646

[31] Joiner KA. Vacuolar membranes surrounding intracellular pathogens: Where do they come from and what do they do? Infectious Agents and Disease. 1993;**2**(4):215-219

[32] Joiner KA, Ganz T, Albert J, Rotrosen D. The opsonizing ligand on salmonella typhimurium influences incorporation of specific, but not azurophil, granule constituents into neutrophil phagosomes. The Journal of Cell Biology. 1989;**109**(6 Pt 1): 2771-2782

[33] Bouvier G, Benoliel AM, Foa C, Bongrand P. Relationship between

phagosome acidification, phagosome-lysosome fusion, and mechanism of particle ingestion. Journal of Leukocyte Biology. 1994;**55**(6):729-734

[34] Flannagan RS, Jaumouille V, Grinstein S. The cell biology of phagocytosis. Annual Review of Pathology. 2012;**7**:61-98

[35] Dale DC, Boxer L, Liles WC. The phagocytes: Neutrophils and monocytes. Blood. 2008;**112**(4):935-945

[36] Mottola G. The complexity of Rab5 to Rab7 transition guarantees specificity of pathogen subversion mechanisms. Frontiers in Cellular and Infection Microbiology. 2014;**4**:180

[37] Cabrera M, Ungermann C. Guiding endosomal maturation. Cell. 2010;**141**(3):404-406

[38] Peters NC, Egen JG, Secundino N, Debrabant A, Kimblin N, Kamhawi S, et al. In vivo imaging reveals an essential role for neutrophils in leishmaniasis transmitted by sand flies. Science. 2008;**321**(5891):970-974

[39] Liu D, Uzonna JE. The early interaction of Leishmania with macrophages and dendritic cells and its influence on the host immune response. Frontiers in Cellular and Infection Microbiology. 2012;**2**:83

[40] von Stebut E, Tenzer S. Cutaneous leishmaniasis: Distinct functions of dendritic cells and macrophages in the interaction of the host immune system with Leishmania major. International Journal of Medical Microbiology. 2018;**308**(1):206-214

[41] Zenian A, Rowles P, Gingell D. Scanning electron-microscopic study of the uptake of Leishmania parasites by macrophages. Journal of Cell Science. 1979;**39**:187-199

[42] Rotureau B, Morales MA, Bastin P, Spath GF. The flagellum-mitogen-activated protein kinase connection in trypanosomatids: A key sensory role in parasite signalling and development? Cellular Microbiology. 2009;**11**(5):710-718

[43] Beverley SM, Turco SJ. Lipophosphoglycan (LPG) and the identification of virulence genes in the protozoan parasite Leishmania. Trends in Microbiology. 1998;**6**(1):35-40

[44] Puentes SM, Da Silva RP, Sacks DL, Hammer CH, Joiner KA. Serum resistance of metacyclic stage Leishmania major promastigotes is due to release of C5b-9. Journal of Immunology. 1990;**145**(12):4311-4316

[45] Davies CR, Cooper AM, Peacock C, Lane RP, Blackwell JM. Expression of LPG and GP63 by different developmental stages of Leishmania major in the sandfly Phlebotomus papatasi. Parasitology. 1990;**101**(Pt 3):337-343

[46] Kelleher M, Moody SF, Mirabile P, Osborn AH, Bacic A, Handman E. Lipophosphoglycan blocks attachment of Leishmania major amastigotes to macrophages. Infection and Immunity. 1995;**63**(1):43-50

[47] Pimenta PF, Saraiva EM, Sacks DL. The comparative fine structure and surface glycoconjugate expression of three life stages of Leishmania major. Experimental Parasitology. 1991;**72**(2):191-204

[48] Talamas-Rohana P, Wright SD, Lennartz MR, Russell DG. Lipophosphoglycan from Leishmania mexicana promastigotes binds

to members of the CR3, p150,95 and LFA-1 family of leukocyte integrins. Journal of Immunology. 1990;**144**(12):4817-4824

[49] Mosser DM, Edelson PJ. Activation of the alternative complement pathway by Leishmania promastigotes: Parasite lysis and attachment to macrophages. Journal of Immunology. 1984;**132**(3):1501-1505

[50] Blackwell JM, Ezekowitz RA, Roberts MB, Channon JY, Sim RB, Gordon S. Macrophage complement and lectin-like receptors bind Leishmania in the absence of serum. The Journal of Experimental Medicine. 1985;**162**(1):324-331

[51] Cooper A, Rosen H, Blackwell JM. Monoclonal antibodies that recognize distinct epitopes of the macrophage type three complement receptor differ in their ability to inhibit binding of Leishmania promastigotes harvested at different phases of their growth cycle. Immunology. 1988;**65**(4):511-514

[52] Da Silva RP, Hall BF, Joiner KA, Sacks DL. CR1, the C3b receptor, mediates binding of infective Leishmania major metacyclic promastigotes to human macrophages. Journal of Immunology. 1989;**143**(2):617-622

[53] Brittingham A, Morrison CJ, McMaster WR, McGwire BS, Chang KP, Mosser DM. Role of the Leishmania surface protease gp63 in complement fixation, cell adhesion, and resistance to complement-mediated lysis. Journal of Immunology. 1995;**155**(6):3102-3111

[54] Russell DG. The macrophage-attachment glycoprotein gp63 is the predominant C3-acceptor site on Leishmania mexicana promastigotes. European Journal of Biochemistry. 1987;**164**(1):213-221

[55] Chang KP. Leishmania donovani-macrophage binding mediated by surface glycoproteins/antigens: Characterization in vitro by a radioisotopic assay. Molecular and Biochemical Parasitology. 1981;**4**(1-2):67-76

[56] Russell DG, Talamas-Rohana P, Zelechowski J. Antibodies raised against synthetic peptides from the Arg-Gly-asp-containing region of the Leishmania surface protein gp63 cross-react with human C3 and interfere with gp63-mediated binding to macrophages. Infection and Immunity. 1989;**57**(2):630-632

[57] Guy RA, Belosevic M. Comparison of receptors required for entry of Leishmania major amastigotes into macrophages. Infection and Immunity. 1993;**61**(4):1553-1558

[58] Wilson ME, Pearson RD. Roles of CR3 and mannose receptors in the attachment and ingestion of Leishmania donovani by human mononuclear phagocytes. Infection and Immunity. 1988;**56**(2):363-369

[59] Chakraborty R, Chakraborty P, Basu MK. Macrophage mannosyl fucosyl receptor: Its role in invasion of virulent and avirulent L. donovani promastigotes. Bioscience Reports. 1998;**18**(3):129-142

[60] Rizvi FS, Ouaissi MA, Marty B, Santoro F, Capron A. The major surface protein of Leishmania promastigotes is a fibronectin-like molecule. European Journal of Immunology. 1988;**18**(3):473-476

[61] Brittingham A, Chen G, McGwire BS, Chang KP, Mosser DM. Interaction of Leishmania gp63 with cellular receptors for fibronectin. Infection and Immunity. 1999;**67**(9):4477-4484

[62] Culley FJ, Harris RA, Kaye PM, McAdam KP, Raynes JG. C-reactive protein binds to a novel ligand on Leishmania donovani and increases uptake into human macrophages. Journal of Immunology. 1996;**156**(12):4691-4696

[63] Campos MA, Almeida IC, Takeuchi O, Akira S, Valente EP, Procopio DO, et al. Activation of toll-like receptor-2 by glycosylphosphatidylinositol anchors from a protozoan parasite. Journal of Immunology. 2001;**167**(1):416-423

[64] Kropf P, Freudenberg MA, Modolell M, Price HP, Herath S, Antoniazi S, et al. Toll-like receptor 4 contributes to efficient control of infection with the protozoan parasite Leishmania major. Infection and Immunity. 2004;**72**(4):1920-1928

[65] Holm A, Tejle K, Magnusson KE, Descoteaux A, Rasmusson B. Leishmania donovani lipophosphoglycan causes periphagosomal actin accumulation: Correlation with impaired translocation of PKCalpha and defective phagosome maturation. Cellular Microbiology. 2001;**3**(7):439-447

[66] Channon JY, Roberts MB, Blackwell JM. A study of the differential respiratory burst activity elicited by promastigotes and amastigotes of Leishmania donovani in murine resident peritoneal macrophages. Immunology. 1984;**53**(2):345-355

[67] Assreuy J, Cunha FQ, Epperlein M, Noronha-Dutra A, O'Donnell CA, Liew FY, et al. Production of nitric oxide and superoxide by activated macrophages and killing of Leishmania major. European Journal of Immunology. 1994;**24**(3):672-676

[68] Ilg T, Stierhof YD, McConville MJ, Overath P. Purification, partial characterization and immunolocalization of a proteophosphoglycan secreted by Leishmania mexicana amastigotes. European Journal of Cell Biology. 1995;**66**(2):205-215

[69] Ramet M, Pearson A, Manfruelli P, Li X, Koziel H, Gobel V, et al. Drosophila scavenger receptor CI is a pattern recognition receptor for bacteria. Immunity. 2001;**15**(6):1027-1038

[70] Gomes IN, Palma LC, Campos GO, Lima JG, TF DEA, JP DEM, et al. The scavenger receptor MARCO is involved in Leishmania major infection by CBA/J macrophages. Parasite Immunology. 2009;**31**(4):188-198

[71] Minero MA, Chinchilla M, Guerrero OM, Castro A. Infection of skin fibroblasts in animals with different levels of sensitivity to Leishmania infantum and Leishmania mexicana (Kinetoplastida: Trypanosomatidae). Revista de Biología Tropical. 2004;**52**(1):261-267

[72] Rittig MG, Bogdan C. Leishmania-host-cell interaction: Complexities and alternative views. Parasitology Today. 2000;**16**(7):292-297

[73] Bogdan C, Donhauser N, Doring R, Rollinghoff M, Diefenbach A, Rittig MG. Fibroblasts as host cells in latent leishmaniosis. The Journal of Experimental Medicine. 2000;**191**(12):2121-2130

[74] Holbrook TW, Palczuk NC. Leishmania in the chick embryo. IV. Effects of embryo age and hatching, and behavior of L. donovani in cultures of chick fibroblasts. Experimental Parasitology. 1975;**37**(3):398-404

[75] Cavalcante-Costa VS, Costa-Reginaldo M, Queiroz-Oliveira T, Oliveira ACS, Couto NF, Dos Anjos DO,

et al. Leishmania amazonensis hijacks host cell lysosomes involved in plasma membrane repair to induce invasion in fibroblasts. Journal of Cell Science. 2019;**132**(6):1-16

[76] Fernandes MC, Cortez M, Flannery AR, Tam C, Mortara RA, Andrews NW. Trypanosoma cruzi subverts the sphingomyelinase-mediated plasma membrane repair pathway for cell invasion. The Journal of Experimental Medicine. 2011;**208**(5):909-921

[77] Corrotte M, Castro-Gomes T. Lysosomes and plasma membrane repair. Current Topics in Membranes. 2019;**84**:1-16

[78] Vergne I, Chua J, Singh SB, Deretic V. Cell biology of mycobacterium tuberculosis phagosome. Annual Review of Cell and Developmental Biology. 2004;**20**:367-394

[79] Jutras I, Desjardins M. Phagocytosis: at the crossroads of innate and adaptive immunity. Annual Review of Cell and Developmental Biology. 2005;**21**:511-527

[80] Veras PS, de Chastellier C, Rabinovitch M. Transfer of zymosan (yeast cell walls) to the parasitophorous vacuoles of macrophages infected with Leishmania amazonensis. The Journal of Experimental Medicine. 1992;**176**(3):639-646

[81] Alexander J, Russell DG. The interaction of Leishmania species with macrophages. Advances in Parasitology. 1992;**31**:175-254

[82] De Souza LS, Lang T, Prina E, Hellio R, Antoine JC. Intracellular Leishmania amazonensis amastigotes internalize and degrade MHC class II molecules of their host cells. Journal of Cell Science. 1995;**108**(Pt 10):3219-3231

[83] Desjardins M, Descoteaux A. Survival strategies of Leishmania donovani in mammalian host macrophages. Research in Immunology. 1998;**149**(7-8):689-692

[84] Tait A, Sacks DL. The cell biology of parasite invasion and survival. Parasitology Today. 1988;**4**(8):228-234

[85] Batista MF, Najera CA, Meneghelli I, Bahia D. The parasitic intracellular lifestyle of trypanosomatids: Parasitophorous vacuole development and survival. Frontiers in Cell and Development Biology. 2020;**8**:396

[86] Chang KP, Dwyer DM. Multiplication of a human parasite (Leishmania donovani) in phagolysosomes of hamster macrophages in vitro. Science. 1976;**193**(4254):678-680

[87] Rabinovitch M, Topper G, Cristello P, Rich A. Receptor-mediated entry of peroxidases into the parasitophorous vacuoles of macrophages infected with Leishmania Mexicana amazonensis. Journal of Leukocyte Biology. 1985;**37**(3):247-261

[88] Antoine JC, Prina E, Jouanne C, Bongrand P. Parasitophorous vacuoles of Leishmania amazonensis-infected macrophages maintain an acidic pH. Infection and Immunity. 1990;**58**(3):779-787

[89] Desjardins M, Descoteaux A. Inhibition of phagolysosomal biogenesis by the Leishmania lipophosphoglycan. The Journal of Experimental Medicine. 1997;**185**(12):2061-2068

[90] Antoine JC, Prina E, Lang T, Courret N. The biogenesis and properties of the parasitophorous vacuoles that harbour Leishmania in murine macrophages. Trends in Microbiology. 1998;**6**(10):392-401

[91] Gagnon E, Duclos S, Rondeau C, Chevet E, Cameron PH, Steele-Mortimer O, et al. Endoplasmic reticulum-mediated phagocytosis is a mechanism of entry into macrophages. Cell. 2002;**110**(1):119-131

[92] Canton J, Ndjamen B, Hatsuzawa K, Kima PE. Disruption of the fusion of Leishmania parasitophorous vacuoles with ER vesicles results in the control of the infection. Cellular Microbiology. 2012;**14**(6):937-948

[93] Dermine JF, Scianimanico S, Prive C, Descoteaux A, Desjardins M. Leishmania promastigotes require lipophosphoglycan to actively modulate the fusion properties of phagosomes at an early step of phagocytosis. Cellular Microbiology. 2000;**2**(2):115-126

[94] Verma JK, Rastogi R, Mukhopadhyay A. Leishmania donovani resides in modified early endosomes by upregulating Rab5a expression via the downregulation of miR-494. PLoS Pathogens. 2017;**13**(6):e1006459

[95] Courret N, Frehel C, Gouhier N, Pouchelet M, Prina E, Roux P, et al. Biogenesis of Leishmania-harbouring parasitophorous vacuoles following phagocytosis of the metacyclic promastigote or amastigote stages of the parasites. Journal of Cell Science. 2002;**115**(Pt 11):2303-2316

[96] Veras PST, de Menezes JPB, Dias BRS. Deciphering the role played by autophagy in Leishmania infection. Frontiers in Immunology. 2019;**10**:2523

[97] Lang T, Hellio R, Kaye PM, Antoine JC. Leishmania donovani-infected macrophages: Characterization of the parasitophorous vacuole and potential role of this organelle in antigen presentation. Journal of Cell Science. 1994;**107**(Pt 8):2137-2150

[98] Veras PS, de Chastellier C, Moreau MF, Villiers V, Thibon M, Mattei D, et al. Fusion between large phagocytic vesicles: Targeting of yeast and other particulates to phagolysosomes that shelter the bacterium Coxiella burnetii or the protozoan Leishmania amazonensis in Chinese hamster ovary cells. Journal of Cell Science. 1994;**107**(Pt 11):3065-3076

[99] Veras PS, Topilko A, Gouhier N, Moreau MF, Rabinovitch M, Pouchelet M. Fusion of Leishmania amazonensis parasitophorous vacuoles with phagosomes containing zymosan particles: Cinemicrographic and ultrastructural observations. Brazilian Journal of Medical and Biological Research. 1996;**29**(8):1009-1018

[100] Wilson J, Huynh C, Kennedy KA, Ward DM, Kaplan J, Aderem A, et al. Control of parasitophorous vacuole expansion by LYST/beige restricts the intracellular growth of Leishmania amazonensis. PLoS Pathogens. 2008;**4**(10):e1000179

[101] Okuda K, Tong M, Dempsey B, Moore KJ, Gazzinelli RT, Silverman N. Leishmania amazonensis engages CD36 to drive Parasitophorous vacuole maturation. PLoS Pathogens. 2016;**12**(6):e1005669

[102] Pessoa CC, Reis LC, Ramos-Sanchez EM, Orikaza CM, Cortez C, de Castro Levatti EV, et al. ATP6V0d2 controls Leishmania parasitophorous vacuole biogenesis via cholesterol homeostasis. PLoS Pathogens. 2019;**15**(6):e1007834

[103] Ribeiro-Gomes FL, Otero AC, Gomes NA, Moniz-De-Souza MC, Cysne-Finkelstein L, Arnholdt AC, et al. Macrophage interactions with neutrophils regulate Leishmania major infection. Journal of Immunology. 2004;**172**(7):4454-4462

[104] Afonso L, Borges VM, Cruz H, Ribeiro-Gomes FL, DosReis GA, Dutra AN, et al. Interactions with apoptotic but not with necrotic neutrophils increase parasite burden in human macrophages infected with Leishmania amazonensis. Journal of Leukocyte Biology. 2008;**84**(2):389-396

[105] van Zandbergen G, Solbach W, Laskay T. Apoptosis driven infection. Autoimmunity. 2007;**40**(4):349-352

[106] Laskay T, van Zandbergen G, Solbach W. Neutrophil granulocytes--Trojan horses for Leishmania major and other intracellular microbes? Trends in Microbiology. 2003;**11**(5):210-214

[107] Love DC, Mentink Kane M, Mosser DM. Leishmania amazonensis: The phagocytosis of amastigotes by macrophages. Experimental Parasitology. 1998;**88**(3):161-171

[108] Kane MM, Mosser DM. Leishmania parasites and their ploys to disrupt macrophage activation. Current Opinion in Hematology. 2000;7(1):26-31

[109] Wanderley JL, Moreira ME, Benjamin A, Bonomo AC, Barcinski MA. Mimicry of apoptotic cells by exposing phosphatidylserine participates in the establishment of amastigotes of Leishmania (L) amazonensis in mammalian hosts. Journal of Immunology. 2006;**176**(3):1834-1839

[110] Real F, Florentino PT, Reis LC, Ramos-Sanchez EM, Veras PS, Goto H, et al. Cell-to-cell transfer of Leishmania amazonensis amastigotes is mediated by immunomodulatory LAMP-rich parasitophorous extrusions. Cellular Microbiology. 2014;**16**(10):1549-1564

[111] Bray RS, Heikal B, Kaye PM, Bray MA. The effect of parasitization by Leishmania mexicana mexicana on macrophage function in vitro. Acta Tropica. 1983;**40**(1):29-38

[112] De Almeida MC, Cardoso SA, Barral-Netto M. Leishmania (Leishmania) chagasi infection alters the expression of cell adhesion and costimulatory molecules on human monocyte and macrophage. International Journal for Parasitology. 2003;**33**(2):153-162

[113] Carvalhal DG, Barbosa A Jr, D'El-Rei Hermida M, Clarencio J, Pinheiro NF Jr, Veras PS, et al. The modelling of mononuclear phagocyte-connective tissue adhesion in vitro: Application to disclose a specific inhibitory effect of Leishmania infection. Experimental Parasitology. 2004;**107**(3-4):189-199

[114] Pinheiro NF Jr, Hermida MD, Macedo MP, Mengel J, Bafica A, dos-Santos WL. Leishmania infection impairs beta 1-integrin function and chemokine receptor expression in mononuclear phagocytes. Infection and Immunity. 2006;**74**(7):3912-3921

[115] Figueira CP, Carvalhal DG, Almeida RA, Hermida M, Touchard D, Robert P, et al. Leishmania infection modulates beta-1 integrin activation and alters the kinetics of monocyte spreading over fibronectin. Scientific Reports. 2015;**5**:12862

[116] Rocha MI, Dias F, Resende M, Sousa M, Duarte M, Tomas AM, et al. Leishmania infantum enhances migration of macrophages via a phosphoinositide 3-kinase gamma-dependent pathway. ACS Infect Dis. 2020;**6**(7):1643-1649

[117] Bogdan C. Macrophages as host, effector and immunoregulatory cells in leishmaniasis: Impact of tissue micro-environment and metabolism. Cytokine X. 2020;**2**(4):100041

[118] Rossi M, Fasel N. How to master the host immune system? Leishmania parasites have the solutions! International Immunology. 2018;**30**(3):103-111

[119] Gantt KR, Goldman TL, McCormick ML, Miller MA, Jeronimo SM, Nascimento ET, et al. Oxidative responses of human and murine macrophages during phagocytosis of Leishmania chagasi. Journal of Immunology. 2001;**167**(2):893-901

[120] Murray HW, Rubin BY, Rothermel CD. Killing of intracellular Leishmania donovani by lymphokine-stimulated human mononuclear phagocytes. Evidence that interferon-gamma is the activating lymphokine. The Journal of Clinical Investigation. 1983;**72**(4):1506-1510

[121] Douvas GS, Looker DL, Vatter AE, Crowle AJ. Gamma interferon activates human macrophages to become tumoricidal and leishmanicidal but enhances replication of macrophage-associated mycobacteria. Infection and Immunity. 1985;**50**(1):1-8

[122] Carneiro MB, Vaz LG, Afonso LCC, Horta MF, Vieira LQ. Regulation of macrophage subsets and cytokine production in leishmaniasis. Cytokine. 2021;**147**:155309

Chapter 10

Shifting Macrophage Phenotypes in Leishmaniasis

Natália S. Vellozo, Flávia L. Ribeiro-Gomes and Marcela F. Lopes

Abstract

Macrophage phenotypes, such as macrophage (M) 1 (classically activated macrophage) and M2 (alternatively activated macrophage), determine the macrophage role as an effector immune cell or as a permissive host for the intracellular pathogenic protozoan *Leishmania* spp. *Leishmania* parasites and the host immune system shape macrophage phenotypes, which in turn can help parasite control or promote infection. Here, we discussed how shifting macrophage phenotypes might change disease outcome in leishmaniasis, by addressing: (1) macrophage phenotypes in leishmaniasis; (2) the functional phenotypes of resident and inflammatory macrophages; (3) the interplay with neutrophils modulates macrophage function; (4) the crosstalk with T cells shapes macrophage phenotypes; and (5) potential therapeutic tools to skew macrophage phenotypes and disease outcomes.

Keywords: macrophage phenotypes, M1 and M2 macrophages, neutrophils, T cells, potential therapeutic tools, *Leishmania*

1. Introduction

Leishmaniasis is a neglected tropical disease caused by more than 20 different species of protozoan parasites belonging to the genus *Leishmania* [1]. About 1 billion people live in endemic areas of leishmaniasis in 92 countries. Currently, 11 million people are infected, with an estimated 1.5 million new cases each year [2]. The clinical manifestations of the disease range from localized skin lesions to disseminated or visceral forms [1], depending on the *Leishmania* species, host features, and the type and magnitude of the immune responses [3]. Cutaneous leishmaniasis (CL) is the most common clinical manifestation, with 700,000 to 1 million new cases worldwide annually. Other disease forms include mucocutaneous leishmaniasis (MCL), diffuse cutaneous leishmaniasis (DCL), and the aggressive and more lethal form of the disease, visceral leishmaniasis (VL), which can progress to post-kala-azar dermal leishmaniasis (PKDL) [4, 5]. *Leishmania* species responsible for the cutaneous clinical forms include the *Leishmania mexicana* complex (*L. mexicana, L. amazonensis, and L. venezuelensis*), the *Leishmania Viannia* complex [*L.* (*V.*) *braziliensis*, *L.* (*V.*) *guyanensis*, *L.* (*V.*) *panamensis*, and *L.* (*V.*) *peruviana*], *Leishmania tropica*, *Leishmania major*, and *Leishmania aethiopica*. Some of these species are also responsible for the MCL and DCL forms. *Leishmania donovani*, *Leishmania infantum*, and *Leishmania chagasi* mainly cause VL and PKDL [5].

Leishmania spp. parasites can induce distinct immune responses, depending on species-specific parasite components and/or the type and strength of the host immunity [3]. Early upon infection, the interactions between *Leishmania* parasites and neutrophils, dendritic cells (DCs), and macrophages shape the type of acquired immune response, crucial for disease progression or control of infection [6, 7] (**Figure 1**). Macrophages are permissive host cells for *Leishmania* parasites, but once activated, they can destroy intracellular parasites. Therefore, macrophages play a key role in innate immunity and in the development of acquired immune response, ultimately leading to the resolution of infection or disease progression.

Macrophages can assume a plethora of functional phenotypes, ranging from M1 to M2, depending on the signals provided by the environment, including Th1 and Th2 cytokines [8–10]. Whereas M1 designates macrophages that eliminate intracellular parasites, at the M2 opposite pole, macrophages can sustain *Leishmania*

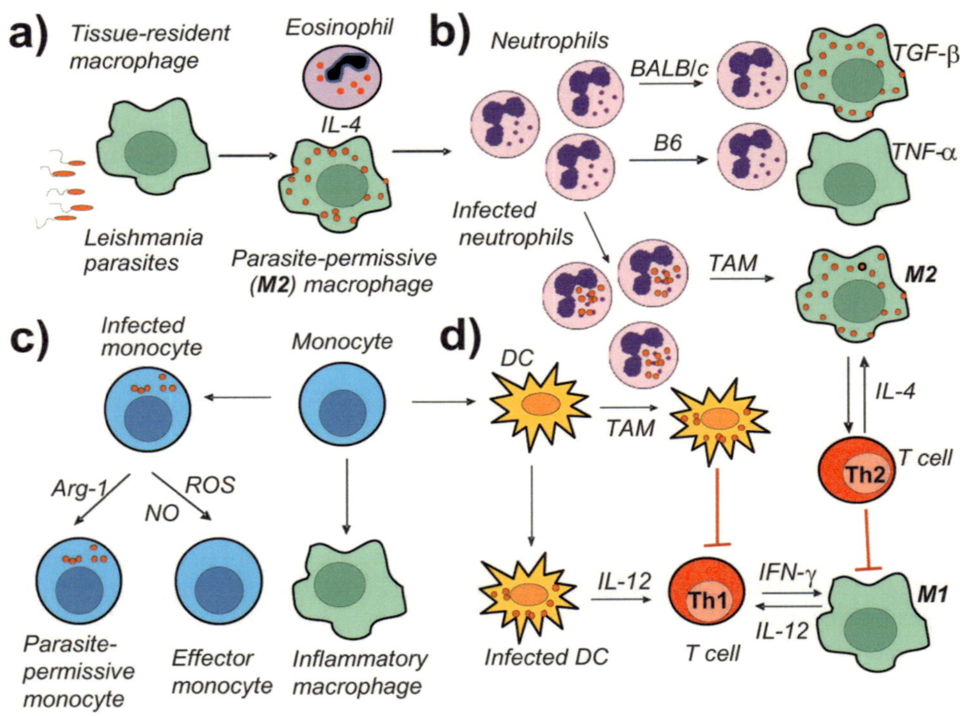

Figure 1.
Macrophages play a key role in immunity to Leishmania *spp.* Leishmania *parasites infect (a) macrophages, (b) neutrophils, (c) monocytes, and (d) dendritic cells (DCs). (a) Dermal-resident M2 are parasite-permissive host cells, maintained by eosinophil-derived IL-4. (b) Neutrophils interact with infected macrophages to induce either tumor necrosis factor (TNF)-α-mediated parasite killing or TGF-β-promoted infection in different mouse strains. Infected "trojan horses" neutrophils transfer parasites to macrophages and DC upon TAM-receptor-mediated efferocytosis. (c) Infected monocytes either kill parasites through ROS and NO production or turn into parasite-permissive Arg-1$^+$ host cells. Monocytes can also differentiate into macrophage and DC. (d) Infected DCs secrete IL-12 and induce interferon-γ-(IFN-γ) producing Th1 cells that activate M1 to kill parasites. Otherwise, DCs that interact with apoptotic neutrophils inhibit T cell activation. Upon interaction with apoptotic/infected neutrophils, macrophages became infected and induce IL-4-producing Th2 cells, which alternatively activate (M2) macrophage to perpetuate infection and inhibit M1-mediated parasite killing.*

replication [10]. However, an unbalanced M1 response may lead to exacerbated inflammation and tissue damage [10, 11]. The balance between the microbicidal M1 responses and M2/regulatory macrophages might be the key to successfully overcoming leishmaniasis. Here, we will discuss how the interactions between *Leishmania* parasites and the host immune system affect macrophage phenotypes and how these phenotypical changes determine disease outcomes in leishmaniasis. A better understanding of factors involved in the development of macrophage phenotypes during *Leishmania* infection is important to design therapeutic strategies capable of modulating the pathogenesis of disease.

2. Macrophage phenotypes in leishmaniasis

Although different species of *Leishmania* trigger distinct immune responses [12–14], seminal work catalyzed advances, by employing the experimental *L. major* model of CL, where C57BL/6 (B6) and BALB/c mice are, respectively, resistant and susceptible to infection. In B6 mice, the Th1 cytokine interferon-γ (IFN-γ) induces classically activated macrophages (M1), which express induced nitric oxide synthase (iNOS) and produce NO (nitric oxide) to kill *L. major* parasites [8, 15–17]. By contrast, in BALB/c mice, the Th2 cytokine IL-4 [18] induces alternative activation of macrophages (M2), characterized by arginase-1 expression and pro-infection activity [19]. While the Th1 versus Th2 paradigm explains relatively well macrophage phenotypes in murine *L. major* infection, a more complex picture emerges from infections with different *Leishmania* spp [20, 21]. Whereas *L. major*-infected macrophages rely on T cell cytokines to control infection, *L. braziliensis* directly activates macrophages for parasite killing [22]. Moreover, despite the intrinsic phenotypical differences in B6 and BALB/c macrophages [8], both mouse strains are resistant to *L. braziliensis* infection [23]. Likewise, *L. braziliensis*, but not *L. major* parasites, induces M1 phenotype in inflammatory macrophages from both B6 and BALB/c mice [24]. In human peripheral blood mononuclear cells (PBMCs), *L. braziliensis* induces CXCL10 proinflammatory cytokine, a M1 feature [25]. Furthermore, ML caused by *L. braziliensis* and *L. panamensis* is characterized by Th1-type responses that produce pro-inflammatory cytokines and the presence of macrophages with low parasitism [26]. Accordingly, the induction of M1 macrophages *in vivo* may underlie host resistance following *L. mexicana* and *L. braziliensis* infection [27].

Recently, M1 and M2 macrophages were analyzed in skin biopsies from patients infected with several *Leishmania spp*. M1 macrophages were detected in *L. chagasi* infection, whereas more M2 macrophages were observed in patients infected with *L. amazonensis* than in *L. braziliensis* lesions [14]. In agreement with these findings, DCL caused by *L. (L.) amazonensis* is characterized by a Th2-type immune response with production of anti-inflammatory cytokines associated with highly parasitized macrophages [26, 28, 29]. Moreover, the enhanced survival of intracellular parasites has been correlated with the M2 phenotype [10, 30–32]. Likewise, in PKDL caused by *L. donovani*, there is a decrease in the production of radical oxygen species (ROS) and NO by macrophages that express CD206 and arginase-1, indicating that M2 macrophages are deleterious [33].

Other studies also suggest that preferential infection in M2 cells plays a role in the severity of CL, DCL [30, 31, 34, 35], and VL [36–40]. Intrinsic characteristics of the parasites that result in enhanced survival within human macrophages, such as resistance to NO [41] or, otherwise, increased expression of IL-4 and arginase-1 [42] have been associated with defective parasite control, larger lesions, and longer disease duration. The results discussed here suggest that the polarization of macrophages to M1 or M2 phenotypes following infection with different *Leishmania* species might underlie the disease outcomes.

3. The phenotypes of resident and inflammatory macrophages

Tissue-resident macrophages maintain homeostasis, carry out immunological surveillance, and act in the initiation and resolution of inflammation, depending on environmental factors that induce activation and gene expression [43]. In addition, tissue-resident M2 macrophages promote tissue repair [43, 44].

Dermal-resident M2 macrophages are preferentially infected by *L. major* Seidman (LmSd) strain, isolated from a patient with nonhealing skin lesions. The eosinophil cytokines IL-4 and IL-10 maintain the M2 phenotype [45], even in the Th1-biased B6 mice. Furthermore, dermal-resident M2 macrophages, characterized by high expression of arginase-1 and mannose receptor, are not replaced by inflammatory macrophages after infection [31]. Remarkably, M2 macrophages use mannose receptor, a M2 hallmark, to internalize *Leishmania* parasites [31]. Dermal-resident M2 macrophages were also the predominant cell type infected with the *L. major* Ryan strain at 1 hour and 24 hours after sand fly bite [46]. The preferential parasite growth in resident M2 macrophages may correlate with oxidative deficiency compared to that of inflammatory macrophages [19, 47]. Likewise, liver-resident Kupffer cells have defective ROS generation after infection with *L. donovani in vivo* or *in vitro* compared to monocyte-derived macrophages [48, 49].

After recognition of the pathogen, resident macrophages drive neutrophil and monocyte influx from the blood. The importance of resident macrophages in the initiation of inflammatory responses is evident after their depletion, which affects the production of chemokines and, consequently, the influx of neutrophils and monocytes [50]. The number of recruited cells exceeded the number of resident cells by 500-fold 14 days after B6 mice infection with *L. amazonensis* [51]. Similarly, $F4/80^{hi}$ peritoneal macrophages were replaced by $CD11b^{+}Ly6C^{+}F4/80^{int}$ monocytes 1–2 days after peritoneal infection with *L. major* or *L. braziliensis* [24].

At the beginning of *L. major* infection, parasites are observed inside immature monocytes recruited to the site of infection both in susceptible BALB/c and resistant B6 mice [52]. Over the first few days, inflammatory monocytes become the main infected cells [53]. However, as the infection progresses, monocytes eliminate the parasites while they differentiate into macrophages [52, 54]. In B6 mice, inflammatory monocytes recruited at 4 h post intraperitoneal infection with *L. major* efficiently kill parasites via ROS [55]. In addition, inflammatory monocytes recruited 24 h after *L. major* infection show NO-dependent leishmanicidal activity [56]. Furthermore, *in vivo* injection of these cells at the time of infection helped infected B6 mice to control skin lesions and reduce parasite burden [56]. Therefore, B6 inflammatory monocytes are effector cells against *L. major* parasites [55, 56].

Leishmania parasites that infect resident macrophages or inflammatory monocytes may have different fates, depending on the different stages of maturation and functional profiles of their host cells. In *L. major* infection, immature inflammatory macrophages fail to induce an M1 response in BALB/c mice. By contrast, in *L. braziliensis* infection, both B6 and BALB/c convert inflammatory macrophages to M1 ($IL\text{-}12^{+}$ and $iNOS^{+}$) phenotype and reduce arginase-1 expression [24]. Overall, these results agree with the idea that resistance to *Leishmania* infection correlates with inflammatory macrophage maturation into M1 in a mouse strain and *Leishmania* spp.-dependent fashion.

Nonetheless, monocytes may stand as a highly permissive niche for replication of *Leishmania* parasites in the dermis [51, 57, 58]. CD11b$^+$Ly6C$^+$ CCR2$^+$ monocytes acquire an alternatively activated phenotype (CD206$^+$arginase-1$^+$) and provide a primary reservoir for parasite replication during the first few weeks of *L. amazonensis* infection, in spite of a strong Th1 response [51]. The dichotomy between the studies can be explained by the difficulty of identifying the resident or inflammatory macrophages, as well as the use of different mouse lineages, sites of infection, and *Leishmania* species (and strains), which can preferentially infect distinct host cells. Further investigation is required to address the functional phenotypes of resident and inflammatory macrophages and their consequences on parasite replication and the outcome of leishmaniasis.

4. The interplay with neutrophils shapes macrophage phenotypes

The interactions between macrophages and neutrophils may regulate the course of *Leishmania* infection (**Figure 1**) [7]. There is a rapid recruitment of neutrophils to the site of infection with several *Leishmania* species in mice and hamsters [52, 59–62]. Neutrophils can modulate the development of an anti-*Leishmania* immune response by secreting cytokines, chemokines, and granule contents, and by interacting with inflammatory monocytes, macrophages and DCs at the infection site [53, 63–66]. The presence of neutrophils at the site of infection may contribute to the induction of a Th2-M2 response and correlate with susceptibility to *L. major* infection in BALB/c mice, where the percentage of neutrophils is maintained high and stable for weeks in the inoculated footpad. Accordingly, the depletion of neutrophils 6 h before challenge with *L. major* promotes partial resistance [63]. By contrast, neutrophils are only transiently recruited to the infection site in resistant B6 mice, while mononuclear phagocytes become the predominant cell population (80%) [52]. Nonetheless, by using the sandy fly model of *L. major* infection, the images obtained from the infection site revealed that many parasites are phagocytosed by neutrophils [62] and that dermal-resident macrophages became infected via phagocytosis of parasitized neutrophils [46]. These studies provide *in vivo* evidence for the "Trojan Horse" hypothesis in leishmaniasis, whereas the silent entry of the parasite into macrophages through the phagocytosis of infected and apoptotic neutrophils had been observed *in vitro* [67, 68].

Other studies that employed cocultured neutrophils and infected macrophages suggest that the interactions between these cells can have different consequences in *L. major* infection in a mouse strain-dependent manner [7, 65]. Neutrophil interaction with infected macrophages from B6 mice reduces parasite burden by activating macrophages to a leishmanicidal and tumor necrosis factor (TNF)-α-producing phenotype via a TLR4 and neutrophil elastase (NE)-dependent pathway [64]. On the other hand, phagocytosis of apoptotic neutrophils by infected BALB/c macrophages promotes parasite growth [65]. Interestingly, B6 neutrophils release 2–3 times more NE than BALB/c neutrophils [64]. These results suggest that recruited B6 neutrophils shape macrophage phenotype to control parasite infection. However, if the clearance of B6 apoptotic neutrophils occurs prior to macrophage infection, it imprints an M2 regulatory phenotype (IL-12^{low}IL-10^{high}), which is permissive to *L. major* replication and helps to establish infection [69]. It is conceivable that neutrophils might interact with macrophages both prior and after their infection with *Leishmania* parasites, leading to opposite outcomes.

Several receptors, including the Tyro-3, Axl, and Mer (TAM) receptors, contribute to the phagocytosis of apoptotic cells or efferocytosis. The TAM Axl and Mer receptors may play a role in the efferocytosis of infected apoptotic neutrophils and parasite transfer to macrophages and DCs in *Leishmania* infection [46, 70]. In addition, dermal-resident macrophages from Axl- and Mer-deficient mice showed reduced frequency of arginase-1^+ cells and increased expression of iNOS. Therefore, the efferocytosis via TAM receptors polarizes dermal-resident macrophages to an M2 phenotype and contributes to early infection [46]. $Axl^{-/-}Mertk^{-/-}$ mice also exhibited reduced parasite loads but had more severe pathology after sand fly-borne *L. major* infection [46].

The phenotypes of macrophages after interacting with neutrophils may also depend on the parasite species. Neutrophils and macrophages cooperate in *L. braziliensis* infection by promoting resistance in infected B6 and BALB/c mice [71]. In BALB/c experimental model, the depletion of neutrophils leads to a significant increase in the parasite load [72]. In addition, BALB/c mice inoculated with parasites and neutrophils exhibited lower parasite load at the site of infection and draining lymph nodes. *In vitro*, it was observed that neutrophils significantly reduced the parasite load in macrophages from BALB/c mice infected with *L. braziliensis*, an effect associated with an increase in TNF-α and superoxide production [72]. This outcome differs from the previous mentioned studies with *L. major* infection, where the interaction of infected BALB/c macrophages with apoptotic neutrophils favors the multiplication of the parasite [63, 65].

Neutrophils can also intervene in the macrophage phenotype by indirectly influencing the T cell response after interacting with DCs. DCs infected through efferocytosis of apoptotic and infected neutrophils fail to activate T cells in lymph nodes [53] and probably delay the Th1 responses that would activate M1 macrophages. There are other factors that can regulate macrophage phenotype during interaction with neutrophils. In natural *Leishmania* infection, sand fly saliva is inoculated in the dermal site of infection. The saliva components accelerate the apoptosis of inflammatory neutrophils [73] and upregulate the Th2 response while downregulating the Th1 response during *L. major* infection [74]. In addition, sand fly saliva components positively interfere with the production of prostaglandin E2 and IL-10 which can inhibit macrophage activation and reduce the production of TNF-α, NO, and H2O2, leading to a M2-parasite-permissive phenotype [75].

5. The crosstalk with T cells modulates macrophage phenotypes

Many studies have characterized the participation of CD4 and CD8 T cells in both protection and pathology in *Leishmania* infection in mice and humans. M1 (classically activated) and M2 (alternatively activated) macrophages have been studied in the context of the Th1-Th2 paradigm [76]. The crosstalk between T cells and macrophages has been correlated with resistance *versus* susceptibility in models involving different *Leishmania* species and animal strains. While some studies demonstrate that Th1/M1 responses mediate immunity to *L. major* parasites in resistant B6 mice, Th2/M2 cells underlie susceptibility to *L. major* infection in BALB/c mice [10, 77]. The Th2 cytokines IL-4, IL10, and IL-13 produced during infection with *L. amazonensis* and *L. panamensis* can drive macrophage polarization toward the M2 phenotype, via activation of the enzyme arginase-1 and production of L-ornithine, favoring the survival and growth of *Leishmania* in macrophages, as well as disease progression [10, 32, 78]. In *L. major*-susceptible mice, arginase activity is directly related to parasite growth [79, 80] and the inhibition of its activity reduces parasite load [80, 81]. *In vitro* studies have already shown that *L. amazonensis*-infected BALB/c macrophages show increased L-arginine uptake and arginase expression [82].

The correlation between Th1-IFN-γ and macrophage-NO is reinforced in studies showing that mice deficient for the expression of IFN-γ or IFN-γ receptor in macrophages do not produce NO in response to various stimuli, suggesting that IFN-γ is a key inducer of iNOS [83, 84]. In addition, mice otherwise resistant to *L. major* infection that were deficient for the gene encoding iNOS [85] or treated with an iNOS enzyme inhibitor [86] became susceptible to infection. Similarly, other studies link the Th2-IL-4 and macrophage-arginase-1 axis to *Leishmania* susceptibility [87]. Although the role of IL-4 in *Leishmania* infection remains overall controversial [7, 20, 88–90], Holscher *et al.* have shown that interleukin-4 receptorα (IL-4Rα) deficiency in phagocytes results in a delay in the progression of leishmaniasis [87], probably by blocking alternative macrophage activation.

Finally, type 1 immune responses are not always beneficial to the host. An exacerbated Th1 cytokine response may contribute to the pathology in mucocutaneous leishmaniasis, for example during *L. braziliensis* infection [91, 92]. Interestingly, the IFN-γ produced by Th1 cells early during *L. amazonensis* infection mediates the expansion and recruitment of $CCR2^+$ inflammatory monocytes that provide, at the site of infection, a reservoir of parasite-permissive cells that undergo alternative activation [51]. Therefore, the paradigm that establishes that resistance *versus* susceptibility correlates with macrophage activation is not absolute and needs further studies. Part of the problem relies on the need of complex subtyping of intermediate phenotypes lying between the extreme poles (M1 and M2) of macrophage activation [93].

6. Tools for skewing M1 and M2 phenotypes and disease outcome

Leishmaniasis represents a major challenge for Public Health owing to the lack of vaccines, toxicity of available CL treatment, and their incomplete effectiveness [94]. Multiple factors can explain the difficult in generating new effective vaccines and lower toxic therapies, mainly the diversity of *Leishmania* species and the complexity of the host immune responses [95]. As an obligate intracellular parasite, residing inside macrophages, *Leishmania* evolved in contact with the host immune system, developing mechanisms to evade or modulate the immune response, which further hamper the development of vaccines [17, 33]. New avenues for the development of therapies aimed at the regulation, activation, or polarization/repolarization of macrophages bring hope for the treatment of leishmaniasis. Here, we discuss some studies (2011–2020) that show the potential use of therapies targeting M1/M2 plasticity in different *Leishmania* spp. infection and how each one can directly modulate macrophage phenotypes.

In PKDL caused by *L. donovani*, there is a decrease in the production of ROS and NO by monocytes and an increase in the expression of CD206 and arginase-1, which are hallmarks of M2 macrophages [33]. However, after chemotherapy with anti-leishmanial drugs, macrophages show an M1 profile, indicating that M2 to M1 repolarization can be considered as a therapeutic approach [33].

Macrophages infected with *L. donovani* acquire an M2 phenotype through the mammalian Target of Rapamycin (mTOR) pathway, as demonstrated in experiments where mTOR inhibition reduced M2 macrophages and parasite load. *In vivo*, the blockade of mTOR pathway increased NO, IL-12, and IFN-γ and reduced IL-10 and arginase-1 and parasite burden in the spleen [39]. Likewise, the treatment of *L. amazonensis*-infected macrophages with the snake venom component crotoxin increased the production of NO, IL-6, and TNF-α, which are hallmarks of M1 activation profile associated with leishmanicidal activity [96].

The alteration of miRNA expression in parasite infection has been studied in the context of macrophage plasticity. *L. donovani*, *L. major*, and *L. amazonensis* induce alterations of miRNA profiles in infected human and murine macrophages [32, 97, 98]. Inhibition of miR-294 or miR721/Nos2 interactions increased iNOS expression and NO production and reduced *L. amazonensis* infection. The role of miR-294 and miR-721 in the regulation of iNOS expression during *Leishmania* replication in infected macrophages points to miRNAs as targets for drug development [32]. Thus, microRNAs control macrophage plasticity, as mechanisms that sustain or impair the expression of M1/M2 genes, with the redirection of macrophage phenotype according to environmental signals [99].

In vitro activation of glucose-6-phosphate dehydrogenase (G6PDH) in *L. major*-infected macrophage regulates macrophage function, by increasing NO production and parasite killing [100]. The modulation of host metabolism during infection may represent a potential therapeutic target for treating leishmaniasis, and metabolic reprogramming of immune cells such as macrophages and monocytes could dictate their ability as effector cells or parasite-permissive reservoirs [101].

Recent studies showed that B6 peritoneal macrophages express the receptor RANK and the M2 markers CD301 (MGL) and CD206. The treatment of B6 macrophages with the T cell cytokines RANKL and IFN-γ induced M1 macrophages capable of producing IL-12, TNF-α, and NO but reduced MGL and arginase-1 expression. In addition, RANKL and IFN-γ increased NO production by BALB/c macrophages. Therefore, RANKL helps IFN-γ to induce a shift in macrophage phenotype from M2 to a M1 profile that is effective in controlling *L. major* infection [102].

By contrast, treatment of bone-marrow-derived macrophages with ATRA (all-*trans* retinoic acid) prevented the induction of M1 macrophages, promoting a shift from M1 to M2 phenotype [24]. After treatment with ATRA, inflammatory macrophages from B6 mice lost their ability to eliminate *L. major* parasites [24, 56]. In addition, mice treated with ATRA developed increased footpad lesions and parasite burden in draining lymph nodes [56]. After intraperitoneal injection, ATRA reduced pro-inflammatory cytokines, iNOS expression, NO production, and increased parasite infection in macrophages [24]. Possibly, ATRA downregulates inflammatory responses, by reducing the activation of nuclear factor-κB (NF-κB) in macrophages [103], whereas RANKL, in turn, induces the NF-κB signaling pathway and M1 responses [102]. Therefore, the NF-κB pathway might be at the crossroads of M1-M2 regulation and stands as a potential therapeutic target to potentiate immunity to infection or otherwise to reduce inflammation [103]. Whereas manipulation of macrophage phenotypes is a new perspective to direct the development of therapeutic strategies to intervene in multiple diseases, care is advised, considering the potential side effects on inflammation and host susceptibility to intracellular pathogens.

DOI: http://dx.doi.org/10.5772/intechopen.105571

7. Conclusion

The studies discussed here show that different manifestations caused by *Leishmania* infection rely on parasite-host cell interface. We also discussed how interactions with different species of *Leishmania*, innate cells, and adaptive immunity during infection generate changes in macrophage phenotypes and how this change of phenotype can alter the disease outcome in leishmaniasis. *Leishmania* species and different virulence factors may have an immunomodulatory effect on macrophages, leading to polarization toward an M2 phenotype, thus circumventing the host microbicidal mechanisms to favor their proliferation. On the other hand, M1 macrophages equilibrate between beneficial microbicidal activity and deleterious inflammatory response that can exacerbate lesions. The key to prevent pathogenesis in *Leishmania* infection may lie in a balance between resident and inflammatory macrophage phenotypes, particularly early in the infection, aiming to provide the best outcome to the host. Further studies will unveil the details involved in the complex balance between parasites and macrophages, providing new targets for future treatments and vaccines that shape macrophage phenotypes and control the pathogenesis of leishmaniasis. Finally, as immune responses against different types of leishmaniasis are multifactorial and distinct, we agree that the generation of different treatments or vaccines may be more effective than a single solution for leishmaniasis [17].

Acknowledgements

The authors' work cited here was supported by the Brazilian National Research Council (Conselho Nacional de Desenvolvimento Científico e Tecnológico, CNPq, Brazil), the Rio de Janeiro State Science Foundation (Fundação Carlos Chagas Filho de Amparo à Pesquisa do Estado do Rio de Janeiro, FAPERJ), the American Association of Immunologists (AAI), and the Oswaldo Cruz Foundation (Fundação Oswaldo Cruz, FIOCRUZ).

Conflict of interest

The authors declare no conflict of interest.

Author details

Natália S. Vellozo[1*†], Flávia L. Ribeiro-Gomes[2†] and Marcela F. Lopes[1]

1 Carlos Chagas Filho Institute of Biophysics, Federal University of Rio de Janeiro (UFRJ), Rio de Janeiro, Brazil

2 Oswaldo Cruz Institute, Oswaldo Cruz Foundation (FIOCRUZ), Rio de Janeiro, Brazil

*Address all correspondence to: nataliavellozo@biof.ufrj.br

† These authors contributed equally to this work.

References

[1] Burza S, Croft SL, Boelaert M. Leishmaniasis. Lancet. 2018;**392**:951-970

[2] Alvar J, Velez ID, Bern C, Herrero M, Desjeux P, Cano J, et al. Leishmaniasis worldwide and global estimates of its incidence. PloS One. 2012;7:e35671

[3] Scott P, Novais FO. Cutaneous leishmaniasis: Immune responses in protection and pathogenesis. Nature Reviews in Immunology. 2016;**16**:581-592

[4] Chappuis F, Sundar S, Hailu A, Ghalib H, Rijal S, Peeling RW, et al. Visceral leishmaniasis: What are the needs for diagnosis, treatment and control? Nature Reviews in Microbiology. 2007;**5**:873-882

[5] Pace D. Leishmaniasis. The Journal of Infection. 2014;**69**(Suppl 1):S10-S18

[6] Liu D, Uzonna JE. The early interaction of *Leishmania* with macrophages and dendritic cells and its influence on the host immune response. Frontiers in Cellular and Infection Microbiology. 2012;**2**:83

[7] Lopes MF, Costa-da-Silva AC, DosReis GA. Innate immunity to *Leishmania* infection: Within phagocytes. Mediators Inflammation. 2014;**2014**:754965

[8] Mills CD, Kincaid K, Alt JM, Heilman MJ, Hill AM. M-1/M-2 macrophages and the Th1/Th2 paradigm. Journal of Immunology. 2000;**164**:6166-6173

[9] Murray PJ, Allen JE, Biswas SK, Fisher EA, Gilroy DW, Goerdt S, et al. Macrophage activation and polarization: Nomenclature and experimental guidelines. Immunity. 2014;**41**:14-20

[10] Tomiotto-Pellissier F, Bortoleti B, Assolini JP, Goncalves MD, Carloto ACM, Miranda-Sapla MM, et al. Macrophage polarization in leishmaniasis: Broadening horizons. Frontiers in Immunology. 2018;**9**:2529

[11] Laskin DL, Sunil VR, Gardner CR, Laskin JD. Macrophages and tissue injury: Agents of defense or destruction? Annual Review of Pharmacology and Toxicology. 2011;**51**:267-288

[12] Mendonca SC. Differences in immune responses against *Leishmania* induced by infection and by immunization with killed parasite antigen: Implications for vaccine discovery. Parasites & Vectors. 2016;**9**:492

[13] Silveira FT. What makes mucosal and anergic diffuse cutaneous leishmaniases so clinically and immunopathogically different? A review in Brazil. Transactions of the Royal Society of Tropical Medicine and Hygiene. 2019:trz037

[14] Sandoval Pacheco CM, Araujo Flores GV, Gonzalez K, de Castro Gomes CM, Passero LFD, Tomokane TY, et al. Macrophage polarization in the skin lesion caused by neotropical species of *Leishmania* sp. Journal of Immunology Research. 2021;**2021**:5596876

[15] Assreuy J, Cunha FQ, Epperlein M, Noronha-Dutra A, O'Donnell CA, Liew FY, et al. Production of nitric oxide and superoxide by activated macrophages and killing of *Leishmania major*. European Journal of Immunology. 1994;**24**:672-676

[16] Mantovani A, Sozzani S, Locati M, Allavena P, Sica A. Macrophage polarization: Tumor-associated

macrophages as a paradigm for polarized M2 mononuclear phagocytes. Trends in Immunology. 2002;**23**:549-555

[17] Rossi M, Fasel N. How to master the host immune system? *Leishmania* parasites have the solutions! International Immunology. 2018;**30**:103-111

[18] Chatelain R, Varkila K, Coffman RL. IL-4 induces a Th2 response in *Leishmania major*-infected mice. Journal of Immunology. 1992;**148**:1182-1187

[19] Pessenda G, da Silva JS. Arginase and its mechanisms in *Leishmania* persistence. Parasite Immunology. 2020;**42**:e12722

[20] Alexander J, Bryson K. T helper (h)1/Th2 and *Leishmania*: Paradox rather than paradigm. Immunology Letters. 2005;**99**:17-23

[21] McMahon-Pratt D, Alexander J. Does the *Leishmania major* paradigm of pathogenesis and protection hold for New World cutaneous leishmaniases or the visceral disease? Immunological Review. 2004;**201**:206-224

[22] Scott P, Sher A. A spectrum in the susceptibility of leishmanial strains to intracellular killing by murine macrophages. Journal of Immunology. 1986;**136**:1461-1466

[23] Rocha FJ, Schleicher U, Mattner J, Alber G, Bogdan C. Cytokines, signaling pathways, and effector molecules required for the control of *Leishmania (Viannia) braziliensis* in mice. Infection and Immunity. 2007;**75**:3823-3832

[24] Vellozo NS, Pereira-Marques ST, Cabral-Piccin MP, Filardy AA, Ribeiro-Gomes FL, Rigoni TS, et al. All-trans retinoic acid promotes an M1- to M2-phenotype shift and inhibits macrophage-mediated immunity to *Leishmania major*. Frontiers in Immunology. 2017;**8**:1560

[25] Vargas-Inchaustegui DA, Hogg AE, Tulliano G, Llanos-Cuentas A, Arevalo J, Endsley JJ, et al. CXCL10 production by human monocytes in response to *Leishmania braziliensis* infection. Infection and Immunity. 2010;**78**: 301-308

[26] Silveira FT, Lainson R, De Castro Gomes CM, Laurenti MD, Corbett CE. Immunopathogenic competences of *Leishmania (V.) braziliensis* and *L. (L.) amazonensis* in American cutaneous leishmaniasis. Parasite Immunology. 2009;**31**:423-431

[27] Diaz-Gandarilla JA, Osorio-Trujillo C, Hernandez-Ramirez VI, Talamas-Rohana P. PPAR activation induces M1 macrophage polarization via cPLA(2)-COX-2 inhibition, activating ROS production against *Leishmania mexicana*. BioMed Research International. 2013;**2013**:215283

[28] Afonso LC, Scott P. Immune responses associated with susceptibility of C57BL/10 mice to *Leishmania amazonensis*. Infection and Immunity. 1993;**61**:2952-2959

[29] Ji J, Sun J, Soong L. Impaired expression of inflammatory cytokines and chemokines at early stages of infection with *Leishmania amazonensis*. Infection and Immunity. 2003;**71**:4278-4288

[30] Farrow AL, Rana T, Mittal MK, Misra S, Chaudhuri G. *Leishmania*-induced repression of selected non-coding RNA genes containing B-box element at their promoters in alternatively polarized M2 macrophages. Molecular and Cellular Biochemistry. 2011;**350**:47-57

[31] Lee SH, Charmoy M, Romano A, Paun A, Chaves MM, Cope FO, et al. Mannose receptor high, M2 dermal macrophages mediate nonhealing *Leishmania major* infection in a Th1 immune environment. Journal of Experimental Medicine. 2018;**215**:357-375

[32] Muxel SM, Laranjeira-Silva MF, Zampieri RA, Floeter-Winter LM. *Leishmania (Leishmania) amazonensis* induces macrophage miR-294 and miR-721 expression and modulates infection by targeting NOS2 and L-arginine metabolism. Scientific Reports. 2017;7:44141

[33] Mukhopadhyay D, Mukherjee S, Roy S, Dalton JE, Kundu S, Sarkar A, et al. M2 polarization of monocytes-macrophages is a hallmark of indian post kala-azar dermal leishmaniasis. PLoS Neglected Tropical Diseases. 2015;**9**:e0004145

[34] Franca-Costa J, Van Weyenbergh J, Boaventura VS, Luz NF, Malta-Santos H, Oliveira MC, et al. Arginase I, polyamine, and prostaglandin E2 pathways suppress the inflammatory response and contribute to diffuse cutaneous leishmaniasis. The Journal of Infectious Diseases. 2015;**211**:426-435

[35] Abebe T, Hailu A, Woldeyes M, Mekonen W, Bilcha K, Cloke T, et al. Local increase of arginase activity in lesions of patients with cutaneous leishmaniasis in Ethiopia. PLoS Neglected Tropical Diseases. 2012;**6**:e1684

[36] Chan MM, Adapala N, Chen C. Peroxisome proliferator-activated receptor-gamma-mediated polarization of macrophages in *Leishmania* infection. PPAR Research. 2012;**2012**:796235

[37] Abebe T, Takele Y, Weldegebreal T, Cloke T, Closs E, Corset C, et al. Arginase activity - a marker of disease status in patients with visceral leishmaniasis in ethiopia. PLoS Neglected Tropical Diseases. 2013;**7**:e2134

[38] Silva RL, Santos MB, Almeida PL, Barros TS, Magalhaes L, Cazzaniga RA, et al. sCD163 levels as a biomarker of disease severity in leprosy and visceral leishmaniasis. PLoS Neglected Tropical diseases. 2017;**11**:e0005486

[39] Kumar A, Das S, Mandal A, Verma S, Abhishek K, Kumar A, et al. *Leishmania* infection activates host mTOR for its survival by M2 macrophage polarization. Parasite Immunology. 2018;**40**:e12586

[40] Roy S, Mukhopadhyay D, Mukherjee S, Moulik S, Chatterji S, Brahme N, et al. An IL-10 dominant polarization of monocytes is a feature of Indian Visceral Leishmaniasis. Parasite Immunology. 2018;**40**:e12535

[41] Giudice A, Camada I, Leopoldo PT, Pereira JM, Riley LW, Wilson ME, et al. Resistance of *Leishmania (Leishmania) amazonensis* and *Leishmania (Viannia) braziliensis* to nitric oxide correlates with disease severity in Tegumentary Leishmaniasis. BMC Infectious Diseases. 2007;7:7

[42] Costa DL, Carregaro V, Lima-Junior DS, Silva NM, Milanezi CM, Cardoso CR, et al. BALB/c mice infected with antimony treatment refractory isolate of *Leishmania braziliensis* present severe lesions due to IL-4 production. PLoS Neglected Tropical Diseases. 2011;**5**:e965

[43] Davies LC, Jenkins SJ, Allen JE, Taylor PR. Tissue-resident macrophages. Nature Immunology. 2013;**14**:986-995

[44] Wynn TA, Vannella KM. Macrophages in tissue repair,

regeneration, and fibrosis. Immunity. 2016;**44**:450-462

[45] Lee SH, Chaves MM, Kamenyeva O, Gazzinelli-Guimaraes PH, Kang B, Pessenda G, et al. M2-like, dermal macrophages are Maintained via IL-4/ CCL24-mediated cooperative interaction with eosinophils in cutaneous leishmaniasis. Science Immunology. 2020;**2016**:eaaz4415

[46] Chaves MM, Lee SH, Kamenyeva O, Ghosh K, Peters NC, Sacks D. The role of dermis resident macrophages and their interaction with neutrophils in the early establishment of *Leishmania major* infection transmitted by sand fly bite. PLoS Pathogens. 2020;**16**:e1008674

[47] Locksley RM, Heinzel FP, Fankhauser JE, Nelson CS, Sadick MD. Cutaneous host defense in leishmaniasis: Interaction of isolated dermal macrophages and epidermal Langerhans cells with the insect-stage promastigote. Infection and Immunity. 1988;**56**:336-342

[48] Lepay DA, Nathan CF, Steinman RM, Murray HW, Cohn ZA. Murine Kupffer cells. Mononuclear phagocytes deficient in the generation of reactive oxygen intermediates. Journal of Experimental Medicine. 1985;**161**:1079-1096

[49] Kausalya S, Kaur S, Malla N, Ganguly NK, Mahajan RC. Microbicidal mechanisms of liver macrophages in experimental visceral leishmaniasis. APMIS : Acta Pathologica, Microbiologica, et immunologica Scandinavica. 1996;**104**:171-175

[50] Cailhier JF, Partolina M, Vuthoori S, Wu S, Ko K, Watson S, et al. Conditional macrophage ablation demonstrates that resident macrophages initiate acute peritoneal inflammation. Journal of Immunology. 2005;**174**:2336-2342

[51] Carneiro MBH, Lopes ME, Hohman LS, Romano A, David BA, Kratofil R, et al. Th1-Th2 cross-regulation controls early *Leishmania* infection in the skin by modulating the size of the permissive monocytic host cell reservoir. Cell Host Microbes. 2020;**27**:752-768

[52] Beil WJ, Meinardus-Hager G, Neugebauer DC, Sorg C. Differences in the onset of the inflammatory response to cutaneous leishmaniasis in resistant and susceptible mice. Journal of Leukocyte Biology. 1992;**52**:135-142

[53] Ribeiro-Gomes FL, Peters NC, Debrabant A, Sacks D. Efficient capture of infected neutrophils by dendritic cells in the skin inhibits the early anti-*Leishmania* response. PLoS Pathogens. 2012;**8**:e1002536

[54] Sunderkotter C, Kunz M, Steinbrink K, Meinardus-Hager G, Goebeler M, Bildau H, et al. Resistance of mice to experimental leishmaniasis is associated with more rapid appearance of mature macrophages in vitro and in vivo. Journal of Immunology. 1993;**151**:4891-4901

[55] Goncalves R, Zhang X, Cohen H, Debrabant A, Mosser DM. Platelet activation attracts a subpopulation of effector monocytes to sites of *Leishmania major* infection. Journal of Experimental Medicine. 2011;**208**:1253-1265

[56] Pereira WF, Ribeiro-Gomes FL, Guillermo LV, Vellozo NS, Montalvao F, Dosreis GA, et al. Myeloid-derived suppressor cells help protective immunity to *Leishmania major* infection despite suppressed T cell responses. Journal of Leukocyte Biology. 2011;**90**:1191-1197

[57] Romano A, Carneiro MBH, Doria NA, Roma EH, Ribeiro-Gomes FL, Inbar E, et al. Divergent roles for

Ly6C+CCR2+CX3CR1+ inflammatory monocytes during primary or secondary infection of the skin with the intra-phagosomal pathogen *Leishmania major*. PLoS Pathogens. 2017;**13**:e1006479

[58] Heyde S, Philipsen L, Formaglio P, Fu Y, Baars I, Hobbel G, et al. CD11c-expressing Ly6C+CCR2+ monocytes constitute a reservoir for efficient *Leishmania* proliferation and cell-to-cell transmission. PLoS Pathogens. 2018;**14**:e1007374

[59] Wilson ME, Innes DJ, Sousa AD, Pearson RD. Early histopathology of experimental infection with *Leishmania donovani* in hamsters. The Journal of Parasitology. 1987;**73**:55-63

[60] Pompeu ML, Freitas LA, Santos ML, Khouri M, Barral-Netto M. Granulocytes in the inflammatory process of BALB/c mice infected by *Leishmania amazonensis*. A quantitative approach. Acta Tropica. 1991;**48**:185-193

[61] Hurrell BP, Schuster S, Grun E, Coutaz M, Williams RA, Held W, et al. Rapid sequestration of *Leishmania mexicana* by neutrophils contributes to the development of chronic lesion. PLoS Pathogens. 2015;**11**:e1004929

[62] Peters NC, Egen JG, Secundino N, Debrabant A, Kimblin N, Kamhawi S, et al. In vivo imaging reveals an essential role for neutrophils in Leishmaniasis transmitted by sand flies. Science. 2008;**321**:970-974

[63] Tacchini-Cottier F, Zweifel C, Belkaid Y, Mukankundiye C, Vasei M, Launois P, et al. An immunomodulatory function for neutrophils during the induction of a CD4+ Th2 response in BALB/c mice infected with *Leishmania major*. Journal of Immunology. 2000;**165**:2628-2636

[64] Ribeiro-Gomes FL, Moniz-de-Souza MC, Alexandre-Moreira MS, Dias WB, Lopes MF, Nunes MP, et al. Neutrophils activate macrophages for intracellular killing of *Leishmania major* through recruitment of TLR4 by neutrophil elastase. Journal of Immunology. 2007;**179**:3988-3994

[65] Ribeiro-Gomes FL, Otero AC, Gomes NA, Moniz-De-Souza MC, Cysne-Finkelstein L, Arnholdt AC, et al. Macrophage interactions with neutrophils regulate *Leishmania major* infection. Journal of Immunology. 2004;**172**:4454-4462

[66] Charmoy M, Megnekou R, Allenbach C, Zweifel C, Perez C, Monnat K, et al. *Leishmania major* induces distinct neutrophil phenotypes in mice that are resistant or susceptible to infection. Journal of Leukocyte Biology. 2007;**82**:288-299

[67] van Zandbergen G, Klinger M, Mueller A, Dannenberg S, Gebert A, Solbach W, et al. Cutting edge: Neutrophil granulocyte serves as a vector for *Leishmania* entry into macrophages. Journal of Immunology. 2004;**173**:6521-6525

[68] Gueirard P, Laplante A, Rondeau C, Milon G, Desjardins M. Trafficking of *Leishmania donovani* promastigotes in non-lytic compartments in neutrophils enables the subsequent transfer of parasites to macrophages. Cellular Microbiology. 2008;**10**:100-111

[69] Filardy AA, Pires DR, Nunes MP, Takiya CM, Freire-de-Lima CG, Ribeiro-Gomes FL, et al. Proinflammatory clearance of apoptotic neutrophils induces an IL-12(low) IL-10(high) regulatory phenotype in macrophages. Journal of Immunology. 2010;**185**:2044-2050

[70] Ribeiro-Gomes FL, Romano A, Lee S, Roffe E, Peters NC, Debrabant A, et al. Apoptotic cell clearance of *Leishmania major*-infected neutrophils by dendritic cells inhibits CD8(+) T-cell priming in vitro by Mer tyrosine kinase-dependent signaling. Cell Death Diseases. 2015;**6**:e2018

[71] Carlsen ED, Jie Z, Liang Y, Henard CA, Hay C, Sun J, et al. Interactions between neutrophils and *Leishmania braziliensis* amastigotes facilitate cell activation and parasite clearance. Journal of Innate Immunity. 2015;**7**:354-363

[72] Novais FO, Santiago RC, Bafica A, Khouri R, Afonso L, Borges VM, et al. Neutrophils and macrophages cooperate in host resistance against *Leishmania braziliensis* infection. Journal of Immunology. 2009;**183**:8088-8098

[73] Prates DB, Araujo-Santos T, Luz NF, Andrade BB, Franca-Costa J, Afonso L, et al. *Lutzomyia longipalpis* saliva drives apoptosis and enhances parasite burden in neutrophils. Journal of Leukocyte Biology. 2011;**90**:575-582

[74] Mbow ML, Bleyenberg JA, Hall LR, Titus RG. Phlebotomus papatasi sand fly salivary gland lysate down-regulates a Th1, but up-regulates a Th2, response in mice infected with *Leishmania major*. Journal of Immunology. 1998;**161**:5571-5577

[75] Brodie TM, Smith MC, Morris RV, Titus RG. Immunomodulatory effects of the *Lutzomyia longipalpis* salivary gland protein maxadilan on mouse macrophages. Infection and Immunity. 2007;**75**:2359-2365

[76] Muraille E, Leo O, Moser M. TH1/TH2 paradigm extended: Macrophage polarization as an unappreciated pathogen-driven escape mechanism? Frontiers in Immunology. 2014;**5**:603

[77] Sacks D, Noben-Trauth N. The immunology of susceptibility and resistance to *Leishmania major* in mice. Nature Reviews in Immunology. 2002;**2**:845-858

[78] da Silva MF, Zampieri RA, Muxel SM, Beverley SM, Floeter-Winter LM. *Leishmania amazonensis* arginase compartmentalization in the glycosome is important for parasite infectivity. PloS One. 2012;**7**:e34022

[79] Iniesta V, Carcelen J, Molano I, Peixoto PM, Redondo E, Parra P, et al. Arginase I induction during *Leishmania major* infection mediates the development of disease. Infection and Immunity. 2005;**73**:6085-6090

[80] Kropf P, Fuentes JM, Fahnrich E, Arpa L, Herath S, Weber V, et al. Arginase and polyamine synthesis are key factors in the regulation of experimental leishmaniasis in vivo. FASEB Journal: Official Publication of the Federation of American Societies for Experimental Biology. 2005;**19**:1000-1002

[81] Schleicher U, Paduch K, Debus A, Obermeyer S, Konig T, Kling JC, et al. TNF-mediated restriction of arginase 1 expression in myeloid cells triggers Type 2 NO synthase activity at the site of infection. Cell Reports. 2016;**15**:1062-1075

[82] Muxel SM, Aoki JI, Fernandes JCR, Laranjeira-Silva MF, Zampieri RA, Acuna SM, et al. Arginine and POLYAMINES FATE in *Leishmania* infection. Frontiers in Microbiology. 2017;**8**:2682

[83] Dalton DK, Pitts-Meek S, Keshav S, Figari IS, Bradley A, Stewart TA. Multiple defects of immune cell function in mice with disrupted interferon-gamma genes. Science. 1993;**259**:1739-1742

[84] Huang S, Hendriks W, Althage A, Hemmi S, Bluethmann H, Kamijo R, et al. Immune response in mice that lack the interferon-gamma receptor. Science. 1993;**259**:1742-1745

[85] Wei XQ, Charles IG, Smith A, Ure J, Feng GJ, Huang FP, et al. Altered immune responses in mice lacking inducible nitric oxide synthase. Nature. 1995;**375**:408-411

[86] Stenger S, Donhauser N, Thuring H, Rollinghoff M, Bogdan C. Reactivation of latent leishmaniasis by inhibition of inducible nitric oxide synthase. Journal of Experimental Medicine. 1996;**183**:1501-1514

[87] Holscher C, Arendse B, Schwegmann A, Myburgh E, Brombacher F. Impairment of alternative macrophage activation delays cutaneous leishmaniasis in nonhealing BALB/c mice. Journal of Immunology. 2006;**176**:1115-1121

[88] Biedermann T, Zimmermann S, Himmelrich H, Gumy A, Egeter O, Sakrauski AK, et al. IL-4 instructs TH1 responses and resistance to *Leishmania major* in susceptible BALB/c mice. Nature Immunology. 2001;**2**:1054-1060

[89] Radwanska M, Cutler AJ, Hoving JC, Magez S, Holscher C, Bohms A, et al. Deletion of IL-4Ralpha on CD4 T cells renders BALB/c mice resistant to *Leishmania major* infection. PLoS Pathogens. 2007;**3**:e68

[90] Hurdayal R, Nieuwenhuizen NE, Revaz-Breton M, Smith L, Hoving JC, Parihar SP, et al. Deletion of IL-4 receptor alpha on dendritic cells renders BALB/c mice hypersusceptible to *Leishmania major* infection. PLoS Pathogens. 2013;**9**:e1003699

[91] Gaze ST, Dutra WO, Lessa M, Lessa H, Guimaraes LH, Jesus AR, et al. Mucosal leishmaniasis patients display an activated inflammatory T-cell phenotype associated with a nonbalanced monocyte population. Scandinavian Journal of Immunology. 2006;**63**:70-78

[92] Giudice A, Vendrame C, Bezerra C, Carvalho LP, Delavechia T, Carvalho EM, et al. Macrophages participate in host protection and the disease pathology associated with *Leishmania braziliensis* infection. BMC Infectious Diseases. 2012;**12**:75

[93] Mosser DM, Edwards JP. Exploring the full spectrum of macrophage activation. Nature Review in Immunology. 2008;**8**:958-969

[94] Caridha D, Vesely B, van Bocxlaer K, Arana B, Mowbray CE, Rafati S, et al. Route map for the discovery and pre-clinical development of new drugs and treatments for cutaneous leishmaniasis. International Journal for Parasitology Drugs and Drug Resistance. 2019;**11**:106-117

[95] Kaye PM, Cruz I, Picado A, Van Bocxlaer K, Croft SL. Leishmaniasis immunopathology-impact on design and use of vaccines, diagnostics and drugs. Seminars in Immunopathology. 2020;**42**:247-264

[96] Farias LHS, Rodrigues APD, Coelho EC, Santos MF, Sampaio SC, Silva EO. Crotoxin stimulates an M1 activation profile in murine macrophages during *Leishmania amazonensis* infection. Parasitology. 2017;**144**:1458-1467

[97] Frank B, Marcu A, de Oliveira Almeida Petersen AL, Weber H, Stigloher C, Mottram JC, et al. Autophagic digestion of *Leishmania major* by host macrophages is associated with differential expression of BNIP3, CTSE, and the miRNAs miR-101c, miR-129, and miR-210. Parasites & Vectors. 2015;**8**:404

[98] Mukherjee B, Paul J, Mukherjee S, Mukhopadhyay R, Das S, Naskar K, et al. Antimony-resistant *Leishmania donovani* exploits miR-466i to deactivate host MyD88 for regulating IL-10/IL-12 levels during early hours of infection. Journal of Immunology. 2015;**195**:2731-2742

[99] Locati M, Curtale G, Mantovani A. Diversity, mechanisms, and significance of macrophage plasticity. Annual Review in Pathology. 2020;**15**:123-147

[100] Zamani S, Hoseini AZ, Namin AM. Glucose-6-phosphate dehydrogenase (G6PD) activity can modulate macrophage response to *Leishmania major* infection. International Immunopharmacology. 2019;**69**:178-183

[101] Ferreira C, Estaquier J, Silvestre R. Immune-metabolic interactions between *Leishmania* and macrophage host. Current Opinion in Microbiology. 2021;**63**:231-237

[102] Rigoni TS, Vellozo NS, Cabral-Piccin MP, Fabiano-Coelho L, Lopes UG, Filardy AA, et al. Rank ligand helps immunity to leishmania major by skewing M2-like into M1 macrophages. Frontiers in Immunology. 2020;**11**:886

[103] Hong K, Zhang Y, Guo Y, Xie J, Wang J, He X, et al. All-trans retinoic acid attenuates experimental colitis through inhibition of NF-kappaB signaling. Immunology Letters. 2014;**162**:34-40

Chapter 11

Macrophage as the Game Changer of the (Future) Therapeutic Paradigm

Ranjan Bhadra

Abstract

Macrophages, the executioner of phagosome maturation, are central to coordinate and cooperate as the bridge between innate and acquired immunity. Mice primed with attenuated *Leishmania* promastigote showed host defense, such as total protection against LPS-induced endotoxic shock and, diarrhoeagenic *E. coli* lethal infection. Cell-based empirical preparations and isolated lipids, sphingolipids and lipoproteins were made out of the promastigotes. Host macrophage-mediated enhancement of microbicidal actions, non-specific and specific host immunity boosting and mitigation of antomicrobial resistance by the empirical preparations and, the cancer cell apoptosis, resolution of sepsis, combating autoimmune disease by isolated chemical constituents were evident, respectively. Macrophage phagosome maturation is the key factor of all these changes and indeed the attenuated *Leishmania* promastigote was found as an efficient agent for such maturation. To assess clinical impact of the studies, the therapeutic aspects of isolated total promastigote lipid were investigated on the synovial fluid mononuclear cells of RA (rheumatoid arthritis) patient as a case study including an animal model of the disease in parallel. The use of the attenuated *Leishmania* promastigote to produce human therapeutic vaccines that served Indian people for decades (1954–2005) by a nearly unknown Kolkata (India) based firm (IBL) was rediscovered recently.

Keywords: *leishmania* promastigote, macrophage, therapeutics

1. Introduction

'There is at bottom only one genuinely scientific treatment for all diseases, and that is to stimulate the phagocytes'. Gorge Bernard Shaw in '*The Doctor's Dilemma*' (1906).The human host and other mammals are continuously exposed to the environment along with numerous microorganisms, including disease-causing dreadful infectious pathogens. Before the advent of the age of antibiotics, human host defended against the infection with his own in-built immune system or through its modulation and, possibly traditionally experience-based useful therapeutic agents. The miraculous success of the penicillin and other antibiotics to combat the bacterial pathogens primarily made an impact of historical significance. More so when the dominant dogma ruled the world that diseases are originated essentially from a germ. If the germs are not identified, would be identified in future course of time. Pasteur's discovery of vaccine and diseases of especially bacterial pathogen originated ones have been combated profoundly by useful and effective antibiotics. So the clinical world was on the verge of declaring that war against infection has been won. But slowly at a creeping mode, the pathogens developed strategies to defeat the assault of antibiotics and what it is now is an emerging threat of antibiotic-resistant pathogens. So it is time to pay attention to the old guard 'the host own immune-mediated defence' for the betterment of health care or the mode of treatment paradigm.

An attenuated *Leishmania donovani* or *L. donovani* (UR-6MHOM/1978) was maintained over decades in the institute, Indian Institute of Chemical Biology, where the author joined as an independent investigator way back in the 80s of the last century. The protozoan parasite being attenuated lacks disease-producing capacity. It can infect host cell macrophage but in the next generation, it ceased to survive. The author out of curiosity planned to see whether the promastigote as a heat-killed preparation would be capable to modulate the immune response of the host. He administered it into healthy normal BALB/c mice to monitor the changes that might take place in the host immune system. He chose bacterial LPS or endotoxin to induce shock in the host as the host macrophage is the target to interact with both the LPS and the promastigote. After 3 days of priming the mice could withstand lethal blow of LPS, indicating that the macrophage had a real change in the responsiveness. After 1 month of priming, the mice showed the development of delayed type of hypersensitivity (DTH) indicating macrophages not only acquired protecting ability against LPS but also had undergone fundamental functional changes that included the changes in T-cell repertories. The mice displayed antibody raising ability against an antigen when the promastigote was used as an adjuvant [1]. The principal effectors of DTH reactions are Th1 lymphocytes mediated events where macrophages function as APC. The antibody raising capacity of a host acquired by B-lymphocyte maturation and APC mediated antigen presentation along with helper Th2 cells in case of protein antigen. Therefore, the priming of the mice with the promastigote of attenuated *Leishmania* had a profound effect on the overall functional changes of the macrophages, to a larger extent in the entire immune system. It must be mentioned that attenuated promastigotes of *Leishmania* have been tried for vaccine development of mammals as a vaccine candidate. Over the decades, it has been extensively tried, but no adversity was reported though no acceptable vaccine candidate fulfilled all the criteria to make one a successful vaccine. It was however not explored to develop any therapeutic item or an adjunct therapy exploring the attenuated promastigote till then.

1.1 The attenuated *leishmania* promastigote and watery diarrhoea control

The bacteria *E. coli* colonize the infant gastrointestinal tract within hours of life, and thereafter, it remains harmless usually deriving mutual benefit with the host. But the barrier of the gastrointestinal tract may be breached under conditions of immune suppression or other debilitating attacks resulting in damage or leakage.
Then, it can cause infection even being harmless 'non-pathogenic'. Several distinct diarrheal syndromes accompanying the bacterial infection including diarrhoeagenic *E. coli* infection are very often faced by clinicians. One such strain was available in our laboratory and the organism caused diarrhoea in mouse when injected through the intraperitoneal (i.p.) route. The animal succumbs within 3–4 days after the infection. The infected animal showed profuse watery diarrhoea. It is documented that

Enteropathogenic *E. coli* (EPEC) infection rapidly modulates electrolyte transport and induce watery diarrhoea [2]. The hallmark of this bacterial pathogenic infection is the development of an A/E (adhesion/effacing) lesion in the intestinal lumen. The Payer's patch (PP), lamina propria (LPr) like immune organs lay as an embedded component below the mucosal surface constituted by the enterocyte monolayer and play a very important role in the regulation of immune response to resolve injury such as A/E lesion. LPr macrophages participate in the sampling of luminal content, via extension of transepithelial dendrites and phagocytose transgressing pathogens. By priming the mice with the attenuated *Leishmania* promastigote and after 2–3 days they were infected with this diarrhoeagenic bacterial pathogen. These animals instead of developing lethal diarrhoeal assault and dying found unaffected and protected completely [3]. The mechanism remained to be elucidated but constitutive IL-10, anti-inflammatory cytokine production by the intestinal macrophage and apoptosis induction could be proposed and that might have an impact in this case.

Intestinal macrophages inherently produce both pro-and ant-inflammatory cytokines including the anti-inflammatory IL-10. Macrophages are M1 phenotype when coming in contact with attenuated *Leishmania* promastigote or promastigote at first with immediate encounter causing the release of pro-inflammatory cytokines. Gradually, it alters to M2 phenotype, especially when promastigotes after being degraded release its constituent lipids, proteins etc. along with resultant anti-inflammatory cytokine release. So the resolution of enteropathogenic *E. coli* infection-mediated damage could be assumed due to the therapeutic aspects of macrophage response modification towards homeostasis attainment [4, 5].

1.2 Role of empirical preparations of the attenuated *Leishmania* promastigote on non-specific host defence

The preparations were made of 10^6–10^7 promastigote per ml. cell count based on six different lots and then used for macrophage stimulation in an *in vitro* system. The designed preparations were IC (intact cell), CH (cell homogenate), CD (cell debris) and CS (cell soup obtained after CD collection by centrifugation). Mouse peritoneal macrophage, human monocyte–macrophage, a permanent murine cell line macrophage J.774 and mouse splenocytes were the test cells. TNF-α, LPS, BCG and an immune suppressor betamethasone were selected as the test compounds or specimen as well documented macrophage response modifier.

The parasite *Leishmania* has two important ligands, gp63 and LPG (lipophosphoglycan) to interact with host macrophage but the LPG moiety was devoid of this strain. Only its gp63 moiety as a well-recognized ligand to interact with the host macrophage was present. Macrophage MR (mannose receptor) is presumably the most efficient among others such as CR1, CR3 and fibronectin receptors for its response modifying interaction.

Cell homogenate or CH appeared most potent than the IC (intact cell). The macrophage response modulation by the IC, CH and CD resulted in generation of both the reactive oxygen species, ROS and nitrogen intermediate NO significantly but not as high as that of LPS or TNF-α associated induction. The LPS stimulation was very sharp and massive compared to IC and CH effect. However, these were not as sharp as the action of LPS in terms of TNF-α release and time kinetics. When the LPS response was suppressed in combination with IC or CH preparations, the ultimate product formation to TNF-α was blocked somewhere at an intermediate step before reaching the penultimate step. But the effect of externally added TNF-α along with IC or CH, in terms of total cytokine release, indicated an additive effect. This observation was of critically significant because once the LPS response attained its ultimate manifestation to TNF-α, its formation has not interfered further with respect to the presence of promastigote components. Macrophages pre-treated with IC, CH and CD did not respond to NO generation by LPS stimulation. The fraction CD or cell debris possibly contained DNA, RNA, insoluble membrane glycoprotein, glycolipids, lipids and lipoprotein, primarily a combined mixture of all these. DNA has no stimulatory or response modifying effect on LPS activity so the blocking of LPS action on macrophage activity by lipids and/or lipoprotein might be proposed and it was indeed the case as was evident subsequently.

IC, CH and CD pre-exposed macrophages showed higher phagocytic activity and intracellular killing of bacteria. This was confirmed by demonstrating in the IC mediated enhanced phagocytosis using engulfed GFP-*E. coli* (Green Fluorescence Protein expressing *E. coli*) bacteria. But such phagocytic up take by CH pre-exposed macrophages was slightly higher. In respect of antibiotic or drug resistance or even multidrug resistant clinical isolates of both Gram-positive and Gram-negative bacterial pathogens, no marked discriminatory action was noted apparently.

The *in vivo* study was conducted taking live animals (mice) such as BALB/c, Swiss, CBA/j and a wild strain. They all were primed with most of the promastigote preparations and after 5 days of priming challenged with lethal doses of *E. coli*^{R} (drug resistant), *S. aureus*^{R} (drug resistant) and *E. coli K-13* (the diarrhoeagenic strain). The unprimed and carrageenan treated groups were also challenged in parallel. The differences in survival rate between the two groups, primed and unprimed was remarkable as the primed groups showed considerable improvement (80–30% or 50% higher). The preparation CH was used for priming of BALB/c mice mainly with multiple (seven arbitrarily chosen) doses at an interval of 4–5 days, and then challenged with diarrhoeagenic *E. coli* K13. It is not known how far the attenuated leishmania promastigote lipoprotein(s) relates to bacterial outer membrane protein. Whether it functionally correlated and arguably induce protection for a long time against the bacterial infections remained as a guess. But the effect of multiple doses priming of mouse with IC showed absolutely safe and acquirement of long-term protection. One of the interesting findings was that the spleen cells of multiple doses of CH primed mouse when cultured in the presence of CH or CH coupled *E. coli K-13*, the culture soup demonstrated the presence of IL-2, and confirming Th1 cell-mediated immunity or CMI development. The protective ability is acquired even by priming with one or two doses. Multiple doses and the frequencies of administration with respect to time gap made a remarkable difference in the protection profiles, namely using CH, IC and lipoprotein (LP), but a safe gap of 3 days is desirable between two injections of the promastigote preparation [6]. The impact of phagosome maturation and over all immune response modulation by the host is possibly most critical in view of macrophage as a game changer, and now IC, the intact promastigote of the attenuated *Leishmania donovani* (UR-6MHOM/1978)-mediated phagosome maturation would be dealt in details.

2. Phagosome maturation by the attenuated Leishmania donovani (UR-6 MHOM/ 1978) promastigote

Phagosome maturation is essentially the most crucial biological process that performs the engulfment of the microbial pathogens and then degrades it to clear the infection. Macrophages are the key effector cells to furnish all the jobs successfully through the orchestration of its phagosome functions. Thus, the macrophages carry out two functions, one is phagocytosis as the 'housekeeping' or scavenging function and the other one is meant for host defence. Particularly the same macrophage has to perform both the functions to achieve a successful host defence strategy. There is also another aspect of phagosome maturation, the maintenance of tissue homeostasis, a determinant to recon as the basic function of macrophage assigned to the fulfilment of phagosome maturation. The removal of apoptotic cells and other extracellular component derived as by-products are a daunting task that is to be completed by macrophages. These are also the responsibilities of mature phagosomes and occur during the process of maturation. In case of the apoptotic cells, they display well known 'eat me' signals which recognizes various type of collectins, scavenger receptors, integrins and bridging molecules that link the surface structures to the macrophage receptors. The viable cells express specialized receptor such as CD47 that acts to inhibit the phagocytosis through receptors such as SIRP-α as apoptotic cell undergo silent absorption instead of degradation and elimination.

Thus, the phagocytosis of both microbes and apoptotic cell is carried by the same macrophage but there is a fundamental difference. The apoptotic cell phagocytosis by macrophage is trigged by anti-inflammatory responses, such as through the production of growth factor (TGF)-β while, in contrast the microbial cell phagocytosis occurs upon triggering the inflammatory response through production of TNF-α, IL-1 and IL-6 and make alert to the infection. The objective of the phagosome maturation by intact promastigote of attenuated *Leishmania* was described for the first time implicating the role of macrophage to act as infection eradicating agent. The maturation indeed undergoes, a full range of changes and it progresses through subsequent modification out of sequential fusion with endosomes when the microbe already is inside the macrophage.

2.1 Phagocytic phase of the phagosome maturation by attenuated *Leishmania* promastigote

This is the demonstration of the phagocytosis associated events that were described with the empirical preparations of the attenuated *Leishmania* promastigotes. Here described possibly the more documented evidence. The parasite *Leishmania* ensures their survival by inhibiting macrophage phagolysosomal fusion and so maturation is imperfect through a complex enzymatic process and reorganization of cytoskeleton structure, accumulating peri-phagosomal actin and reducing the recruitment of late phagosomal marker Rab7 and delaying recruitment of LAMP1 probably. Other strategies include modulation of macrophage for lower NO generation, reduced ROS, IL-12 and TNF-α production, NF-kB and AP-1 activation. The resolution of microbial infection, in contrast, depends on the arms of inflammatory response but at the later stage, it necessitates the induction of the anti-inflammatory cytokines such as IL-10, TGF-β and IL-4, the Th2 type cytokines. Activated protein kinase (MAPK) plays also a critical role because activation of p-44/42 MAPK leads to IL-10 production and p38 MAPK downregulation results in abrogated IL-12 production. This is now clear that within the same macrophage phagocytosis of microbial agents assigned to the destruction through the association with pro-inflammatory macrophage effector function and its apoptotic cell resolution requires anti-inflammatory or silent absorption. These are the characteristic feature of pathogenic *Leishmania* to establish infection, but its counterpart attenuated Leishmania strain was reported as a booster of respiratory burst and TNF-α production [7]. In the latest study, it was reported that attenuated strain of leishmania simultaneously induces both the forms of the cytokines to accomplish the jobs.

The macrophage exposed to the heat-killed intact attenuated *L.* (*L.* stands for *Leishmania*) promastigotes showed augmentation of ROS and NO generation, the former develops in a steady state with a gradual increase up to 24 hrs. to reach the peak while NO production was also time-dependent but noticed at 24 hrs. Both the species were highly microbicidal in action the attributes to combat the infection with bacterial pathogens. Macrophage phagosome membrane-associated gp91 phox and iNOS or induced nitric oxide synthase are instrumental behind the ROS and NO generation As already mentioned, the phagocytic uptake was significantly enhanced by latex particles, which were really non-physiological but provider of an index to mark the extent of response. *E. coli*-GFP (green fluorescence protein) expressing one was used to confirm the enhancement firmly. The fascinating observation was the enhanced uptake of pathogenic *Leishmania* strain (AG 83), as it is known that such pathogenic parasite usually limits the uptake, thus the action of the attenuated strain surpasses or overpowered the influences of the pathogenic strain-mediated interference. So, the strength of phagocytic engulfment appeared more forceful. It is not known if the time gapped multiple doses priming under *in vivo* would be more effective or force bearing to combat infection. Upon pre-exposure to macrophage with the promastigote, the Th1 type cytokines level raised significantly, such as the level of IL-12, IL-1β, TNF-α and IL-6 were induced markedly. Expression of Th2 cytokine namely TGF-β was lowered but another anti-inflammatory cytokine IL-10 had a significant increase. It might be mentioned that phagocytosis of microbial pathogen and apoptotic cell when to take place in the same macrophage then the former is under the regulatory dictum of pro-inflammatory cytokine while the latter is under the aegis of anti-inflammatory cytokine. It tells us that the clearance of both the microbial infective agents and the apoptotic dead cell is mediated by the macrophage simultaneously. The same macrophages on account of attenuated *L.* promastigote activation carry out the desired functions efficiently.

The heightened level of the expression and translocation of NF-kB and c-Jun, the crucial transcription factors were evident due to the attenuated *L.* promastigote exposure to the macrophages. It provides clearly the effect of the promastigotes, making host responses towards better defence. Both the transcription factors are critical regulators of pro-inflammatory cytokine release. The flow cytometric analysis of the *L.* promastigote pre-exposed macrophage for 4 hrs, confirming the increased accumulation of NF-kBp65 and c-Jun in the nuclear extract of the activated cell. It means that the macrophage function as progress towards the late phagosome with the received cues from within and as the consequences of released constituents of the attenuated *L.* promastigote. For example, as it would be shown later in detail that lipids isolated from the promastigote decrease the accumulation of these nuclear transcription factors in the Synovial Fluid Mononuclear Cell (SFMCs) of RA patients implicating benefit to the patients.

The increase in pro-inflammatory cytokine activity was mediated through p38MAPK and p44/42 MAPK activation. The enrichment of the attenuated promastigote exposed macrophage-mediated release of Th1 type cytokine over the Th2 type was observed as indicated by higher level of IL-12 over IL-10 though both the MAPK were involved here simultaneously. Other markers of the phagosome maturation are indicated by the co-localization of Rab7, Lysosomal Associated Membrane Protein-1, Cathepsin D, Rab 9 and V-ATPase. Inhibition of V-ATPase was found to cause significant hindrance in phagosome maturation. Acidification and phagosome maturation, a coupled phenomenon occurs in unison in the attenuated promastigote exposed macrophages ([8] and ref. therein). Thus, the achievements of macrophage phagosome maturation, the crucial functional attainment have been well documented with crucial manoeuvring capability using the promastigotes of attenuated *Leishmania*.

3. Impact of phagosome maturation as a macrophage game changer

Phagosome maturation is considered the end of the phagocytic process. In this process macrophages, the classical phagocytes, among others if properly activated, the efficient clearance is ensured. As it has already been evidenced that attenuated *L.* promastigote is highly efficient in achieving this feat. The internalized particulate matter both apoptotic cell and bacteria or any other microbial pathogen are regarded as garbage for clearance. They must be degraded and digested or defects in degradation have a number of consequences. For example, the lack of degradation (of DNA during apoptosis) or lysis of the apoptotic cell within macrophage results in autoimmune disease [9]. Neutrophil-mediated killing is hampered by the slow or inadequate phagosome maturation and certain pathogens seem to use the phagocytic machinery to enter and/or live within the host, all these have the better opportunity to survive in the context of knowing the various steps of cargo handling by macrophages. However, the attenuated *L.* promastigote exposure to macrophages caused its activity modulation to a great height. It might lead to the attainment of the homeostasis of immune system by way of providing optimum and therapeutic attributes.

The macrophages, as the pivotal host cells whose response modification through *L.* promastigote-mediated phagosome maturation, have been described elaborately. Properly time gapped multidose administration of this promastigote-derived material could lead to the repeated response modification of macrophages in sequences. It can act as a disease combating agent after attaining appropriately stimulated physiological state without damaging the host. The intact cell (promastigote) or its preparations were empirical but there is provision to use it for the disease cure. However, such macrophage activity changes could be manoeuvred using its identified individual component(s). In view of this total lipids and sphingolipids were isolated and examined for i) the potentiality of the compounds to treat human diseases in future and ii) the compatibility of their use in humans. The attenuated heat-killed promastigote is unique in the sense that it did not elicit any harmful consequences and its safety is assured through the vaccine trial.

4. Leishmanial lipid, macrophages and rheumatoid arthritis, an autoimmune disease

A cohort of patients in the department of Rheumatology, Calcutta Medical College, Kolkata, India, have fulfilled the criteria of RA (Rheumatoid Arthritis) as per the American College of Rheumatology [10] were selected for study. After approval of the medical college ethical committee and having patients' consent Synovial Fluid (SF) collection was made from the patients showing knee joint swelling with signs of active synovitis. The adherent Synovial Fluid Mononuclear Cells (SFMCs) were then prepared and cultured in presence of total lipids isolated from the attenuated *Leishmania* promastigote, the working material here. The lipids isolated by Bligh and Dyer [11] method showed six spots upon TLC analysis following standard technique.

The pathophysiological and therapeutic eventuality involving inflammation and cartilage destruction are of crucial significance of activated macrophages associated with the synovial membrane and knee joint. Permanent joint damage prompted a critical re-evaluation of therapeutic regimens currently used with anti-inflammatory and disease-modifying treatments for RA.

One of the major targets is the regulation of proinflammatory cytokines released by the monocytes –macrophage in Rheumatoid Arthritis or RA. TNF-α, here acts as pleiotropic cytokine reported to have an inductive effect on the enhanced expression of other cytokines, adhesion molecules etc. but mostly produced by macrophages in the synovial membrane. It is a proximal cytokine in the inflammatory cascade and the degree of expression depends on the histological configuration.

The leishmanial lipids were used to modulate responses of the macrophage of RA patients with a view to the resolution of the disease. In presence of the leishmanial total lipids, the aggravated inflammatory condition of SFMC was down-regulated showing its responses modification distinctly as if it was acting like a response modifying therapeutic agent. The response modifying, in terms of TNF-α release primarily was assayed experimentally both in an *in vitro* and *in vivo* system, in the latter case using animal models.

The pro-inflammatory cytokines, namely TNF-α, IL-1β and reactive nitrogen intermediate NO (nitric oxide) and enzymes are abundantly released by the synovial tissue lining cell, synovial fluid cell and infiltrating monocyte–macrophage involved in driving the inflammatory response and joint destruction mainly [12]. So the study included estimation of the release of TNF-α, IL-1β and NO production by adherent SFMC, primarily the infiltrating monocytes-macrophage after treatment with the leishmanial lipids. An anti-inflammatory cytokines IL-10 was also induced by macrophage as it was evidenced during phagosome maturation and found to be released by the macrophage. So it was also included to be monitored whether countering the effect of the pro-inflammatory cytokines also takes place or not or could be quantifiable. During phagosome maturation, such anti-inflammatory cytokine, IL-10 release was observed by the intact attenuated *L.* promastigote treatment so its level was thought to be determined to have an overall picture. Then, the changes in the level of NF-kB p65 in the nuclear extract of the SFMCs were determined to substantiate the basis of the effect of the lipids for lowering of the release of proinflammatory cytokines. SFMCs were a heterogeneous cell population composed of primarily monocyte–macrophage, fibroblast and synovial cells whose hyperplasia was a characteristic feature of the disease RA. So apoptotic cell death of the viable SFMCs was also used as a parameter to monitor the other aspect of the leishmanial lipids action. Currently, therapeutic intervention includes the treatment of RA patients with biological such as infliximab or etanercept and those are highly clinically efficient for RA suggesting that the neutralization of the TNF-α is the primary target of the disease control. These treatments were also found to delay joint destruction. So the treatment is to be targeted to the suppression of TNF-α release rather than neutralization and simultaneously to decrease the NF-kB p65 level both in extent and translocation parameter by the lipids. A rat model of Rheumatoid Arthritis developed by collagen-adjuvant induced RA was also used in parallel to see effect of leishmanial lipids.

The adherent SFMCs, primarily monocyte-macrophage were stimulated with human gamma interferon (IFN-γ) or phorbol myristate acetate (PMA) before exposure to leishmanial lipids. The decreased release of the cytokine, TNF-α in the culture media confirmed the effect of leishmanial lipids as a suppressor. The distinctly diminished release of IL-1β and decreased NO production were found in parallel. The changes were observed with the lipids in a dose- and time-dependent manner. But an increased IL-10 release was established clearly as the effect of the promastigote lipids, demonstrating the leishmanial lipids functioned as an anti-inflammatory cytokine-releasing agents in a dose-dependent manner. Both the anti- and pro-inflammatory cytokine release were affected, though the release of the former increased while decreased secretion of the later favoured the relief or resolution of the disease. Thus, at the cytokine level, the lipid action was highly therapeutic in nature. With respect to the status of the transcription factor NF-kBp65 of SFMCs, a decrease in its level was evident in a dose-dependent manner. Thus, it was clear that the transcription factor expression in SFMCs of RA was also highly specific or sensitive to the presence of leishmanial lipids. The cytosolic protein content level was also suppressed by the leishmanial lipids in a dose-dependent manner.

The total viable cells present in adherent SFMCs of the RA patient as determined by MTT assay showed dramatic reduction of the viability in a dose- and time-dependent manner upon exposure to the leishmanial lipids. Sphingolipids comprise 5–10% of the leishmanial membrane lipids and it was shown that a sphingolipid-enriched preparation obtained from this attenuated *L.* promastigote induced apoptosis of both mouse and human melanoma [13, 14]. In this case of RA patients, the total lipid-mediated apoptosis of SFMCs was nearly 70% and 22–25% at a dose of 100 μg and 50 μg /ml of total leishmanial lipids for 48 hrs. Treatment. It was reported that normal peripheral mononuclear cells obtained from healthy donors suffered no significant cytotoxicity at a dose of 100 μg/ml. It might be referred that normal melanocytes were not vulnerable to leishmanial sphingolipids unlike its cancer counterpart, melanoma. The leishmanial lipids acted probably as an apoptosis inducer in a wider spectrum of cells other than cancerous one. Cells functionally altered due to pathological changes found susceptible to apoptosis after being treated with the attenuated *L.* promastigote lipids, but normal cells did not suffer such cytotoxicity (unpublished observation). Because the dead SFMCs cells revealed all the signatures of the apoptosis; the activation of caspase-3 and -9 and Bax, DNA fragmentation, cytochrome c release along with the alteration of mitochondrial membrane potential and downregulation of Bcl-2 [13, 14]. All these observations indicated and supported strongly that leishmanial lipids are a powerful suppressor of cytokine expression in relation to RA pathogenesis. It was further interesting to note that the effect of the leishmanial lipids was probably at the nuclear induction level rather than an individual constituent level such as neutralization of TNF-α or TNF-α receptor blocker level or anti-proliferative action provider like methotrexate, a drug used for RA management.

It has been reported that a higher expression of tm-TNF-α (transmembrane TNF-α) in RA patient resulted in an increase in apoptosis by tm-TNF-α, compared with healthy donors. After infliximab treatment, the tm-TNF-α binding was proposed as a regulator of the reverse signalling to improve the pathological condition and also as a result of cell-targeted therapeutic action [15]. Thus, the effect of leishmanial lipids was comparable to a cell-targeted therapeutic action in case of SFMCs of RA but no confirmed interaction could be proposed with tm-TNF-α binding. The advantage of higher dose (a dose 100μgm/ml) of leishmanial lipid could be exploited when higher (76–78%) apoptotic cell death of SFMCs of RA patients was observed indicating better recovery. SFMCs were diseased cells and not per say cancerous cells, and they acted as the target of leishmanial lipids.

Taking RA as representative case, the *in vitro* studies have been illustrated here but for *in vivo* studies, rats were used to conduct the experimentation in an animal model. Here, RA was induced by collagen-adjuvant (FCA)-mediated procedure with confirmation of paw swelling in 14 days. The rat serum level of TNF-α, IL-1β, and NO produced was reduced after the treatment with the leishmanial lipids. The paw swelling was reduced on 16th days returning close to normal. But it was interesting to observe that normal healthy mouse not having induced AR if treated with leishmanial lipids showed a higher levels of serum TNF-α and IL-1β but not show any detrimental consequences, compared with control (lipid untreated). It was possibly due to enhanced nonspecific host defence [16].

5. Macrophage, lipids of attenuated *Leishmania donovani* promastigote, sepsis attenuation

The macrophage-mediated therapeutic applications based on the *L.* promastigote-derived bioactive molecules namely lipids, sphingolipids and lipoprotein and the intact promastigote itself have been described here briefly. As the clinical studies are far away from the concept and so organized studies are to be focused to compare some old experience-based therapies and a prospective experimental therapy.

5.1 The case of sepsis

Prospective experimental therapy vs. **experience**-based therapy (or therapeutic vaccine or **vaccine in bed**).

An experimental therapy of sepsis has taken at first for discussion:

Mice not treated with pLTL (pathogenic Leishmanial Total Lipid) but challenged with LPS lethal shock had a survival rate of 41% and 9% at 24 hr. and 48 hrs, respectively, but displayed total death within 72 hrs. Mice primed for 3 consecutive days with pLTL at doses, 50 and 25 mg/ml and exposed to lethal dose of LPS had 78.8% and 53.8% survival without further loss of life. The reduced cytokine release was evident due to pTLT priming and factors [(IL-12p40, IL-17, IFN-γ, MIP-2, KC and RANTES (C–K)] were further included to prove its existence and they were detected by ELISA based assay. High dose pLTL, 50 mg/ml pre-treated animals showed the reduction of the vascular permeability factors, such as VEG, and suppressed the expression of cell adhesion molecules, including ICAM-1, VCAM-1, PECAM-1, P-selectin and E-selectin, compared with its level in liver of septic mice. Thus, endotoxin associated liver damage was improved considerably in the pLTL treated group.

Macrophages, the key regulators of the host immune response expression, play an important role in the pathogenesis of inflammation. They secrete quite a large number of inflammatory mediators such as prostaglandins, reactive oxygen and nitrogen species, inflammatory cytokines including tumour necrosis factor-alpha (TNF-α), interleukin-1 (IL-1), interleukin-6 (IL-6), interleukin-12 (IL-12), and interleukin-17 (IL-17), chemokines, including macrophage inflammatory protein (MIP), and bioactive lipids. These are regulated by the ubiquitous transcription factor, nuclear factor B (NF-kB). The consequences of complex immune reactions are described as sepsis that represents an uncontrolled inflammatory outburst from harmful host responses to infection, causing disruption and damage to several cells and tissues. IkB appears to function as a strong negative feedback mechanism elicitor that allows a fast turn-off of the NF-kB response to control inflammation-associated diseases. But identification of new therapeutic targets for the management of septic shock remains imperative as all investigational therapies, including anti-tumour necrosis factor (TNF-α) and anti-interleukin (IL-1) agents, have uniformly failed to lower the mortality of critically ill patients with severe sepsis. Though different bacteria have been identified as causative organisms in sepsis, gram-negative bacteria like *Escherichia coli* remain as one of the most common pathogens (up to 60%) in intraperitoneal infections with high mortality rates. Moreover, the recognition of CD14-TLR4 complex by cell wall components of Gram-negative bacteria *(E. coli)* may lead to activation of the inflammatory responses. The overproduction of inflammatory cytokines generates systemic activation which affects vascular permeability and gives rise to metabolic changes that can lead to tissue injury and eventually to the failure of various major organs to induce mortality. Infectious inflammatory stimuli elicit acute lung distress which may be perceived as the most fatal cause affecting the initiation of various cellular cascades. It may also lead, firstly, to pre-eminence of inflammatory cells in the interstitium and alveolar spaces and, secondly, to an increase in PMN-derived proteases and oxidative metabolites in the bronchoalveolar lavage fluid (BALF). Local inflamed cells in the lung interstitium activate the pulmonary capillary endothelium culminating in the expression of adhesion molecules on the endothelial cell. Strategies aimed at preventing such cell activation, and thus attenuating systemic inflammation relevant to lung injury are proposed to control the sepsis.

To decipher the molecular approaches by which LTL (Leishmania Total Lipids of attenuated promastigote) inhibits the inflammatory responses of Gram-negative bacterial sepsis, attempts were made to evaluate the survival rate and body weight improvement of mice in the *E. coli* challenged murine sepsis model. The inhibition of production of serum cytokines including TNF-α, IL-1β, IL-6, IL-12 and IL-17 and of the chemokine MIP-2, was achieved by administering LTL. In the *in vitro* culture of macrophages, such inhibition of the sepsis mediators by LTL was evidenced after *E. coli* induced stimulated release of the cytokines and chemokines. TNF-α and IL-1β are known as signature cytokines that initiate an acute inflammatory cascade to cause inflammatory injury leading to the recruitment of inflammatory cells to the affected organ. TNF-α a pleiotropic cytokine plays a central role to regulate other cytokines especially IL-17 and IL-12 that are rapidly generated in bacterial *E. coli* infection. LTL showed attenuation of the systemic inflammatory reactions and multiple organ failures associated with abdominal sepsis syndrome. It is well known that *E. coli* provokes the signalling through its receptor cluster involving CD14 and TLR4. The activation of the IκB kinase complex (IKK) led to phosphorylating the inhibitory IκB proteins that is necessary for ubiquitination and degradation leading to the release and subsequent translocation of NF-κB p65 from the nucleus. TNF-α and IL-1β, macrophage induced cytokines stimulate the production of a variety of chemokines, namely, macrophage-inflammatory protein-2 (MIP-2), this was attenuated by LTL together with functional effectors in the bronchoalveolar lavage fluid (BALF).

The recruitment of leukocytes at the inflammatory site required coordinated expression of specific combination of adhesion molecules and those are diverse in nature, sequentially develop to organize the pathophysiological condition with epithelial cells. The main endothelial CAMs(cell adhesion molecules cascade) involved in the inflammatory response are E-selectin and two members of the Ig-gene superfamily, intercellular adhesion molecule (ICAM)-1 and vascular cell adhesion molecule (VCAM)-1 that are expressed sequentially, but LTL addition alters the sequences of events towards attenuation. The study referred to is possibly the first evidence that attenuated leishmanial total lipid contributes to host defence during bacteremic sepsis caused by *E. coli*. And this was proposed by the observation that combating the inflammatory response to infection and exaggerated inflammation related to tissue injury have been successfully compromised. In the present case, lung injury was reduced by the suppression of the expression of macrophage cytokine-induced cell adhesion molecules. Thus, macrophage functional modulation improved the survivability with alteration of pathological changes in mice with septic mice lungs [17, 18].

5.2. The case of an experience-based therapy or a therapeutic vaccine for sepsis

It is said that if there is sepsis, an infection must be sought at a first instance. Then why there would be no vaccine? The term therapeutic vaccine means to get a patient vaccinated while in bed. The question is how it could be possible? The first dose would begin with 0.1 ml of the vaccine. This was a verified approach and practised over the decades.

The doctor who developed it was an M.D. degree awardee trained abroad (possibly in Germany) and provided it for treatment way back in early 40s of the last century and set up the first biomedical research institute in India. His name is **Dr. J.C. Ray M.D.** and became the first director, as a founder director of the renowned biomedical research institute of India, currently Indian Institute of Chemical Biology, Kolkata, India.

The author became interested in the vaccine because it works on the basis of macrophage functional modulation. This vaccine served the people here (India) for over 50 years (1954–2005) as per the document available. Name of the producer firm is **I**mmuno **B**iological **L**aboratories or **IBL** and the product is named **ANASEPSIN (IBL)** but technically *Streptococcus* and *Staphylococcus* Anti pyogenic Vaccine. Besides the two mentioned microorganisms, others included were *Pneumococcus, E. coli* (*B. coli* as described at that time) and *Pseudomonas aeruginosa* (*pyocyaneus* as described at the then time).

The documents were reached to the author in 2007, after 2 years of his retirement and **Dr. J.C. Ray M.D.** passed away in the late seventies (1975) of the last century. The author joined to Indian Institute of Chemical Biology in 1984 as an independent investigator. So, no scope of communication was possible with the great **Scientist** who saved lives over the decades. For not complying with the GMP norms, the unit remained closed since 2005, but few documents were made available to the author as stated.

What were in the vaccines? The above bacteria, especially pathogenic but non-pathogenic types were also picked up and heat-killed preparations were made up. Then respective count was made by O.D. measuring against standard count in a spectrophotometer or any convenient equipment. Initial cell count was stated 100 to 10 million of the different bacteria and then suspended in homogenized leishmania promastigote (it was made of the promastigote of attenuated *Leishmania* as per available information). The injection begins at 0.1 ml, then 0.2, 0.4, 0.6, 0.8 and 1 ml dose subcutaneously and progressively at an interval of 3 or 4 days. Then doses with higher count containing killed bacteria were used and time gapped injections were scheduled enhancing to 4–5 days interval.

This is a crude type of vaccine (based on whole cell) prepared long back and used till 2005 as per the documents available, and no detailed clinical data were recorded systematically. This is a separate chapter with the potential to revive the products though it was very primitive, but as per hearsay, it was very efficacious and affordable financially for commoners.

6. Cues to the manoeuvrability of macrophage function to be a game changer

Macrophages are capable of integrating an enormous and impressive amount of information regarding the identity and virulence of pathogens, as well as endogenous cues present in their microenvironment, in order to modulate the immune response to best protect the host. Over 30 years of extensive studies that advanced our understanding that the NF-kB signalling module consists of five NF-kB monomers (RelA/p65, RelB, cRel, NF-kB1 p50 and NF-kB2 p52) which can dimerize to form up to 15 unique transcription factors and interact with the kB consensus motif found in many gene promoters, as well as five inhibitory proteins (IkBα, β, ε, γ and δ) that make up the IkB protein family. What the author is trying to focus on is that so many genes involved in the functional manoeuvrability of the macrophage have been deciphered but any control or more precisely in the domain of therapeutic regulatory aspects are yet to be discussed, except the revelation of the *Leishmania* promastigote-mediated events and more defined the lipids of this parasite promastigote covered very recently. The 'promastigote tricks' were discovered and explored way back in the early 50s of the last century by **Dr. J.C. Ray, M.D.** founder director of present Indian Institute of Chemical Biology, Kolkata, India. The lack of publicity and scientific exposition might be the reasons other than meeting the fund crunch for his research endeavour **Dr. Ray**, kept the firm (IBL) in a kind of obscurity about his novel and great service as a developing **giant** of *therapeutic vaccine*. But recently, the disclosure of the lipids of the said promastigote and some scientific endeavour made it possible to indicate that the changes in functional aspects of the macrophage are possible to manoeuvre its activities during the NF-kB nuclear transcription factor expression dynamics. What is more pertinent is the non-haematopoietic cell of bone marrow origin possibly lung epithelial cell, after having been injured, was also found to have remedial fate during the leishmanial lipid's exposure to it under *in vivo* system. The author has discussed the promastigote and lipids already and mentioned the attributes to the effect of leishmanial lipoproteins in host defence, especially protection against LPS threat. But the severe downregulation of the expression of LPS induced cytokine release in terms of TNF-α production and survival improvement after infecting the lipoprotein primed mice with the bacterial pathogens have been described as a phenomenon of host protection and an example of macrophage-mediated defence.

Negative regulation of NF-kB signalling was stated in an interesting mode. The synthesis of new IkB proteins or modules and subsequent reactivation of the pathway can lead to a periodic oscillation of active NF-kB translocation between the nucleus and cytosol. The newly synthesized IkB proteins bind to active NF-kB dimmers and remove from DNA binding and shuttling back to the cytoplasm where the complex can be reactivated and IkB can again be ubiquitinated and degraded via the proteasome. This is a powerful negative feedback loop. The balance of positive and negative feedback signals has a profound impact on the transcriptional outcome of NF-kB activation. Recent studies showed that immune cells challenged with traditional immune stimuli showed substantial and significant variations in the NF-kB response dynamics in the different contexts of at different times in the cell cycle. The positive feedback and sustained NF-kB nuclear occupancy was also proposed and described as dose-dependently induced by LPS action. Recurrent NF-kB oscillations between the cytosol and nucleus are linked to gene expression and studied at the single-cell level to decipher the transcription dynamics. But in case of an individual cell and its effect it is segregated, the body system during illness undergoes multi-cellular cross-talk based events. The NF-kB activation, transcription dynamics and gene expression studies in a single cell might result in better outcome of multiple NF-kB, IkB and IKK genes functioning to monitor or perturb or to better investigate how they can be controlled to interact between macrophages and other immune cells. Central to this ability, there are ways in which NF-kB signalling is modulated based on shifting thresholds of activation, capacity of various classes of the PRR to integrate information acquired and keeping over all tight regulation of transcription through rigorous positive and negative feedback loops. Fitting of these components together in the diverse context and how we may be able to modulate or interfere with them to the benefit of patients is an important field of research as envisaged. In this context, the interference to the action of leishmanial lipids to the NF-kB expression control, the mechanisms involved thereby needs to be demonstrated in an experimental set-up. But so long the beneficial aspects could be exploited and if it is proved to be satisfactory then therapeutic application would be well come. It is therefore imperative how we can harness the benefit of the leishmanial lipids or the preparations based on the use of the whole promastigote. The reader may go through the review [19] for a better and more detailed understanding.

The lipid(s) like the ones isolated from attenuated strain showed no toxicity at a dose of 500 mg per kg of body weight and no body weight loss treating at a dose 50 mg per kg. body weight in mice. The macrophage cell, RAW264 stimulated by LPS (bacterial endotoxin) showed ROS production and enhancement of active phagocytic uptake but upon treatment with leishmanial lipid both the stimulatory responses were reduced to more than half.

7. Antimicrobial resistance, attempted mitigation, *Leishmania* promastigote nonspecific host defence

Antibiotic resistance has become one of the greatest threats in human health care set-ups dealing with the issues for successful prevention and treatment of persistent infections. Misuse and overuses of antibiotics including in the agriculture sectors and allied fields have made a tremendous impact in the field of antibiotic resistance development. But spontaneity of environmental evolution, enormous mutational ability of bacteria and the capacity for passing the resistant genes through horizontal gene transfer system created significant impending factors to antimicrobial resistance mitigation. Multifactorial threats of antimicrobial resistance have posed numerous complex issues affecting countries across the globe. However, three categories have come out remarkably as patients, health care and economics to name them succinctly. At present, 'Stewardship' has been objectively imposed to get out of the problem to the rescue in the situation.

Israel, one of the most advanced countries in the world, whose health care system run wholly by the state, imposed the best possible 'Stewardship' in 2007–2008 by the introduction of containment for the country-wide outbreak of antibiotic-resistant *Klebsiella pneumonia* (CRE—carbapenam-resistant *Enetrobacteriaceae*) in her 27 hospitals, as a nationally implemented intervention strategy. The incidence of nosocomial CRE was significantly reduced from 55.5 to 11.7 cases per 100,000 patient days [20]. But total prevention or mitigation of the problem of antibiotic resistance remains at a level of concern.

There was another study that reported that the faecal, oral and skin bacterial microbiome and antibiotic resistome of the members of an isolated Yanomami Amerindian village in Venezuela were analysed with the revelation of very interesting observations. Their ancestors arrived in South America more than 11,000 years ago and had no known exposure to antibiotics till at the time of this investigation. In their microbiome, they carry bacteria that harbour functional antibiotic resistance genes, including those that confer resistance to synthetic antibiotics [21]. Thus, it appears that functional AR genes occur as a feature of human microbiome even in the absence of exposure to commercial antibiotics. Thus, overexposure to or misuse of antibiotics does not essentially poise the dangers of antibiotic resistance though it is a factor no doubt.

The report described in 1992 that most of the bacteria associated as a contaminant with *Leishmania major* lesion was eliminated during parasite treatment. Only *Klebsiella* and *E. coli* were retained when treated even with paromomycin and were considered antibiotic-resistant contaminants. Surprisingly, total elimination of these antibiotic-resistant contaminants was evidenced only during the healing process and took 20 days following the completion of the parasite removal by treatment [22]. It implicated that as a consequence of parasite clearance the host immune system was altered and acquired the capacity of resolving the resistant bacteria.

In another study in Iran, among the 84 (patients) studied, 65 (77.4%) had a positive culture of bacteria in the *L. major* lesions indicating of secondary bacterial infection. The infections are usually treated with antibiotics but there were controversies about whether any positive gain of antibiotic treatment is rendered by antibiotics. Here, the treatment of cutaneous lesion with glucantine not only resolves the lesions but also cured the secondary infection in the presence or absence of antibiotics for selected groups. It clearly implicated that during the treatment and cure of cutaneous leishmaniasis the host immune response has been modulated and that helped the patients get rid of secondary bacterial infection even in the absence of antibiotics. It led to suggest that the secondary bacterial infection associated with lesions of cutaneous leishmaniasis was cleared (irrespective of sensitive or resistant varieties of bacterial pathogens) due to immunomodulation resulting upon curing the parasitic disease [23].

Lastly in the laboratory of the author, the mice were primed with attenuated *Leishmania* promastigote (heat-killed) preparations remained unaffected after 3 days of priming, if challenged with the pathogenic as well as drug-resistant clinical isolates [6].

Immuno Biological Laboratories or **IBL** described a curative vaccine with the heat-killed typhoid germs, namely *Salmonella typhi., S. typhi A* and *S. typhi B* in a colloidal preparation of attenuated *Leishmania* promastigote and claimed as an useful item for enteric fever treatment and sold for years (over 50 years). It was an excellent typhoid bacterial antigen mix capable of generating specific antibodies, stated by the product [IMMUNO-T.A.B(IBL) curative vaccine for the treatment of enteric fevers] literature. The company also described that the patients' recovery was quicker and no relapse was noticed even though there were reports of chloramphenicol resistance in regular treatment with the antibiotic. This was probably the case because the phagosome maturation and innate immune response enhancing in the presence of promastigote-derived substances, all kinds of host-mediated events would be elicited towards enhanced pinocytosis, endocytosis and phagocytosis either sequentially or overlapping simultaneously. As the events are host-mediated and (heat-killed) *Leishmania* cell-mediated phenomenon where immune responses were never detrimental on the contrary it was to attain the condition of homeostasis upon curing.

The questions of anti-immunology, one of the fundamentals, need to be addressed in the view of AMR (antimicrobial resistance). The pathogenic bacteria, virus and even fungal cellular constituent conventionally exert their anti-immunology strategies through their first encounter with the host macrophage after invasion. Here, the surface molecules of the interacting species, the macrophages and the invading agents must have direct molecular encounter. The antigenic/pathogenic component of the infectious agent having been masked with the promastigote-derived molecules supposedly, would surely be blocked to interact with the host cell (macrophages presumably). The pathogen would have very limited scope to make open the strategic options to compromise with the host cell. Again within 2–3 days, if there is any opportunity the pathogen could have to interact, a fresh injection (progressively) with a higher dose would result in the contact between the leishmanial constituents and host intracellular components along with antigens. By that time, their effective co-localization would result through fusion of late phagosome and lysosomal entities within macrphages. The lipoprotein acting as the pro-inflammatory cytokine inducer or lipids of the promastigotes acting as anti-inflammatory cytokines producing agents might have a regulatory role. For example, *Salmonella*, an intracellular pathogen undergoes apoptosis in a macrophage with cell death, instead of escape when apoptosis is regulated by promastigote factors. There are two options of the host macrophage—either enhance the apoptosis in such a way that the pathogen gets involved in the apoptosis-mediated clearance and the other one is to face the detrimental phagocytic assault that the pathogen may suffer by degradation in a necrotic fashion. The promastigote sphingolipids are strong apoptosis inducers or powerful phagocytic assault creators by their capacity of proinflammatory cytokine/oxidative species release. So, it is apparently suggestive that the claim of the company, **Immuno Biological Laboratories** that no relapse of the *Salmonella* infection might be valid. The pathogen covered/sealed within the promastigote material could be engulfed by macrophages easily and such enclosed invader hardly has any opportunity to escape, but experimental demonstration demands to prove it.

8. Leishmanial promastigote Sphingolipids, apoptosis, and cancer

Attenuated leishmanial sphingolipids induce apoptosis in Sarcoma 180 cancer cells through the regulation of tumour development *via* angiogenic switchover. These bioactive leishmanial agents induce human A375 melanoma cell death *via* both caspase-dependent and independent cell death pathways or apoptosis. Both mouse and human melanoma *in vitro* displayed antineoplastic impact in tumour survival and heat-killed attenuated *Leishmania* promastigotes induces apoptosis of HepG2 cells through ROS-mediated p53-dependent mitochondrial pathway. The sphingolipids isolated from the attenuated promastigote *Leishmania donovani* (UR-6) indicated that their characteristic features might be to destroy the diseased cells of the host. For example, it induced apoptosis not only of cancerous but also of synovial fluid mononuclear cells of RA patients. But normal melanocytes and PMN do suffer any cytotoxicity upon exposure to the attenuated *Leishmania* promastigote or lipids, sphingolipids and lipoprotein derived from it while responding to functioning as expected. Once the apoptosis initiation is sensed, the macrophages come forward to clear the cargo within its sphere of activity. Apoptotic innate immune response is a state of immune-suppressive condition as the death is silent and the molecules in the fluid state of the promastigote preparation manipulate macrophage function through pinocytosis. Regarding melanoma destruction by apoptosis is an unique feature of *Leishmania* sphingolipids as there is no convenient way destined to eliminate these skin cancer cells. Intracutaneous injection starting from a very small dose, one can attempt to treat melanoma through apoptosis induction [24, 25].

As the theme of this chapter is the macrophage as game changer in the future treatment paradigm, the author invented a method for drug delivery system using IgG (intravenous fluid) and a schematic representation of the process has been given in **Figure 1** [26] along with **Figures 2** and **3**. **Figures 2** and **3** described the experience-based therapy or therapeutic vaccine developed by **Immuno Biological Laboratories** and peer-reviewed published works based experimental therapies using the materials derived from attenuated as well as pathogenic *Leishmania* promastigotes characterized at molecular level in **Figure 3** respectively. All schemes are given below.

A glimpse of the products (used by people of India over 50 years) of a local company *Immuno Biological Laboratories or IBL, Kolkata, India [27].*

1. Immuno- T.A.B (curative) vaccine for treating enteric fever or typhoid.

2. Deneurin. A product developed by IBL that included dried substance of cobra venom and neurotropic bacteria. Dedicated to the treatment of cancer patients having

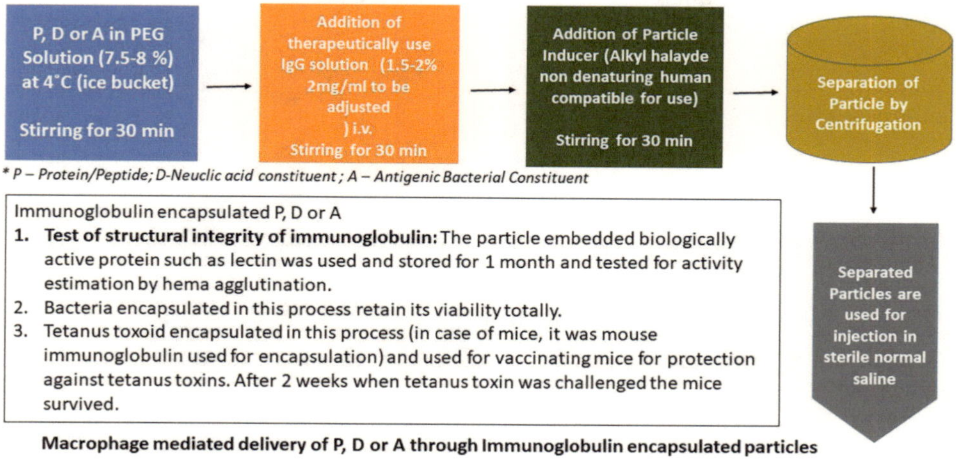

Figure 1.
Macrophage mediated delivery of P, D or a through immunoglobulin encapsulated particles (future treatment paradigm using macrophage as the game changer – Hypothesis).

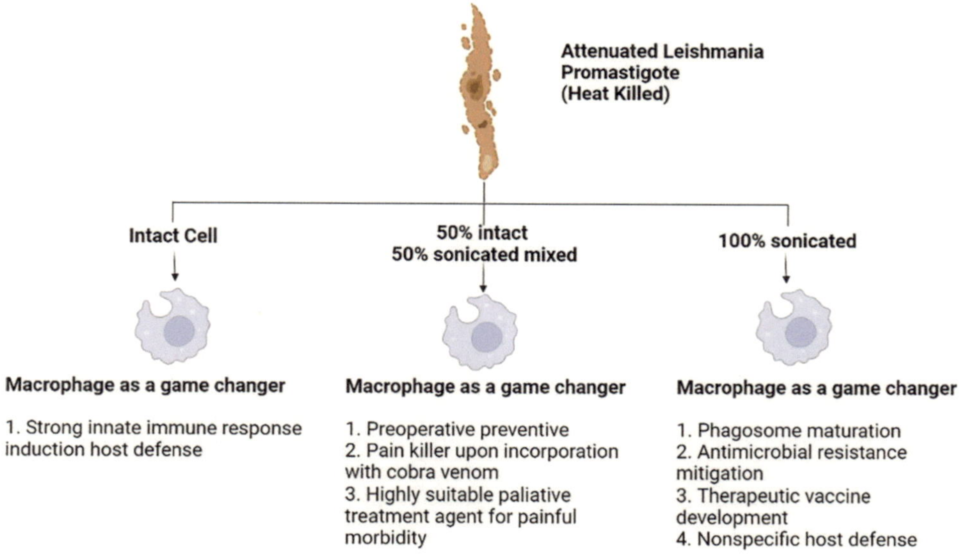

Figure 2.
Proposed treatment paradigm (experience based therapy – IBL evidence linked therapeutic items).

been painful morbidity, a palliative therapy for cancer patient, here pain is compromised with snake venom, but no addiction developed like Morphin. **3. Dellergen**. A product represents combination of specific and heterospecific hyposensitization antigens. Meant for treating the allergy and asthma. **4. Halsidin**. Meant for anti-influenza and catarrhal vaccination. **5. Anasepsin**. Already discussed for the treatment for sepsis. **6. Protodin (IBL).** It is like the adjuvant or the non-specific vaccine can be used alone as an immunomodulator to enhance host immunity, even a patient receiving it at first visit to clinic would have no adversity, but could get time to diagnose properly.

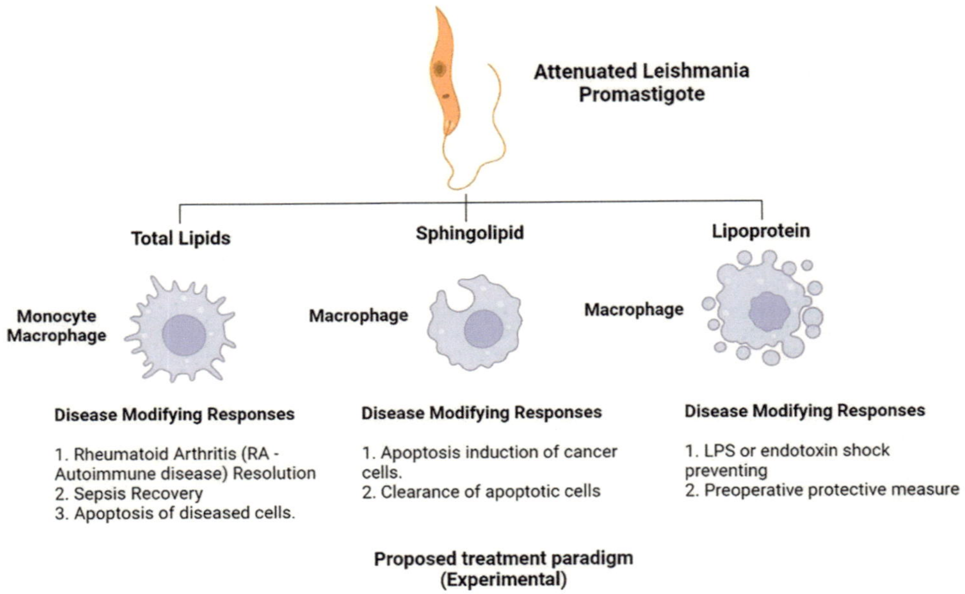

Figure 3.
Proposed treatment paradigm (experimental).

It can be used for boosting immunity in case a patient having milder symptoms or prior to COVID-19 infection as the author envisaged.

All the products are injectable and contained protodin (IBL) as base material. All the information is given on good faith and may need proper clinical evaluation at user end but an expert clinical trial conducting physician valued these items as highly contributory (personal communication).

9. Conclusion

The two figures are the representations of **Figures 2** and **3**, displaying the attenuated *Leishmani*a promastigote-derived molecular constituents and the whole cell-based material-mediated macrophage activity modulation, respectively, towards its game changing parameter. It had been stated as self-explanatory styles with the emphasis of disclosing scientific basis by the peer-reviewed publications (**Figure 3**). This was only for the events not known prior to the experience-based therapeutic vaccine (**Figure 2**) that served people over more than 50 years. The third one or **Figure 1** is a novel strategy envisaged by the author back in 2003 and provided with support for its experimental evidence. The explanation is omnipresent and interesting, as he did not find such an approach over the period since that time and desired exploration by the scientific world.

Author details

Ranjan Bhadra
Division of Immunology, Indian Institute of Chemical Biology, Kolkata, India

*Address all correspondence to: ranjanbhadra9@gmail.com

References

[1] Bhadra R. Prevention against endotoxic shock by immunization with a preparation from *Leishmania donovani* promastigote. In: Bhaduri AN, Basu MK, Sen AK, Kunar S, editors. Current Trends in Leishmania Research. New Delhi, India: CSIR. Govt.of India; 1993. pp. 269-276

[2] Collington GK, Booth IW, Knutton S. Rapid modulation of electrolyte transport in Caco-2 cell monolayers by enteropathogenic *Escherichia coli* (EPEC) infection. Gut. 1998;**42**:200-207

[3] Bhadra R, Das K. A process for the preparation of protozoan cell suspension useful as an immunomodulator for enhancement of host defense. 1679/Del/98 (Indian Patent). 1998

[4] Bain CC, Mowat AM. Macrophages in intestinal homeostasis and inflammation. Immunological Reviews. 2014;**260**:102-117

[5] Ashley MH, P'ng L. Intestinal macrophages in resolving inflammation. Journal of Immunology. 2019;**203**:593-599

[6] Das K. Enhancement of Host Defense by Non-specific Immunomodulation with Leishmanial Proteins [Ph. D. Doctoral thesis]. Kolkata, India: J. U.; 2000.

[7] Mukhopadhya S, Bhattacharyya S, Majhie R, et al. Use of an attenuated leishmanial parasite as an immunoprophylactic immunotherapeutic agent against murine visceral leishmaniasis. Clinical and Diagnostic Laboratory Immunology. 2000;7:233-240

[8] Banerjee S, Bose D, Chatterjee N, et al. Attenuated Leishmania induce pro-inflammatory mediators and influence leishmanicidal activity by p38 MAPK dependent phagosome maturation in *Leishmania donovani* co-infected macrophages. Scientific Reports. 2016;**6**: 22335

[9] Nagata S. Apoptosis and autoimmune diseases. Annals of the New York Academy of Sciences. 2010;**1209**:10-16

[10] Arnett FC, Edworthy SM, Bloch DA, McShane DJ, Fries JF, Cooper NS, et al. The American Rheumatism Association 1987 revised criteria for the classification of rheumatoid arthritis. Arthritis and Rheumatism. 1988;**31**:315-324

[11] Bligh EG, Dyer WJ. A rapid method of total lipid extraction and purification. Canadian Journal of Biochemistry and Physiology. 1959;**37**:911-917

[12] Kennedy A, Fearon U, Veale D, Godson C. Macrophages in synovial inflammation. Frontiers in Immunology. 2011;**2**:52. DOI: 10.3389/fimmu.2011.00052

[13] Ratha J, Majumder KN, Mandal SK, Dhara K, Singh SK, Saha KD, et al. Attenuated Leishmanial sphingolipid induces apoptosisin A375 human melanoma cell via both caspase-dependent and independent pathways. Molecular and Cellular Biochemistry. 2007;**304**:143-154

[14] Ratha J, Majumder KN, Mandal SK, Bera R, Sarkar C, Saha KD, et al. A sphingolipid rich lipid fraction isolated from attenuated *L.donovani* promastigote induces apoptosis in mouse and human melanoma cell *in vitro*. Molecular and Cellular Biochemistry. 2006;**29**:113-123

[15] Horiuchi T, Mitoma H, Harashima S, Tsukamoto H,

Shimoda T. Transmembrane TNF-α: Structure, function and interaction with anti-TNF agents. Rheumatology. 2010;**49**:1215-1228

[16] Majuimdar KN, Banerjee A, Ratha J, Mandal M, Sarkar RN, Das Saha K. Leishmanial lipid supresses tumor necrosis factor α, interleukin-1β and nitric oxide production by adherent synovial fluid mononuclear cells in rheumatoid arthritis patients and induces apoptosis through the mitochondrial-mediated pathways. Arthritis & Rheumatism. 2008;**58**:696-706

[17] Das S, Chatterjee N, Bose D, Banerjee S, Pal P, Jha T, et al. Lipid isolated from a Leishmania donovani strain reduces *Escherichia coli* induced sepsis in mice through inhibition of inflammatory responses. Mediators of Inflammation. 2014;**2014**:409694

[18] Chatterjee N, Das S, Bose D, Banerjee S, Jha T, Saha KD. Leishmanial lipid suppresses the bacterial endotoxin-induced inflammatory response with attenuation of tissue injury in sepsis. Journal of Leukocyte Biology. 2014;**96**:325-336

[19] Dorrington MG, Fraser IDC. NF-κB signaling in macrophages: Dynamics, crosstalk, and signal integration. Frontiers in Immunology. 2019;**09**:1-12

[20] Schwaber MJ, Lev B, Israeli A, et al. Containment of a country-wide outbreak of carbapenem-resistant *Klebsiella pneumoniae* in Israeli Hospitals via a nationally implemented intervention. Clinical Infectious Diseases. 2011;**52**(7): 848-855

[21] Clemente JC, Pehrsson EC, Blaser MJ, et al. The microbiome of uncontacted Amerindians. Science Advances. 2015;**1**(3):e1500183

[22] el-On J, Sneier R, Elias E. *Leishmania major*: Bacterial contamination of cutaneous lesions in experimental animals. Israel Journal of Medical Sciences. 1992;**28**(12):847-851

[23] Layegh P, Ghazvini K, Moghiman T, et al. Bacterial contamination in cutaneous Leishmaniasis: Its effect on the lesions' healing course. Indian Journal of Dermatology. 2015;**60**:211

[24] Das S, Chatterjee N, Bose D, Banerjee S, Jha T, Saha KD. Leishmanial sphingolipid induces apoptosis in Sarcoma 180 cancer cells through regulation of tumour growth via angiogenic switchover. Tumour Biology. 2015;**36**(4):3109-3118

[25] Bose D, Banerjee S, Das S, Chatterjee N, Saha KD. Heat killed attenuated Leishmania induces apoptosis of HepG2 cells through ROS mediated p53 dependent mitochondrial pathway. Cellular Physiology and Biochemistry. 2016;**38**(4):1303-1318

[26] Bhadra, R. A biotechnical process for the delivery of therapeutically active protein, and peptide, various drugs, DNA etc.by encapsulating it with body fluid components based on the formation of hydrogelparticles or microsphere. (a patent drafted in 2003). 2003

[27] Immuno Biological Laboratories or IBL (*nic* name Dr. Ray's Lab.) (1954-2005—the period of regulatory authority approved therapeutic vaccine producer and marketing firm with Valid Drug Licence issued by Govt.), P-91, Lake Road, Calcitta,-29 , India. (owned by Late Aruna Roy, Proprietress and wife of Late Dr. J.C. Ray M.D., the founder director of Indian Institute of Chemical Biology, currently one of the Prime Biomedical Research organization of India)

Section 4

Macrophages in Bacterial Infections

Chapter 12

The Ambiguous Role of Macrophages in Pulmonary Tuberculosis

Dženan Kovačić, Adna Softić, Adna Salihović and Jovana Jotanović

Abstract

Tuberculosis persists among the top 10 causes of death globally; causing 1.7 million deaths and 10 million new infections in 2018. Approximately 1/3 of the global population is infected with *Mycobacterium tuberculosis*; 10% of which are expected to develop active TB at some point in their life. The high burden of tuberculosis in the world is owed to lack of adherence to treatment, diminishment in treatment options and post-infection bacterial metabolic dormancy called latent TB (LTB), along with logistic, financial and political obstacles impeding successful TB control programs globally. Infections with *M. tuberculosis* leave no component of the immune system unengaged, hallmarked with granulomatous pathology as a function of the adaptive immune system. The hallmark of infection is a granulomatous pathological course, with the purpose of containing the difficult-to-kill bacilli, although the nature of the granuloma remains moot. The cells responsible for granuloma formation are professional alveolar macrophages, which seem to have both a beneficial and detrimental role in TB immunopathology. Herein, we discuss relevant immunological intricacies of macrophages in TB, ranging from immunogenetics, receptor-mediated uptake, macrophage-mediated immunopathology and the infamous tuberculosis granuloma.

Keywords: tuberculosis, tuberculosis granuloma, macrophages and tuberculosis, tuberculosis immunopathology, macrophages

1. Introduction

Pulmonary tuberculosis (TB), a severe respiratory infection whose causative agent is *Mycobacterium tuberculosis* (Mtb), persists as one of the top 10 causes of death in the world and has successfully maintained its position as the leading infectious cause of death from a single infectious agent. Approximately one third of the global population (2.3 billion individuals) is considered to be infected with Mtb in a clinically silent manner, although determining the exact number has proven to be quite difficult [1, 2]. Concern regarding this infectious disease is rising due to the emergence of resistant strains that are not adherent to specific geographies [3]. Numerous lineages of Mtb have to date been identified, three of which (lineages 2, 3, and 4) are considered the 'modern lineages' to which the global TB epidemic has been ascribed [3]. Emergence of these severely pathogenic and geographically unanchored lineages occurred due to the loss of theMmpS6/MmpL6-encoding Mtb-specific deletion 1 region (TbD1) throughout the evolutionary course of Mtb [3].

Pulmonary tuberculosis is divided into asymptomatic infection and active TB disease (ATB) [4]. Asymptomatic (latent) TB (LTB) is a clinically dormant form of infection whose mechanisms of activation and physiological maintenance with respect to host-pathogen dynamics are not fully characterized and although advances in imaging and high-throughput approaches have allowed for findings of tremendously higher resolution, details of the intricate dance between Mtb and the host remain moot [5]. Active tuberculosis is characterized with a wide spectrum of clinical manifestations, hallmarked by a purulent, bloody cough that aerosolizes into infectious droplet nuclei containing the pathogen [6, 7]. Although progress has been made in studying the immunogenetics and antimycobacterial mechanisms of the host, developing a broader comprehension of the matter has stagnated due to the underlying complexity of the relationship between the host and Mtb. Regardless, the innate immune response to inhalation of viable Mtb cells has been well studied and characterized with modest comprehensiveness, with a rigorously preserved hypothesis ascribing the most pathological importance to the TB granuloma [8–11]. Whether inhalation of infectious droplet nuclei will result in active TB disease or LTB, depends on a plethora of genetic and external factors, some of which are better understood than others, and research is currently being directed at understanding these issues [12]. One such factor is the natural degree of resistance humans possess to the development of active TB disease upon being infected [8, 9, 13, 14]. Resistance to TB disease, however, is evidently influenced by numerous factors originating from the host, the pathogen and the environment. Innate resistance to the Mtb, however, is not fully understood from the aspect of human immunogenetics, although significant progress has been made in this field [15]. Furthermore, primary and post-primary tuberculosis—two entities of infection with distinct immunopathologic continua—seem to be studied in a disproportionate manner; primary TB is at the forefront of research, whilst the relevance of secondary TB is substantially overlooked [15]. Available evidence, however, suggests that the subsequent initiation of secondary TB is essential for Mtb survival in the host, which may elicit a need for a broadening of research focus within the domain of TB prophylaxis [2, 16, 17]. Regardless, the innate response to Mtb inhalation has been a topic of intense study in the field of immunology. These molecularly-oriented studies have synthesized a rather large number of vaccine candidates, many of which are currently undergoing clinical trials [17, 18]. In fact, nearly each novel human vaccine candidate primarily functions by amplifying the TH1 innate immune response; an approach owed to the general understanding that an insufficient magnitude of TH1 immunity leads to poor control and subsequent proliferation of Mtb; something based in a rather large body of literature [17, 19–21].

Immunization strategies for tuberculosis currently undergoing clinical trials include killed, whole cell mycobacteria (DAR-901, *Mycobacterium vaccae*, MIP), live, attenuated mycobacteria (MTBVAC, VMP-1002); adjuvanted protein vaccines (M72/AS01E, H56:IC31, ID93 + GLA-SE), and viral-vectored vaccines (Ad5Ag85A, ChAdOx185A/MVA85A, TB/FLU-04 L) [2]. Quite prominent emphasis on the obscurity of substantial progress in regards to research and development of immunization methods for TB, is the fact that, in August 2019, there were 14 vaccine candidates being clinically assessed [19]. Ironically, a recent study on macaques concluded that intravenous (iv) administration of the Bacillus Calmette-Guérin (BCG) vaccine—the only clinically approved vaccine for tuberculosis—dramatically improved the efficacy of the vaccine in this animal model [22]. Considering the generally limited efficacy and temporary protection of the BCG vaccine when administered intramuscularly, subcutaneously, orally, and intranasally, this new study has placed the 99-year-old immunization method under the spotlight, once again [19].

This chapter comes at a crucial and exciting epoch in the domain of tuberculosis research, primarily facilitated by the rise of extensively-drug-resistant tuberculosis (XDR TB), multiple-drug-resistant tuberculosis (MDR TB) and totally-drug-resistant TB (TDR TB) across the world, and the diminishment of sensical and safe treatment options for all forms of TB [2, 23]. An imperative to expedite current research efforts directed towards development and discovery of more efficient treatment and diagnostic methods, has even been a topic of discussion by the United Nations, although this did not prove to be as fruitful as initially [2, 24]. Recent studies have incorporated other therapeutics into this treatment protocol, however the results on their efficacy appear to be population and circumstance-specific [23, 25–27]. Thus, tuberculosis is currently categorized as a global health 'emergency' by the WHO. It seems a rather sensical approach to focus research and provide comprehensive reviews on the immunopathologic course of TB and the relevant underlying genetic background that influences the outcome of TB infection.

The scope of this chapter includes the variability of the immune response to Mtb infection, concordant to differences in the immunogenetic profiles of the infected hosts across different populations in the context of immunoreceptors expressed on macrophage surfaces. We aim to present the most relevant findings in TB-related immunopathology and the corresponding implications in treatment and patient outcome in the context of macrophage involvement.

1.1 Immunopathological events of primary infection

Five stages of pulmonary tuberculosis (**Figure 1**) have been distinguished by Lurie's 1964 study on rabbits [5, 12, 18, 28, 29]. The importance of this study is seen in its high degree of fidelity with respect to the natural mode of contagion, which cannot be replicated by in vitro conditions [30]. Upon inhalation of even as few as 10 Mtb cells, the first stage is characterized by the rapid action taken by the innate immune defenses; phagocytosis of Mtb cells by resident macrophages (Mϕs) and other antigen-presenting cells (APCs) such as pulmonary dendritic cells (DCs) [31]. Varying immunopathologic continua may be observed for different phagocytic cells lines that phagocytize Mtb once it reaches the lung tissue upon inhalation, as the pathogen is able to employ different tactics to evade the host's immune defenses and interfere with every involved component of the immune system [7, 13, 32]. The evolutionary battle between the human host and Mtb prompted the pathogen to enhance its entry tactics into phagocytes by engaging a specific set of phagocytic receptors and efficiently modulating and interfering with every immunobiological process that plays a role in TB infection, often with staggering success [7]. Ergo, the ability of Mtb to create a survivability niche within the bactericidal environment of phagocytes is considered essential for bacterial survival and intracellular persistence.

Pattern recognition receptors (PRRs) located on the surface of APCs and respiratory epithelial cells that are engaged by Mtb include complement receptors (CRs), immunoglobulin fragment carrying the constant region of the heavy chain (Fc), C-type lectins (CTLs), toll like receptors (TLRs) and the scavenger receptors (SRs) (Image 1) [29]. Despite several receptors displaying partial redundancy in knockout

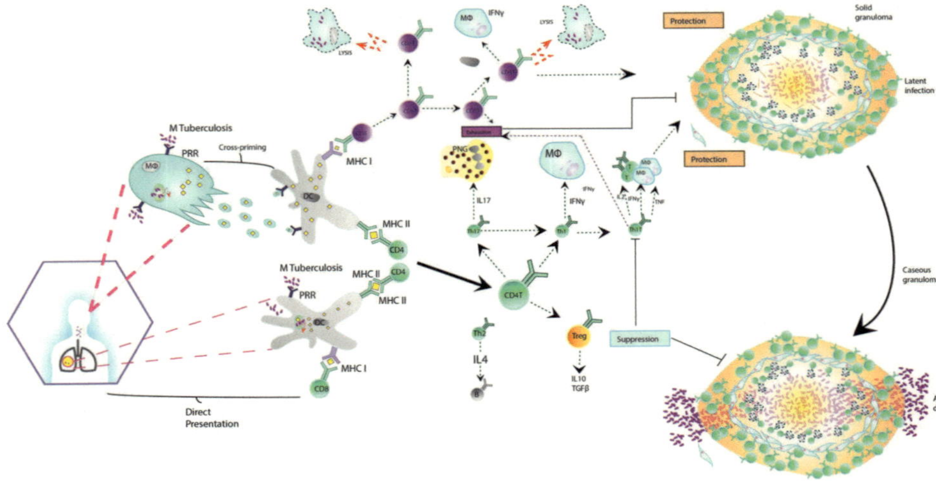

Figure 1.
The immune response to inhalation of Mycobacterium tuberculosis *within the context of Lurie's five stages of pulmonary tuberculosis. Abbreviations: MΦ-macrophage PRR-pattern recognition receptor:* M. tuberculosis*—* Mycobacterium tuberculosis*; DC—dendritic cell; MHC II—major histocompatibility complex type II; CD4—cluster of differentiation 4; CD8—cluster of differentiation 8; CD8T—cytotoxic T; IFNγ—interferon gamma; PNG—polymorphonuclear granulocytes; IL17— interleukin 17; Th17—T helper cells 17; CD4T—T helper cells; Th2—T helper cell type 2; IL4—the interleukin 4; B—B lymphocyte; Treg—regulatory T cells; L10—Interleukin-10; TGFβ—transforming growth factor beta, IL2—Interleukin-2; TNF—tumor necrosis factor; T—T lymphocyte.*

murine models, engagement of each receptor has pathologically relevant implications in TB pathogenesis. For instance, studies on murine models revealed significant reduction in the number of opsonized mycobacteria actively internalized by Mϕs and other phagocytes in the absence of CR3s [28, 33]. C-type lectins located on Mϕs and DCs are likely favored by Mtb since their engagement opens an opportunity for the pathogen to modulate the intensity of the associated inflammatory responses [34]. Specifically, Mtb has the ability to suppress the MR-TLR2-associated pro-inflammatory response by secreting the early secreted antigenic target protein 6 (ESAT-6), which inhibits the activity of NF-kappa (NF-κB) by downregulating reactive oxygen species (ROS) production [26, 35, 36]. Relevant to this discussion is that ESAT-6 is used in the IGRA due to its potency as a T cell antigen; thus, this secretory mycobacterial protein is an important hallmark of TB infection [37]. Fcγ receptors (FcγR) play a role in regulating the intensity of the host immune response and are concordantly divided into activating and inhibiting types. Toll-like receptors (TLRs) play a cardinal role in priming both pro-inflammatory and anti-inflammatory responses [38]. The cytoplasmic domain of these phylogenetically conserved transmembrane proteins is homologous to the interleukin-1 receptor (IL-1R) signaling domain, which links to IL-1R-associated kinase (IRAK) in order to activate transcription factors that will promote cytokine production. Furthermore, phagocytosis of Mtb does not lead to a pro-inflammatory immune response in the absence of TLRs; particularly relevant is the TLR2, although other TLRs have demonstrated notable roles in immunopathology [7, 32]. With regards to an efficient immune response, TLR recognition of Mtb cell wall lipoproteins will induce the secretion of IL-12—a proinflammatory cytokine that promotes maturation of naïve T cells into Th1 cells—by infected phagocytes [7, 13]. Mutations or genetic polymorphisms will likely, therefore, compromise the ability of the human host to mount an appropriately controlled inflammatory response to TB [39–46]. Aforementioned avenues for phagocytic receptor engagement make it all the more sensical that Mtb favors entry routes that seldom elicit a pro-inflammatory response, at least in early stages of infection. Pathways activated through the engagement of these receptors allow for immunobiological modulations that comprise the mycobacterial intracellular and intragranular persistence mechanism [37]. Although the intrinsic potency of Mϕs to kill internalized mycobacteria is evidently high through utilization of a barrage of bactericidal tactics, sufficiently virulent Mtb cells manage to evade or block these mechanisms [4, 47]. Thus, the intrinsic Mϕ competence and mycobacterial virulence significantly influence the course of the infection upon phagocytosis. Mycobacterial cells that evade the intrinsic killing mechanisms of phagocytes trigger an immunopathologic continua designated as the second stage, in which logarithmically multiplying Mtb cells inhibit the process of phagosome maturation and disrupt other incoming immune cells [18, 28, 48–55]. Immature phagocytes infected with multiplying mycobacteria attract monocytes and other inflammatory-oriented immune cells in an attempt to swiftly contain the bacilli [56–58]. Studies conducted on murine models and human monocytic cell lines have somewhat elucidated the process by which Mtb blocks the phagosome maturation process, and are further discussed in the following sections.

Approximately 2–3 weeks after engulfing Mtb, infected phagocytes release cytokines in order to recruit antigen-specific T cells (CD4+) to primary tubercle lesions in order to form adaptive immunity [32, 49, 56]. Activated T cells undergo clonal expansion and initiate the killing mechanisms of Mϕs infected with mycobacteria. Within the Mϕ environment, the third stage commences, whereupon logarithmic Mtb growth is halted through various bacteriostatic mechanisms [26, 37]. Infected Mϕs generally go through apoptosis, a consequence of recruiting the tumor necrosis factor alpha (TNF-α), whose inhibition significantly improves Mϕ survivability in the host lungs [37]. Progressive intragranular apoptosis leads to central solid necrosis, which may be followed by liquification of the caseous foci [26]. Survivability of Mtb in dead phagosomes, however, has been continuously reported throughout the years, as necrosis is an outcome favorable for pathogen dissemination and immune evasion [58–60]. Progression of the solid necrotized lesions containing metabolically dormant bacilli into liquified caseous lesions forms ideal conditions for bacterial re-activation and rapid multiplication [5, 7, 13–15, 61–65]. Although immunocompetent patients are evidently able to suppress the development of TB disease, host genetics and pathogen virulence determine whether dormant Mtb bacilli remain contained in the granuloma, or cause the formation of liquified caseous foci [8, 9, 59]. These foci progress to form cavities in which Mtb extracellularly multiplies, causing subsequent bronchial rupture and migration of the bacilli outside of their containment [10].

2. The innate immune response to *M. tuberculosis*: the pivotal role of macrophages

Perhaps the most direct evidence of constitutional human resistance to TB infection and disease may be extrapolated from the 1926 Lübeck disaster, in which 251 neonates were orally administered a large dose of live, virulent *M. tuberculosis* [22]. Clinical or radiological signs of infection were detected in 173 infants that were able to survive the infection, whereas 72 died from TB disease [12, 22]. The remarkable ability of the surviving 173 infants to survive the clinical manifestations of TB clearly demonstrates the efficacy and undisputable relevance of the innate immune response to Mtb, a large portion of which belongs to macrophages [12]. Studies spanning over recent decades have shown that development of symptomatic TB does not always occur upon initial infection in humans, cattle, mice and rabbits [12]. Further perplexing is the fact that a relevant portion of close contacts with microbiologically confirmed TB cases displays no diagnostically valuable immunopathologic changes (ex. negative tuberculin skin test (TST) and interferon gamma (IFN-γ) Release Assay (IGRA)) [66]. Interestingly, even data on acquired sensitivity to the TST is inconsistent for individuals considered to be at risk of infection; some develop sensitivity sooner than others [12, 18, 22, 28, 67, 68]. The source of this perplexity may very well be located in the host's immune genes and their functionality rather than the sole virulence of the pathogen, although both factors play relevant roles in TB pathogenesis. Disputed among clinicians and researchers is data suggesting that patients immunized with the standard BCG vaccine test positive for tuberculosis, regardless of the presence of an active or latent infection [66, 68, 69]. Conclusively to the TST cut-off research, an increase in TST cut-off criteria up to >15 mm, as opposed to the standard >5 mm cut-off, has been recommended for BCG-immunized patients; optimally throughout a time interval of 15 years after immunization [70]. Evidently, the response to inhalation of Mtb is not uniform in phenotypic manifestation for all individuals. The aforementioned variability is owed to the immunopathology governed by the host's immunogenetic profile, potential presence of comorbidities, pathogen virulence and prominence of numerous environmental factors, along with factors pertaining to receptor-specific internalization of the bacillus by macrophages [71]. Mutations and polymorphisms in genes coding for phagocytic receptor proteins seem to influence the competency of the host's constitutional resistance to progression from primary infection to primary disease or post-primary symptomatic infection [40, 41, 43, 44]. Significant and perhaps disproportional attention has been given T cell mediated immunity in contrast to humoral immunity. Whether humoral immunity poses a significant role in Mtb immunopathology has not been sufficiently elucidated yet, although there is evidence linking B cell immunity and immune competence in murine models [4].

Innate immunity is critical for early anti-mycobacterial responses, it is also important for the progression of infection and long-term control of Mtb by continually priming and educating adaptive immune responses and by regulating inflammation [28]. The system comprises two components, cellular and humoral, the latter including circulating complement proteins, defensins, cytokines and chemokines secreted by innate immune cells [72]. The cellular component which requires our attention comprises of innate immune cells which consist of epithelial cells, endothelial cells (ECs), granulocytes (neutrophils, basophils, eosinophils, mast cells (MCs)), monocytes, macrophages, natural killer (NK) cells, dendritic cells (DCs), invariant NKT cells (iNKT cells), γδT cells, innate immune T cells called mucosal invariant T cells (MAIT) cells and innate lymphoid cells (ILCs). These cells are crucial for the maintenance of the immune homeostasis and regulation of the adaptive immune system; they act as antigen presenting cells (APCs) as well as provide other signaling molecules/factors required in the effective adaptive immune response in response to infection or chronic inflammatory diseases [72].

In the case of TB, the earliest encounter between the host's immune system and Mtb occurs at the interface between resident lung (alveolar) macrophages and the virulent bacterial cells. These cells are often niches for bacterial replication and Mtb utilizes a myriad of strategies that subvert innate immune responses to establish a chronic infection [4]. During the past several decades, much has been uncovered and mechanisms through which the immune system responds to Mtb are in many ways illuminated, even though much still lingers in the shadows, which will hopefully be cast away over time. The first step is the recognition of mycobacteria as invading pathogens, followed by activation of innate host defense responses, and the subsequent initiation of adaptive immune responses [4]. Knowledge about these processes is crucial for understanding the pathophysiology of tuberculosis and for the development of novel strategies for vaccination and treatment such as immunotherapy.

The initiation process of the innate immune response starts with pattern recognition of microbial structures called pathogen-associated molecular patterns (PAMPs). Recognition of PAMPs is performed by germline-encoded receptors expressed mainly on immune cells termed pattern recognition receptors; in this case, being alveolar macrophages [26].

2.1 Expression levels of cytokines and cytokine receptors influence the extensity of immunopathology

Recruitment of innate immune cells in the early stages of infection is the result of secretion of cytokines and chemokines either by infected phagocytic cells or respiratory lung epithelial cells [56]. Studies have shown that primary lung epithelial cells possess the ability to cross-talk with infected macrophages, which benefits the process of monocyte recruitment. Infected phagocytic cells, inside of which the first stage of Mtb infection commences, may either migrate to the mediastinal lymph nodes in order to prime a T cell response via antigen presentation, or directly prime naïve T cells [73]. In the context of innate immunity, recruitment of polymorphonuclear leukocytes (PMNLs) to the sight of infection seems to be a 'double-edged' sword that either leads to effective control of infection, or damaging inflammation [73]. A mouse study on the recruitment of PMNs by alveolar epithelial cells during early stages of infection, concluded that severely damaging inflammation can occur as a consequence of this process [73]. It was discovered that CXCR2 and CXCL5 significantly contribute to a high influx of PMNLs, which is the mechanism behind the destructive inflammatory response during the initial stages of infection in mice and non-human primates (NHP) [73, 74]. Numerous CXCR2 ligands seem to positively regulate PMNL recruitment in murine models.

With regards to TB in vivo infection, TLR2 recognition of Mtb molecular patterns induces expression of CXCL5 by alveolar epithelial cells, which subsequently recruits PMNLs via CXCR2. Tlr2−/− mutants demonstrated significantly diminished, although not abolished, secretion of CXCL5 in vivo [73, 75]. Considering that alveolar epithelial cells are not the only cells present in the bronchoalveolar space during Mtb infection, and that those cells secrete inflammatory mediators that promote secretion of CXCL5, this finding is not at all surprising. There is an absolute dependency on CXCR5 for recruitment of PMNLs into the bronchoalveolar space during Mtb infection [73]. In contrast, PMNL recruitment induced by CXCL5 was found to account for roughly 60% of PMNLs recruited to the airspaces in vivo [73]. Exacerbated inflammation occurs with an incredibly high degree of dependence to CXCL5 secretion and the dose of Mtb that has infected the host [56, 73]. CXCL5 is not only expressed by alveolar epithelial cells, but rather a variety of other tissue-resident cells, making its role in tissue inflammatory responses well emphasized [76]. Although much work lies ahead in understanding the implications of CXCL5 and CXCR2 in TB immunopathology in the context of innate and acquired immunity, having a better understanding of these pathways could aid in devising treatment approaches that would allow for avoidance of the devastating inflammatory damage seen in certain subpopulations of TB patients. As for these findings corresponding to human immunopathology in TB, the ENA-78 neutrophil attractant secreted by human pulmonary epithelial cells is very similar to murine CXCL5 [77]. Of course, further studies should be conducted in order to comprehensively understand whether the studies on CXCL5 could be translated to human TB. Unfortunately, this particular aspect of Mtb infection in humans has thus far received modest attention, however current research is indicative of this likely being the case.

2.2 The behavior of macrophages infected with *M. tuberculosis*

The continuous development in the field of immunology has established their role in various immunological and non-immunological processes including embryonic development. Along with acting as phagocytic cells involved in the phagocytosis of pathogens, xenobiotics, these cells also secrete various cytokines, chemokines, and growth factors including TNF-α, TGF-β, platelet-derived growth factor (PDGF), endothelial growth factor (EGF), and vascular endothelial growth factor (VEGF) [72].

Alveolar macrophages encounter Mtb within the first 48 hours of infection, thereby representing the primary replicative niche for the bacillus [77]. Once Mtb is recognized by alveolar macrophages, it is engulfed through surface receptors, which leads to phagocytosis of the bacterium into phagosomes, which typically fuses with lysosomes for pathogen eradication and further consequent acidification of the pathogen-containing phagolysosome. Until recently the mechanism behind the establishment of a chronic infection in mammalian primates remained rather obscure; the lung interstitium, however, was definitely known to be the focal point of the infection based on previous studies [77]. In a 2018 study, performed by Cohen et al., discovered that alveolar macrophages transport Mtb from the alveoli to the interstitial tissue, under the influence of interleukin-1 signaling and the Mtb ESX1 secretion system [77]. Furthermore, localization of infected alveolar macrophages to the lung interstitial tissue leads to virulent Mtb cells being introduced to replication-permissive monocytes [13, 78]. Involvement of IL-1 in this process is not surprising considering that Mtb is a potent stimulator of the inflammasome, which regulates IL-1 production [79]. Contextually to recognition of mycobacterial antigens, one of the most important receptors for mycobacteria is the complement receptor 3, while other receptors such as CR1 and CR4, mannose receptor, surfactant protein A receptor, CD14, Fcγ receptor, scavenger receptors, have also been implicated in phagocytosis and internalization of mycobacteria inside the Mϕs [57].

The mycobacterial surface glycoprotein, mannose-capped lipoarabinomannan (Man-LAM) is recognized by the C-type lectins and the macrophage mannose receptor (MMR). An important role of toll-receptors, mainly the TLR2, has been demonstrated for the attachment of mycobacteria to macrophages [57]. Mtb is capable of inhibiting that process of phagosome maturation, as a result of which acidification of the phagosome is compromised, thus avoiding degradation and antigen processing [57]. Mtb is equipped with a variety of mechanisms that enable such form of survival, the key ones of which are stress-adaptive genes that are expressed in Mtb in order to counter the nitrosative, oxidative, hypoxic, and nutrient-diminished phagosome environment [80]. From an evolutionary point of view, it is clear that Mtb has developed alongside humans and thus adapted for a lifestyle inside the Mϕ, employing many strategies to survive within these cells.

Mtb entry intro Mϕs through different receptors can induce the activation of different pathways that can either inhibit or promote bacterial replication. Mϕ defenses include antimicrobial peptides (AMPs), nitrosative stresses, phagolysosome fusion and autophagy and may operate independently of or subsequent to IFN-γ signaling [7]. The overall interaction of multiple receptors and their engagement with Mtb ligands is a complex and dynamic issue. For instance, TLR-2 recognition of mycobacterial ManLAM activates NF-κB and NOS2 gene transcription that leads to antimycobacterial nitric oxide (NO) production, which is strongly associated with resistance to Mtb, even though evidence for that is stronger in mouse models [72, 81]. It has been shown that the reactive nitrogen intermediates (RNI) in mice are toxic to mycobacteria in vitro and by inhibition of NOs in vitro or in vivo infection can be exacerbated [44]. In relation, mice with disrupted NOS2 alleles display exacerbated disease following Mtb infection [44]. As for humans, in vitro studies using human alveolar macrophages and primary monocytes showed no anti-mycobacterial properties for NO, but specific staining for NOS2 in the bronchoalveolar lavage (BAL) of TB patients revealed upregulation in infected individuals compared to healthy controls. Another interesting fact is that mutations in Gp91phox, encoded by CYBB, a subunit of phagocyte oxidase enzyme complex (NADPH), pivotal for ROS (reactive oxygen species) are significantly correlated with reduced risk of TB [44].

In human macrophages, TLR-mediated recognition of Mtb is reported to synergize with the vitamin D pathway to induce the antimicrobial peptide (AMP), cathelicidin [77]. That process happens through calcitriol, a biologically active vitamin D metabolite, which induces the hCAP-18 gene encoding the pro-form of cathelicidin, following TLR ligation of macrophages. Studies have shown that cathelicidin exerts antimicrobial functions by activating transcription of host autophagy genes Beclin-1 and Atg5 [4]. Besides that, the vitamin D pathway also synergizes with IFN-γ secreted by T-cells to induce IL-15 autocrine signaling to promote autophagy and phagosome maturation in Mtb-infected human macrophages [4, 79].

Autophagy also plays a role in promoting phagosome maturation to enhance bacterial killing and it is integrated into the host response to Mtb infection by synergizing with pathogen sensing, phagosome maturation, and IFN-γ inducible pathways to mediate anti-mycobacterial immunity [4]. Autophagy-related proteins are likely to perform multiple functions and care must be taken when interpreting specific knockouts or knockdowns of individual genes. For instance, myeloid cell-specific ablation of Atg5 compromised control of Mtb in mouse studies. Deletion of autophagy-related genes Ulk1, Ulk2, Atg4B, or p62 compromised the ability to induce autophagy, but were dispensable for control of *M. tuberculosis*. Further analysis of lung sections from Mtb-infected mice showed that Atg5 knockout indicated that it may be involved in regulations of neutrophil responses during infection.

The factor responsible for macrophage activation is IFN-γ produced by CD8+ cytotoxic T (Tc1) cells, CD4+ T helper 1 (Th1) T cells, and natural killer (NK) cells. IFN-γ activation leads to conversion of macrophages to potent phagocytotic cells with increased production of reactive oxygen intermediates and reactive nitrogen intermediates, superoxides and proinflammatory cytokines helping the cells to efficiently kill the intracellular pathogens. This type of IFN-γ-mediated activation induces M1 macrophages [57].

On the other hand, T helper 2 (Th2) type of cytokines, IL-4 and IL-13, induce a response different from the one induced by IFN-γ with distinct set of genes being expressed to form what is known as the alternative activation pathway of macrophages, and the cells are named as alternative activated type 2 or M2 macrophages [13, 72].

Various immune complexes, IL-10, vitamin D3 can also contribute to the activation of M2 macrophages [57]. M2 macrophages generally exhibit a higher phagocytic activity, mannose and galactose receptors, produce higher concentration of ornithine and polyamines due to high arginase pathway, secrete high amount of IL-10 and express higher levels of the IL-1 decoy receptor and IL-1RA. Having all these characteristics, M2 macrophages play a crucial role in anti-parasitic immune response [72].

3. Immunoreceptors expressed on macrophages and their role in the immunopathological course of TB

3.1 *M. tuberculosis* is capable of turning macrophages into non-bactericidal environments in an Immunoreceptor-specific manner

Mannose receptors (CD206) play an important role in TB innate immunity due to their efficacy and specificity as endocytic receptor through engagement of virulence-associated mycobacterial cell wall components that contain mannose, particularly glycoproteins and sulphated and non-sulphated polysaccharides [82]. MR-positive immune cells are able to deliver various antigens to sites where humoral and cellular responses occur, therefore playing a role in bridging innate and acquired immunity [83–86]. This CTL is a Ca^{2+}-dependent type I transmembrane glycoprotein contains an extracellular N terminal, cysteine-rich (CR) domain, a fibronectin II (FNII) domain, eight carbohydrate recognition domains, a cytoplasmic tail and a transmembrane domain. The cytoplasmic tail contains 49 amino acids and there is a tyrosine residue on the 18th position that has been heavily implicated in endocytosis [51]. Much has been uncovered about the signaling pathways of CD206 in recent years, implicating this receptor in functions such as M2 macrophage polarization, antigen presentation, entry trafficking, macrophage-associated tumor biology and receptor targeting for therapeutic purposes [71, 79, 87]. CTL signaling is achieved through various adaptor proteins, of which the FcRγ chain is the most common [51]. Although the implications of this remain in question, heat shock proteins (HSP) in unstimulated cells interact with CD206 [88, 89]. Furthermore, it is not fully understood how this alters the structural configuration of MR upon their activation in vivo, although strides have been made in uncovering the significance of actin remodeling in this process, and its implication in phagolysosome maturation [51]. Phagocytosis is an actin-dependent process, therefore MR-mediated phagocytosis requires receptor clustering, recruitment and engagement of various adaptor proteins and activation of the Rho family of small GTPases in order to facilitate cytoskeletal remodeling [51]. Surface localization of CD206 depends on its ability to interact with FcRγ, which likely occurs at the interface of the positively-charged transmembrane region of the receptor [51]. This is where the value of murine models in understanding receptor-related aspects of TB immunopathology in humans sees its shortcomings: the cytoplasmic tail and TM region of the murine MR is neutrally charged, likely leading to reduced FcRγ tail binding and diminished surface MR exposure [51]. In the contest of human macrophages, recruitment and activation of the Src homology region 2 domain-containing phosphatase 1 (SHP-1) is an MR-dependent event that occurs during Mtb infection; SHP-1 phosphorylates and co-localizes with phagosomes containing Mtb [51]. As a consequence of this, SHP-1 reduces the activity of class III PI3P by interfering with the serine/threonine-protein kinase Vps15 and the phosphatidylinositol 3-kinase (PI3) hVPS34 [29, 87, 90]. Inhibition of SHP-1 has been found to lead to enhanced phagolysosome fusion [34].

Once Mtb is phagocytosed through CD206 engagement, subsequent immunomodulation facilitated by mycobacterial cell wall components may lead to the development of active disease. Mycobacterial ManLAM heavily influences several immunobiological processes throughout the continua of the immune response (**Figure 2**) [91]. ManLAM inhibits the process of phagolysosome fusion, which is considered a key aspect of TB infection with regards to mycobacterial intracellular persistence. It does so by blocking a crucial phosphatidylinositol 3-phosphate (PI3P)-regulated pathway involved in transportation of lysosomal and other crucial components from the trans-Golgi network to immature phagosomes; a process required for phagosome maturation [29, 87, 92, 93]. Two rab5 effector hVPS34 and the early endosomal antigen 1 (EEA1) are components crucial for phagosome maturation [32]. EEA1 binds to the membrane-associated PI3P via its FYVE and PX domains, to which ManLAM may competitively bind and thus preclude phagolysosome fusion. It was discovered that Mtb ManLAM interferes with a pathway involving Ca^{2+}, calmodulin and the Ca^{2+}/calmodulin-dependent protein kinase II (CaMKII) [29, 32, 87, 91, 92, 94]. EEA1 and Syntaxin 6 deliver various lysosomal components from the trans-Golgi network to immature phagosomes, making them crucial for phagosome maturation. However, Mtb uses ManLAM to disrupt recruitment of EEA1 to phagosome membranes by inhibiting the rise in cytosolic Ca^{2+}, thus rendering the Ca^{2+}/Calmodulin pathway, impotent [7]. Considering that hVPS34 interacts with calmodulin in order to generate PI3P, physiological maintenance of PI3P on phagosomes and other intracellular membranes requires calmodulin [91]. In summary, Mtb-associated ManLAM

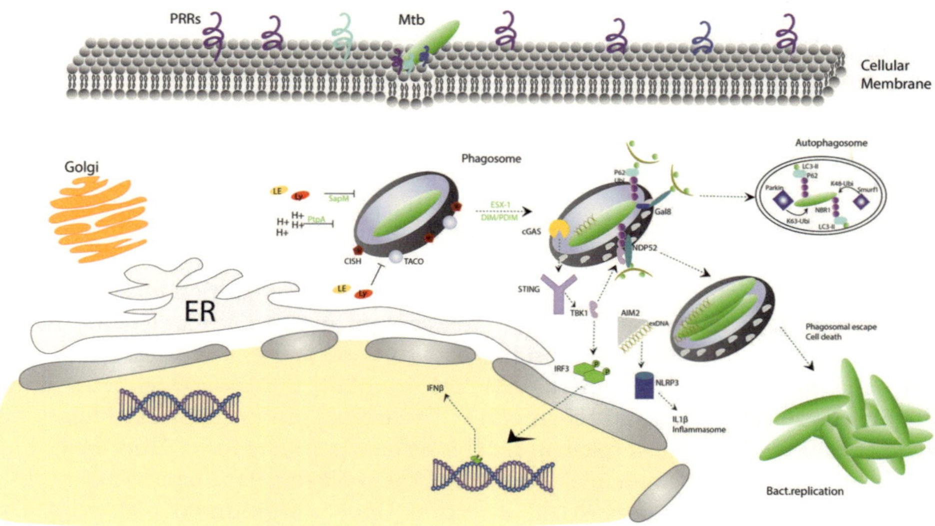

Figure 2.
*The process of successful and unsuccessful phagosome-lysosome fusion during pulmonary tuberculosis. Abbreviations: Golgi—Golgi apparatus, ER—endoplasmic reticulum, PRRs—pattern recognition receptors, Mtb—*Mycobacterium tuberculosis*, PtpA—protein tyrosine phosphatase, SapM—secreted acid phosphatase, CISH—cytokine-inducible SH2-containing protein, TACO—tryptophan-aspartate containing coat protein, IFNβ—interferon beta, IRF3—interferon regulatory factor 3, DIM/PDIM—Phthiocerol dimycocerosate, cGAS—cyclic GMP-AMP synthase, STING—stimulator of interferon genes, TBK1—TANK-binding kinase 1, P62—nucleoporin 62, Ubi—ubiquitin, Gal8—Galectin-8 protein, INDP52—calcium-binding and coiled-coil domain-containing protein 2, AIM2—absent in melanoma 2, NLRP3—NLR family pyrin domain containing 3 inflammasome, IL1β—interleukin 1β, LC3-II—microtubule-associated proteins 1A/1B light chain 3B, parkin—E3 ubiquitin ligase, K63-Ubi—polyubiquitinations K63, K48-Ubi—ubiquitination K48, NBR1—next to BRCA1 gene 1 protein, Smurf1—E3 ubiquitin-protein ligase SMURF1.*

provides a survivability niche within macrophages by blocking the increase in Ca2+ transients, therefore effectively disrupting a Ca^{2+}/Calmodulin associated pathway required for phagosome maturation. Physiological increase in cytosolic Ca^{2+} is heavily influenced by sphingosine kinase (SK), whose signaling pathways is triggered by FcR clustering. Studies suggest that the mechanism by which ManLAM disrupts the increase in cytosolic Ca^{2+} is likely through interference with SK signaling pathways [30].

Cytotoxicity of ManLAM, however, is diminished when dissociated from mycobacterial cells via the activity of the respiratory mucosa [92]. ManLAM debris are incapable of inhibiting the process of phagolysosome fusion, allowing for the attractive assumption that the human respiratory tract evolved in such a way to amplify the immune response to Mtb by creating these highly immunostimulatory debris in the early stages of infection [92]. Despite the evident potency and relevance of this Mtb-associated mechanism, ManLAM-mediated prevention of phagolysosome fusion is but one of the several mechanisms in the arsenal of Mtb, some of which have only been recently discovered [92].

Preferred engagement of the CR and MR-dependent phagocytic pathways was a sensical evolutionary approach by Mtb, since engulfment of microbes via CRs and MRs do not necessarily incite an inflammatory response by the host, and MR-abundant alveolar macrophages act as chaperones that deliver Mtb to replication-permissive cells [26, 30]. The mechanism by which CTLs elicit an anti-inflammatory response is found in the ManLAM-mediated stimulation of a nuclear receptor peroxisome proliferator-activated receptor gamma (PPAR-γ), which in turn triggers such a response. Limited phagosome-lysosome fusion is specific only for monocytes expressing MR, whereupon absence of this receptor on Mϕs and DCs does not lead to the inhibition of phagosome maturation. LAM may be exported from the infected Mϕs and presented to T-cells via the MHC I CD1 molecules [21, 95]. Previous research suggests that Mtb uses LAM to recruit host immune cells whose function it will subsequently modulate in order to facilitate survival.

3.2 Macrophage Toll-like receptors and their implications for tuberculosis

Toll-like receptors are type 1 transmembrane pattern recognition receptors instrumental to animal immunity [96]. They contain an extracellular leucine-rich repeat (LRR) domain—involved in signal transduction and molecular recognition—and intracellular toll/interleukin-1 receptor (TIR) domain, which represents a highly conserved protein-protein module. These receptors are expressed in a wide range of cells, with the most relevant for this discussion being Mϕs. Thus far 10 TLRs have been nominated in humans, with each of them playing cardinal roles in both innate and acquired immunity to Mtb infection. Upon recognition of Mtb molecular patterns via the receptor LRR domain, the Myeloid Differentiation Primary Response 88 (MyD88) is activated, which is utilized by all TLRs lest except for TLR3 (**Figure 3**). A wide spectrum of anti-mycobacterial actions taken by the immune system involve the synergic activity of TLRs and MyD88, leading to the subsequent involvement of IRAK, TNF receptor associated factor 6 (TRAF6), transforming growth factor beta-activated kinase 1 (TAK1) and mitogen-activated protein kinases (MAPK); it should be noted, however, that each TLR alone is capable of initiation a separate immunopathologic continua as means of amplifying the anti-Mtb immune response. Each TLR can bind a specific subset of pathogen-associated molecular patterns (PAMPs), they activate the innate immune system and help with the host protection. TLR2,

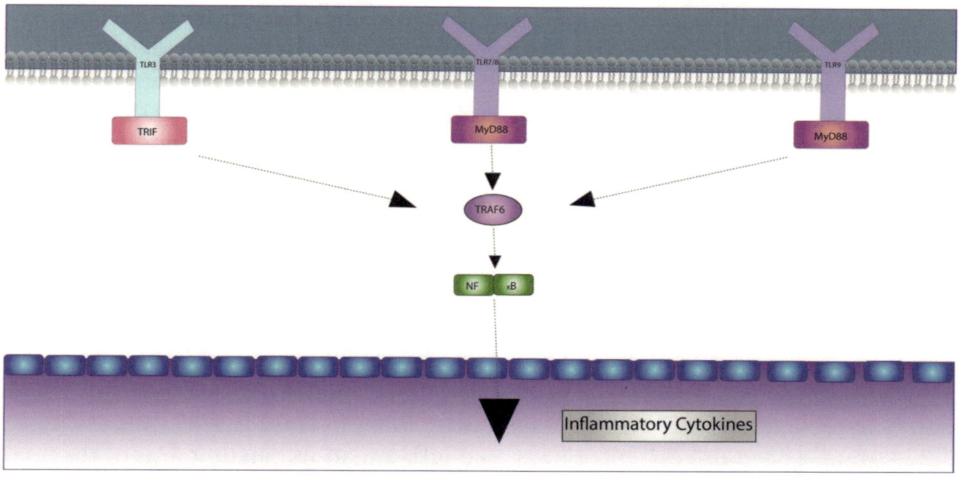

Figure 3.
Schematic representation of toll like (TLR) signaling. NF-κB gets translocated into the nucleus to initiate the transcription of inflammatory cytokine genes. Abbreviations: MyD88—Myeloid differentiation primary response, TRIF—TIR-domain-containing adapter-inducing interferon-β, NF-κB—NF-kappa B.

TLR4, and TLR9 are the most common TLRs that detect Mtb, with TLR2 playing the most important role 5. TLRs recognize Mtb PAMPs, which triggers an intracellular signaling cascade that binds the myeloid differentiation primary response protein 88 (MyD88) to TLRs intracellular domains6. MTB is an acid-fast bacterium because its cell wall is mostly made up of hydrophobic mycolic acids. This is a component of the mycobacterial cell wall that accounts for half of its dry weight. The admission of nutrients is slowed by this thick layer of mycolic acids, causing mycobacteria to proliferate slowly, but it also boosts cellular resistance to lysosomal enzyme destruction. The mycolic acids are typically found in a thick layer on the cell wall's exterior surfaces7. Lipids and polysaccharides make up the mycobacterial wall, which also contains a lot of mycolic acid.

TLR2 and TLR4 are activated by purified cell wall components of mycobacteria [81]. Lipomannan and lipoarabinomannan are two lipoglycans with substantial immunomodulatory properties [30, 38]. TLR2, in conjunction with TLR1, can identify Mtb cell wall lipoprotein antigens, which cause macrophages to produce cytokines. TLR9 is triggered by mycobacterial DNA. The engagement of IL-1 receptor-associated kinases, TNF receptor-associated factor 6, TGF-activated protein kinase 1 and mitogen-activated protein kinase is then enhanced by MyD88 [97]. The transcription factor NF-κB is activated and translocated to the nucleus as a result of this signaling cascade. Multiple pro-inflammatory cytokines, including tumor necrosis factor, interleukin-1 and interleukin-12, are produced as a result [98]. Tumor necrosis factor and interleukin-12 are then secreted, causing nearby natural killer and T cells to produce IFN-y. IFN-y is a key macrophage stimulator and activator of major histocompatibility complex class II molecule production. IFN's importance in the immune system arises from its capacity to directly suppress virus replication, as well as its immunomodulatory properties. IFN-y stimulates macrophages, enhancing antigen presentation and promoting anti-mycobacterial effector mechanisms such as reactive oxygen and nitrogen intermediates, autophagy, phagolysosome fusion and acidification autophagy [99, 100].

For instance, TLR2 has been implicated in regulating T cell trafficking by inducing the production of CCL8, a CD4+ chemokine, and in recruiting regulatory T cells (Treg) to infection foci in order to regulate inflammation. Tampering with the inflammatory response in the context of TLR2 is at least in part owed to the TLR2-induced secretion of CXCL5, considering that PMNL recruitment by this chemokine has the potency to drive destructive inflammation during early stages of infection [81]. Mycobacterial ESAT-6 readily promotes macrophage apoptosis by activating the TLR2/NF-κB [101]. One of the ways that Mtb causes a delay in priming the adaptive immune response is through the activities of mycolic acid and various mycobacterial lipoproteins, which have potency to downregulate MHC II expression and pro-inflammatory responses. Furthermore, TLR2 enhances the expression of vitamin D receptor genes [81, 102–104]. It should be noted that induction of ROS can be achieved through TLR2/dectin-1 cooperation [105]. Induction of a rather wide range of anti-mycobacterial mechanisms is also partly owed to TLR2 [63–65, 106, 107]. TLR2−/− mice have also exhibited increased inflammation, pneumonitis of the interstitial lung tissue and abnormal granuloma morphology, with a very modest increase in bacterial burden [108]. Concordantly to these findings, concluding that TLR2 plays both beneficial and detrimental roles in Mtb infection seems to be rather prudent, as TLR2 signaling is influenced by numerous components of both the immune system and mycobacterial virulence, with notable implications in innate immunity and priming of adaptive immunity.

Functions of TLR4 have been reported to include promotion of CD4 and CD8 T cell recruitment, polarization of T effector cells towards a Th1 cell phenotype and numerous other activities that may be construed as both beneficial and detrimental [81]. Mycobacterial phosphatidyl inositol mannosides can inhibit the production of proinflammatory cytokines and NO by interfering the synergic activity of TLR4 and MyD88. Repressing the host's ability to produce NO is a sensical approach, as low levels of NO have been associated with the activation of dormancy-related genetic programs such as the DosRST regulon [106]. With the recently uncovered detrimental role of alveolar macrophages during early stages of infection, this could be a mechanism used by Mtb to ensure survivability of infected phagocytes in order to be transported to the lung interstitial tissue abundant in replication-permissive monocytes. The Mtb-associated resuscitation-promoting factor B (RpfB) interacts with TLR4 on DCs, activating the synergic signaling of MyD88 and toll/IL-1R homology domain-containing adapter-inducing IFN-β (TRIF), in order to ensure downstream signaling to MAPK and NF-κB [108]. This signaling pathway promotes education of naïve T cells and their subsequent polarization to CD4+ and CD8+, which will secrete IFN-γ and IL-2 [105]. Furthermore, this pathway induces T cell proliferation and polarization in the context of Th1 immunity, further emphasizing the importance of TLR2 signaling in TB immunopathology [105].

Plasmacytoid DCs (pDC), a special subset of DCs, function in close cooperation with TLR9 in such a way as to allow these immune cells to conduct their immune functions, including initiation of the immune response and control of inflammation through the induction of chemokines (**Figure 4**). pDCs are known to play an important role in recruiting NK cells; pDC−/− mice show a drastic reduction in NK cell recruitment upon intraperitoneal injection. Considering that pDCs express the CCR5, CCR2 and the CXCR3 ligand receptors on their surface, this likely translates to diminished binding of chemokines CCL2, CCL3, CCL4, CXCL10 and CXCL9 [109]. Mycobacterial DNA, the unmethylated CpG oligodeoxynucleotide motif in particular, acts as a TLR9 ligand and initiates the signaling pathway that promotes

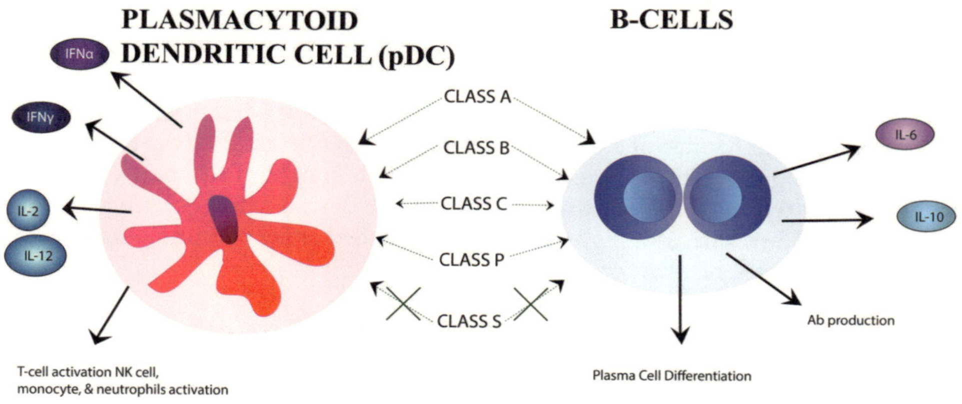

Figure 4.
Plasmacytoid cells in tuberculosis immunopathology. Abbreviations: IFNα/γ—interferon α/γ; IL-2/6/10/12—Interleukin-2/6/10/12, Ab—antibodies, NK cells—natural killer cells.

such pDC activity in Mtb infection [105]. Abrogation of TLR9 in mutant mice leads to higher susceptibility to TB diseases, in contrast to wild-type mice. Interestingly, previous studies on the synergic activity of TLR9 and TLR2 found that TLR9−/− mice demonstrated only mild differences in overall lung histopathology and granuloma formation [105]. However, focal necrosis was seen in TLR9/2−/− mice, a pathological outcome that also occurs for MyD88−/− mice, albeit the lung pathology in MyD88−/− mice is evidently more severe, further emphasizing the importance of MyD88 in TB immunopathology [109]. It should be noted, however, that no relevant difference in susceptibility was discovered in either TLR9−/− or TLR2−/− mice; alterations in granulomatous pathology and TNF-α secretion occur only for high-dose inoculums of Mtb as a consequence of TLR9 deficiency [105]. Considering that pDCs secrete IL-12—a cytokine that induces and controls the production of IFN-γ by CD4+ T cells—the relevance of TLR9-mediated signaling is evidently pivotal in both innate and acquired immunity [110, 111]. It would appear that synergic activity of a minimum of two TLRs is important in the signaling pathways that initiate competent immune responses to TB, although each receptor alone has proven to be relevant in vivo in gene knockout studies conducted on mice. Interestingly, a recent mouse study has concluded that TLR2 and TLR9 signaling is not necessary for vaccine-induced immunity [24, 112]. It should be noted, however, that an immunization strategy based on the combination of enhancement of TLR4, TLR3 and TLR9 signaling and the Mtb antigen Rv2034—a powerful CD4+ cell stimulant—has been successfully explored in mice and guinea pigs [113].

Although certain TLRs are part of signaling pathways relevant to TB immunopathology, they alone are only but a cog in a very complex machinery that comprises the TLR-mediated immune response to Mtb infection. It is attractive to speculate that devising immunotherapies guided towards enhancing TLR signaling due to their pivotal role in priming Th1 immunity through cytokine secretion, could be a fruitful avenue to pursue. Rampant inflammation at the level of innate immunity, influenced by TLR signaling, may also be a target of novel immunotherapies directed at diminishing the violent effects that excess PMNL recruitment has on the lung tissue [33, 105, 108]. However, to infer that enhanced TLR signaling alone would be sufficient in combating tuberculosis, would be rather misinformed. Namely, it was discovered that, in murine models, XDR TB reduces the expression of TLR2 and TLR4 and consequently the production of cytokines that were otherwise abundantly present in mice infected with DS Mtb [114]. The inhibitory effects of XDR strains reduced the overall lung pathology in such a way that alveolar damage was reduced and granulomatous formations were smaller in size, in contrast with the detrimental immunopathologic events that were caused by DS TB. In light of this particular finding, one may infer that XDR TB was less virulent due to its down regulating effects on TLRs than DS strains, although much work is needed to further understand the implications of these results.

3.3 Implications of specific macrophage TLRs in tuberculosis pathogenesis

TLR2 signaling is triggered by heterodimerization with TLR1 or TLR6, and it follows a well-known signaling pathway. The "bridging adaptor" Mal is recruited by dimerized receptors, which aids in the recruitment of MyD88 and the formation of the myddosome complex, which consists of Mal, MyD88, and IRAK proteins. The nuclear translocation of NFkB and AP1 to commence transcription of cytokine and chemokine genes is triggered by the activation of IRAK4 followed by IRAK1/IRAK2 and activation of TRAF6 and TAK112. Mtb produces a vast number of TLR2 ligands [97]. It's secreted antigen 19 kDa lipoprotein (LpqH) was the first *M. tuberculosis* ligand to be demonstrated to signal through TLR2 [115]. TLR2 receptors sense mycobacterial lipoproteins LprA (Rv1270), LprG (Rv1411c), and PhoS113 [98, 116]. TLR2 is usually thought to play a minor function in Mtb immunity [97]. In Mtb infection, TLR2 signaling promotes three functional responses: protection, evasion, and regulation [97]. These responses are not required for the control of acute Mtb infection, but they may be required in chronic infection [81]. TLR2-activated pro-inflammatory cytokines induce protective mechanisms that keep Mtb control, while immune evasion mechanisms allow Mtb to evade antibacterial effector molecules [115–117]. TLR2 signaling is inhibited by immune regulatory pathways that have been activated by the pathogen, much like in the case of MRs. Mtb persists with low immunopathology and collateral harm to host tissue as a result of the multi-factorial functional response's combinatorial effect. In chronic infection, TLR2 signaling benefits both the host and the bacteria [97]. While TLR2 activation in macrophages is critical for controlling Mtb infection, it may not always be advantageous to host cells because Mtb has developed strategies to exploit TLR2 activation for its own gain. TLR2 has the capacity to engage several, structurally unique ligands and elicit different signals, and is one of the few receptors that can heterodimerize with TLR1 or TLR6, and also connect to additional co-receptors like CD14. One theory is that TLR2's interaction different binding partners helps to diversify ligand recognition [104].

TLR4 is best known for recognizing the Gram-negative bacteria's lipopolysaccharide (LPS) [118]. TLR4 detects lipids in cell walls, glycoproteins, and secretory proteins in Mtb [118]. The LAM precursor LM, as previously mentioned, causes macrophages to produce pro-inflammatory cytokines. Because BMDMs produce TNF and reactive nitrogen intermediates (RNI) in a TRL4-dependent manner in the presence of Ac4LM, the tetra-acylated version of LM (Ac4LM) operates as a particular TLR4 activator [119]. TLR4 is activated by a variety of mycobacterial proteins, including several heat shock proteins, Mtb H37Rv 38-kDA glycoprotein and the Mtb 50S ribosomal protein Rv0652. TLR4 stimulation can initiate the MyD88-independent TIR-domain including adapter-inducing IFN-β pathway [118]. It later on increases the expression of IRF3 to generate IFN-β secretion in this route, and both IRF-3 and IFN-β have important parts to play in TB pathogenesis [120]. While some Mtb strains only engage TLR2, others trigger TLR4, resulting in distinct cytokine profiles marked by varied IFN-β production and as a result different bacterial pathogenicity ensues [30, 81].

TLR9 has been found in endosomes and phagolysosomes, where it can be activated by mycobacterial DNA upon pathogen uptake [105]. Thus, TLR9 is an important pattern-recognition receptor that could explain the host resistance to Mtb being dependent on MyD88. It identifies CG motifs (CpG) in bacterial DNA that are undermethylated, including Mtb DNA [121]. CpG sites are DNA areas in which cytosine is followed by guanine in a 5′ → 3′ direction linear sequence of bases. TNF-α, is produced with treatment of primary macrophages which can be inhibited with a TLR9 blocker or DNA methylation [121]. Mtb is a powerful stimulator of TLR9-dependent proinflammatory cytokine production by dendritic cells and macrophages, and these cells' in vitro responses to live mycobacteria are also TLR9-dependent [105]. Furthermore, this suggest that TLR9 is involved in the control of mycobacteria-induced Th1 responses in vivo during Mtb infection [105].

4. Macrophages and their role in tuberculosis granuloma formation

Many have questioned the purpose of the granuloma (**Figure 5**) within the body, but some would argue that the formation of the granuloma by the various white blood cells and macrophages in the body is an attempt by the adaptive immune system to contain the cells already infiltrated by Mtb cells [58]. It is begun as an innate immune system response but evolves in complexity as the adaptive immune system takes over [122]. The granuloma will begin forming as a group of macrophages who have been infiltrated and infected by Mtb, which are then surrounded by other macrophages and white blood cells in order to isolate these infected macrophages with their surrounding environment [123]. The granuloma will then be enclosed by a fibrous cuff and the surrounding area will undergo significant angiogenesis, similar to what

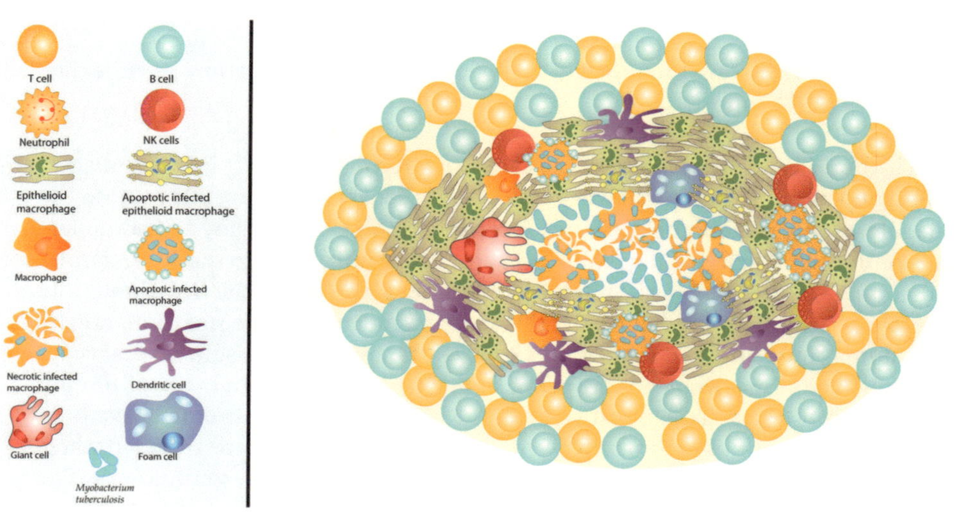

Figure 5.
Graphic illustration of the tuberculosis granuloma.

occurs when a cancerous tumor forms [124]. The macrophages and white blood cells within the granuloma will trigger conditions of hypoxia and lower nutrient availability [122]. Within the granuloma, it is believed that the bacteria do not continue replicating but instead focus their resources on gluconeogenesis to ensure their survival [58].

Of course, this also has a negative effect on the human body's own cells, and can eventually result in a necrotic or caseating granuloma [125]. This is partly due to "foamy" or lipid droplet-containing macrophages, which are formed by increased diffusion of LDL vesicles in the macrophage cells, and whatever is not exported by ATP active transport methods is esterified to convert it into lipid bodies, which give the cell its foamy appearance [123]. These cells are proinflammatory, and the increased presence of them promotes Mtb within the granuloma, enhancing the deteriorating conditions around and inside it and leading to eventual necrosis [55]. Lipid droplets released from the cell in the form of triglycerides can be absorbed by Mtb-infected macrophages, where they are then used by the Mtb bacteria for lipid metabolism [123]. Additionally, superoxide and NO production from the macrophages is severely limited due to the hypoxic conditions, so many times in the case of a granuloma, the best that can be hoped for is an isolated environment containing the bacteria, as bactericidal action by the macrophages becomes more difficult [123]. The most devastating problem presented by the granuloma is Mtb's ability to hijack the process for its own survival. Mtb bacteria have adapted to the formation of the granuloma, and mycobacterial recruitment proteins like ESX-1 release compounds to recruit macrophages to form the granuloma [4]. The reason for this is to provide the bacteria a fresh supply of macrophages for them to infect while simultaneously cutting themselves off from lymphocytes, who have a more pronounced bactericidal action against them [123]. The structure of the granuloma also creates difficulty for penetration by drugs and other therapies, and some have even considered treating the granuloma using similar methods to cancerous tumor treatment [126]. There are various types and stages of the granuloma ranging from primary granulomas to acute caseating granulomas. Caseating granulomas will begin descending into necrosis, releasing the Mtb into the surrounding lung tissue, which can then further infect others by being released in aerosolized droplets [18, 127].

4.1 Macrophages transport living *M. tuberculosis* into replication-permissive interstitial tissue

The bacillus once engulfed by the alveolar macrophage (AM) into the phagolysosome sabotages the lysosomal pathways. By incorporating proton pumps into the phagolysosome membrane, fusion to lysosomes is blocked, as they accommodate the environment suitable for replication and hence polarize into the M2 macrophage phenotype [128, 129]. In later stages, the bacillus may subvert the functional role of lysosome pathways by inducing cell necrosis as a means of dissemination, creating granulomas in the lung interstitium [130, 131]. Granulomas exist in several types wherein diverse macrophages are primary residents, leading to a range of unique microenvironments that are statistically independent of each other in a host body [132]. The outcome of the infection will depend on the phenotype of macrophages present (M1/M2 polarization) altered by the bacillus within the granulomas. The precedent to granuloma establishment—the translocation of the AM from the alveolus to the lung interstitium—depends on several signaling pathways. ESX-1 secretion system is necessary for the bacillus' escape from the AM phagolysosome by potentiating inflammasome (comprised of NLRP3, ASC and caspase-1) activation within the AM and hence interleukin-1β (IL-1β) release, which increases alveolar permeability once bound to IL-1R on the epithelial barrier [133]. The RD1-dependent inflammasome signaling pathway transfers the living Mtb-infected AM whereas the STING pathway facilitates movement across the epithelial barrier by transferring the bacillus from the AM to a *mycobacterium* growth-permissive monocyte for crossing [134]. This is accomplished primarily by the glycolipids on the cell-surface of bacillus. Specifically, the phthiocerol dimycoceroserate (PDIM) lipid prevents recognition of pathogen-associated molecular patterns (PAMPs) by Toll-like receptors (TLRs) [135]. The phenolic glycolipid (PGL) thereon induces chemokine CCL2 via cytosolic signaling pathway STING to recruit growth-permissive monocytes for bacterial transfer by leveraging their CCR2 receptor [135]. STING activation does not induce CCL2 through type 1 IFNs therefore is independent to type 1 IFN involvement in contrast to the RD1-dependent inflammasome signaling pathway [134]. The CCL2 elicited monocytes then play an inflammatory role in the interstitium- however, the monocytes may switch roles to favor the host by offering antigens to pulmonary lymph nodes for T cell response.

5. Conclusions

Human tuberculosis is a tremendously complex infection, leaving no compartment of the immune system spared. Thus, conclusive studies on this disease from an immunological standpoint are difficult to conduct, due to the heterogenicity present within different populations in the context of host immunogenetics and potential previous exposure to pathogenic and non-pathogenic mycobacteria. Though other innate immune cells eventually come into play, macrophages play a pivotal role in the immune response to infections with *Mycobacterium tuberculosis*, as they represent the first professional line of defense against respiratory infections in general. Indeed, macrophages are equipped with the necessary bactericidal mechanisms to effectively destroy infectious agents, however Mtb has successfully developed a barrage of methods by which they may be circumvented, thereby converting the macrophage from a foe into a safe confinement. Macrophages that have failed to eliminate the bacillus tend to shuttle and localize the pathogen in environments that are rich in replication-permissive cells, thereby perpetuating further bacterial replication and dissemination. Failure of macrophages to clear out the infection is primarily rooted in receptor-mediated uptake of Mtb, where the pathogen favors MR-mediated uptake, as it allows for the bacillus to manipulate the intracellular environment in order to avoid destruction in the phagosome by preventing phagosome-lysosome fusion. However, even in the case where infected macrophages shuttle the pathogen the replication-permissive lung interstitium, the cytokines produced by these infected cells recruit novel APCs, seemingly in order to physically entrap Mtb. This results in the formation of a tuberculosis granuloma, characterized by an infected core, surrounded by non-infected APCs such as macrophages, with the granuloma exterior being further supported by T cells. Though these granulomas seem like a sensical and efficient method of preventing further dissemination of the pathogen, mycobacterial survivability within the hypoxic and noxious granuloma environment is enabled through reprogramming of the metabolic profile of Mtb. This reprogramming enables a state of metabolic dormancy, clinically distinguished by the term latent tuberculosis—an asymptomatic form of TB. When in this state, Mtb is capable of utilizing the abundant concentration of lipids, among other molecules, present in foamy macrophages in order to facilitate survival. In spite of this, the human immune system is capable of continuously maintaining the structural integrity of the granuloma and ensure that viable but dormant mycobacterial cells are contained. Whether a dormant infection will become activated depends on the competence of the host's immune system. Erosion of the granuloma leads to rapid activation and replication of the bacillus and its dissemination through the airways. Furthermore, eroded granulomas are characterized by extensive caseous necrosis which leaves radiographically observable lung cavities in TB patients. Thus, professional macrophages that are engaged in combating Mtb infection are difficult to categorize in terms of their efficiency at resolving the infection. It appears that every infection with Mtb, in the very least, leads to latent TB, thereby making the conversation of complete elimination of the bacillus from the immune system, rather improbable. Rather, it is more prudent to understand the immune response to Mtb infection as containment rather than infectant elimination, and this is primarily owed to the ambiguous dual role those professional macrophages play in infectious with Mtb, supplemented by factors that include macrophage immunoreceptors, cytokine expression profiles and the overall virulence of the bacillus itself.

Acknowledgements

The authors would like to thank Dado Latinović from the International Burch University for designing and generating all of the scientific illustrations provided within this work.

Conflict of interest

None to declare.

Notes/thanks/other declarations

We sincerely hope that, with the rapid expansion and improvement of scientific methods, we will eventually understand *M. tuberculosis* as well as it understands us.

Author details

Dženan Kovačić[1]*, Adna Softić[1], Adna Salihović[1] and Jovana Jotanović[2]

1 Faculty of Engineering and Natural Sciences, Department of Genetics and Bioengineering, International Burch University, Sarajevo, Bosnia and Herzegovina

2 Faculty of Natural Sciences and Mathematics, University of Sarajevo, Sarajevo, Bosnia and Herzegovina

*Address all correspondence to: dzenan.kovacic@stu.ibu.edu.ba

References

[1] Houben RM, Dodd PJ. The global burden of latent tuberculosis infection: a re-estimation using mathematical modelling. PLoS Medicine. 2016 Oct 25;**13**(10):e1002152

[2] World Health Organization. Global tuberculosis report 2019. 2019. Recuperado: https://www. who.int/tb/publications/global_report/en. 2020 Apr

[3] Bottai D, Frigui W, Sayes F, di Luca M, Spadoni D, Pawlik A, et al. TbD1 deletion as a driver of the evolutionary success of modern epidemic mycobacterium tuberculosis lineages. Nature Communications. 2020;**11**(1):684. Available from: http://www.nature.com/articles/s41467-020-14508-5

[4] Sia JK, Rengarajan J. Immunology of *Mycobacterium tuberculosis* infections. Microbiology Spectrum. 2019 Jul 12;**7**(4):4-7

[5] Lurie MB. Native and acquired resistance to tuberculosis. The American Journal of Medicine. 1950 Nov 1;**9**(5):591-610

[6] Guerrero Manriquez GG. Immunogenetic and Immunotherapy in Tuberculosis [Internet]. 2019. Available from: www.intechopen.com

[7] Nguyen L, Pieters J. The Trojan horse: Survival tactics of pathogenic mycobacteria in macrophages. Trends in Cell Biology. 2005;**15**:269-276

[8] Abel L, El-Baghdadi J, Bousfiha AA, Casanova JL, Schurr E. Human genetics of tuberculosis: a long and winding road. Philosophical Transactions of the Royal Society B: Biological Sciences. 2014 Jun 19;**369**(1645):20130428

[9] Derek C, Gail C. Novartis Foundation. Genetics and Tuberculosis. Cape Town, South Aftica: Wiley; 1998. p. 269

[10] Pagán AJ, Ramakrishnan L. Immunity and immunopathology in the tuberculous granuloma. Cold Spring Harbor Perspectives in Medicine. 2015 Sep 1;**5**(9):a018499

[11] Kiran D, Podell BK, Chambers M, Basaraba RJ. Host-directed therapy targeting the Mycobacterium tuberculosis granuloma: A review. Seminars in Immunopathology. 2016;**38**:167-183

[12] Cassidy JP, Martineau AR. Innate resistance to tuberculosis in man, cattle and laboratory animal models: Nipping disease in the bud? Journal of Comparative Pathology. 2014;**151**:291-308

[13] Pieters J. Mycobacterium tuberculosis and the macrophage: Maintaining a balance. Cell Host and Microbe. 2008;**3**:399-407

[14] Silva Miranda M, Breiman A, Allain S, Deknuydt F, Altare F. The tuberculous granuloma: an unsuccessful host defence mechanism providing a safety shelter for the bacteria?. Clinical and Developmental Immunology. 2012 Oct;**2012**

[15] Hunter RL, Olsen MR, Jagannath C, Actor JK. Review: Multiple Roles of Cord Factor in the Pathogenesis of Primary, Secondary, and Cavitary Tuberculosis, Including a Revised Description of the Pathology of Secondary Disease [Internet]. 2006. Available from: http://www.granuloma.homestead.com

[16] Behr M, Ellis R, Ernst J, Evans T, Flynn J, Hatherill M, et al.

Developing vaccines to prevent sustained infection with Mycobacterium tuberculosis. Vaccine. 2015 Jun 12;**33**(26):3056-3064

[17] Schrager LK, Harris RC, Vekemans J. Research and development of new tuberculosis vaccines: a review. F1000Research. 2018;7

[18] Hunter R, Actor J. The pathogenesis of post-primary tuberculosis. A game changer for vaccine development. Tuberculosis. 2019;**116**:S114-S117

[19] Darrah PA, Zeppa JJ, Maiello P, Hackney JA, Wadsworth MH, Hughes TK, et al. Prevention of tuberculosis in macaques after intravenous BCG immunization. Nature. 2020;**577**(7788):95-102

[20] Rao M, Valentini D, Poiret T, Dodoo E, Parida S, Zumla A et al. B in TB: B cells as mediators of clinically relevant immune responses in tuberculosis. Clinical Infectious Diseases. 2015 Oct 15;**61**(suppl_3):S225-S235

[21] Steigler P, Verrall AJ, Kirman JR. Beyond memory T cells: mechanisms of protective immunity to tuberculosis infection. Immunology and Cell Biology. 2019 Aug;**97**(7):647-655

[22] Fox GJ, Orlova M, Schurr E. Tuberculosis in newborns: the lessons of the "Lübeck Disaster"(1929-1933). PLoS Pathogens. 2016 Jan 21;**12**(1):e1005271

[23] Migliori GB, Tiberi S, Zumla A, Petersen E, Chakaya JM, Wejse C, et al. MDR/XDR-TB management of patients and contacts: Challenges facing the new decade. The 2020 clinical update by the Global Tuberculosis Network. International Journal of Infectious Diseases. 2020 Mar 1;92:S15-S25

[24] WHO | Technical report on critical concentrations for TB drug susceptibility testing of medicines used in the treatment of drug-resistant TB. WHO. 2018

[25] Shibabaw A, Gelaw B, Gebreyes W, Robinson R, Wang S-H, Tessema B. The burden of pre-extensively and extensively drug-resistant tuberculosis among MDR-TB patients in the Amhara region, Ethiopia. Anupurba S, editor. PLOS ONE. 2020;**15**(2):e0229040. Available from: https://dx.plos.org/10.1371/journal.pone.0229040

[26] van Crevel R, Ottenhoff THM, van der Meer JWM. Innate immunity to mycobacterium tuberculosis. Clinical Microbiology Reviews. 2002;**15**:294-309

[27] Zimri K, Casper R, Hoddinott G, Schaaf HS, Garcia-Prats AJ, Rose PC, et al. A novel approach for eliciting adolescent MDR-TB treatment tolerability: Qualitative data from South Africa. The International Journal of Tuberculosis and Lung Disease: The Official Journal of the International Union against Tuberculosis and Lung Disease. 2020;**24**(1):43-47

[28] Dheda K, Schwander SK, Zhu B, van Zyl-Smit RN, Zhang Y. The immunology of tuberculosis: From bench to bedside. Respirology. 2010;**15**:433-450

[29] Kang PB, Azad AK, Torrelles JB, Kaufman TM, Beharka A, Tibesar E, et al. The human macrophage mannose receptor directs *Mycobacterium tuberculosis* lipoarabinomannan-mediated phagosome biogenesis. Journal of Experimental Medicine. 2005;**202**(7):987-999

[30] Harding C, v., Boom WH. Regulation of antigen presentation by *Mycobacterium tuberculosis*: A role for Toll-like receptors. Nature Reviews Microbiology. 2010;**8**(4):296. Available from: /pmc/articles/PMC3037727/

[31] Russell DG. The evolutionary pressures that have molded *Mycobacterium tuberculosis* into an infectious adjuvant. Current Opinion in Microbiology. 2013;**16**:78-84

[32] Strohmeier GR, Fenton MJ. Roles of lipoarabinomannan in the pathogenesis of tuberculosis. Microbes and Infection. 1999 Jul 1;**1**(9):709-717

[33] Pathak SK, Basu S, Basu KK, Banerjee A, Pathak S, Bhattacharyya A, et al. Direct extracellular interaction between the early secreted antigen ESAT-6 of *Mycobacterium tuberculosis* and TLR2 inhibits TLR signaling in macrophages. Nature Immunology. 2007;**8**(6):610-618

[34] Aderem A, Underhill DM. Mechanisms of phagocytosis in macrophages. Annual Review of Immunology. 1999 Apr;**17**(1):593-623

[35] Medzhitov R, Janeway CA. Innate immunity: Impact on the adaptive immune response. Current Opinion in Immunology. 1997;**9**(1):4-9

[36] Visintin A, Mazzoni A, Spitzer JH, Wyllie DH, Dower SK, Segal DM. Regulation of Toll-like receptors in human monocytes and dendritic cells. The Journal of Immunology. 2001 Jan 1;**166**(1):249-55

[37] Kleinnijenhuis J, Oosting M, Joosten LA, Netea MG, Van Crevel R. Innate immune recognition of Mycobacterium tuberculosis. Clinical and Developmental Immunology. 2011 Oct;**2011**

[38] Brightbill HD, Libraty DH, Krutzik SR, Yang RB, Belisle JT, Bleharski JR, et al. Host defense mechanisms triggered by microbial lipoproteins through toll-like receptors. Science. 1999;**285**(5428):732-736

[39] Selvaraj P, Alagarasu K, Harishankar M, Vidyarani M, Nisha Rajeswari D, Narayanan PR. Cytokine gene polymorphisms and cytokine levels in pulmonary tuberculosis. Cytokine. 2008;**43**(1):26-33

[40] Akahoshi M, Nakashima H, Miyake K, Inoue Y, Shimizu S, Tanaka Y, et al. Influence of interleukin-12 receptor β1 polymorphisms on tuberculosis. Human Genetics [Internet]. 2003;**112**(3):237-243. Available from: http://www.ncbi.nlm.nih.gov/pubmed/12596048

[41] Remus N, El Baghdadi J, Fieschi C, Feinberg J, Quintin T, Chentoufi M, et al. Association of IL12RB1 polymorphisms with pulmonary tuberculosis in adults in Morocco. The Journal of Infectious Diseases [Internet]. 2004;**190**(3):580-587. Available from: https://academic.oup.com/jid/article-lookup/doi/10.1086/422534

[42] Anand SP, Selvaraj P, Jawahar MS, Adhilakshmi AR, Narayanan PR. Interleukin-12B & interleukin-10 gene polymorphisms in pulmonary tuberculosis. Indian Journal of Medical Research. 2007;**126**(2):135-138

[43] Liu C, He T, Rong Y, Du F, Ma D, Wei Y, et al. Association of mannose-binding lectin polymorphisms with tuberculosis susceptibility among Chinese. Scientific Reports. 2016 Nov 4;**6**(1):1-6

[44] Liu Q, Wang J, Sandford AJ, Wu J, Wang Y, Wu S, et al. Association of CYBB polymorphisms with tuberculosis susceptibility in the Chinese Han population. Infection, Genetics and Evolution. 2015;**33**:169-175

[45] Zhang H, Zhou G, Zhi L, Yang H, Zhai Y, Dong X, et al. Association between mannose-binding

lectin gene polymorphisms and susceptibility to severe acute respiratory syndrome coronavirus infection. The Journal of Infectious Diseases [Internet]. 2005;**192**(8):1355-1361. Available from: https://academic.oup.com/jid/article-lookup/doi/10.1086/491479

[46] Ansari A, Hasan Z, Dawood G, Hussain R. Differential combination of cytokine and interferon-γ+ 874 T/A polymorphisms determines disease severity in pulmonary tuberculosis. PLoS One. 2011 Nov 29;**6**(11):e27848

[47] Vergne I, Deretic V. The role of PI3P phosphatases in the regulation of autophagy. FEBS Letters. 2010;**584**: 1313-1318

[48] Kaufmann SHE. How can immunology contribute to the control of tuberculosis? Nature Reviews Immunology. 2001;**1**:20-30

[49] Huang Z, Luo Q, Guo Y, Chen J, Xiong G, Peng Y, et al. *Mycobacterium tuberculosis*-induced polarization of human macrophage orchestrates the formation and development of tuberculous granulomas in vitro. PloS One. 2015 Jun 19;**10**(6):e0129744

[50] Patankar YR, Sutiwisesak R, Boyce S, Lai R, Lindestam Arlehamn CS, Sette A, et al. Limited recognition of *Mycobacterium tuberculosis*-infected macrophages by polyclonal CD4 and CD8 T cells from the lungs of infected mice. Mucosal Immunology. 2020;**13**(1):140-148

[51] Rajaram MVS, Arnett E, Azad AK, Guirado E, Ni B, Gerberick AD, et al. *M. tuberculosis*-initiated human mannose receptor Signaling regulates macrophage recognition and vesicle trafficking by FcRγ-chain, Grb2, and SHP-1. Cell Reports. 2017;**21**(1):126-140

[52] Axelsson-Robertson R, Ju JH, Kim HY, Zumla A, Maeurer M. *Mycobacterium tuberculosis*-specific and MHC class I-restricted CD8+ T-cells exhibit a stem cell precursor-like phenotype in patients with active pulmonary tuberculosis. International Journal of Infectious Diseases [Internet]. 2015;**32**:13-22. Available from: http://www.ijidonline.com/article/S1201971214017342/fulltext

[53] De Martino M, Lodi L, Galli L, Chiappini E. Immune response to *Mycobacterium tuberculosis*: a narrative review. Frontiers in Pediatrics. 2019:350

[54] Moreira-Teixeira L, Mayer-Barber K, Sher A, O'Garra A. Type I interferons in tuberculosis: Foe and occasionally friend. Journal of Experimental Medicine. 2018;**215**(5):1273-1285. DOI: 10.1084/jem.20180325

[55] Russell DG, Barry CE, Flynn JL. Tuberculosis: What we don't know can, and does, hurt us. Science. 2010;**328**:852-856. Available from: https://science.sciencemag.org/content/328/5980/852

[56] Monin L, Khader SA. Chemokines in tuberculosis: The good, the bad and the ugly. Seminars in Immunology. 2014;**26**:552-558

[57] Bhat KH, Yaseen I. *Mycobacterium tuberculosis*: macrophage takeover and modulation of innate effector responses. Mycobacterium-Research and Development. 2018 Jun 20

[58] Ehlers S, Schaible UE. The granuloma in tuberculosis: dynamics of a host–pathogen collusion. Frontiers in Immunology. 2013 Jan 7;**3**:411

[59] Simeone R, Bobard A, Lippmann J, Bitter W, Majlessi L, Brosch R, et al. Phagosomal rupture by *Mycobacterium tuberculosis* results in toxicity and host cell death. PLoS Pathogens.

2012;**8**(2):e1002507. Available from: http://www.ncbi.nlm.nih.gov/pubmed/22319448

[60] Drain PK, Bajema KL, Dowdy D, Dheda K, Naidoo K, Schumacher SG, et al. Incipient and Subclinical Tuberculosis: A Clinical Review of Early Stages and Progression of Infection [Internet]. 2018. Available from: http://cmr.asm.org/

[61] Denholm J. The use of anti-tuberculosis therapy for latent TB infection. Infection and Drug Resistance. 2010;**3**:63. Available from: /pmc/articles/PMC3108738/?report=abstract

[62] Denholm JT, Street AC. Diagnosis and management of latent tuberculosis infection. Medicine Today. 2010;**11**:72-76

[63] Leistikow RL, Morton RA, Bartek IL, Frimpong I, Wagner K, Voskuil MI. The *Mycobacterium tuberculosis* DosR regulon assists in metabolic homeostasis and enables rapid recovery from nonrespiring dormancy. Journal of Bacteriology. 2010;**192**(6):1662-1670

[64] Mehra S, Foreman TW, Didier PJ, Ahsan MH, Hudock TA, Kissee R, et al. The DosR regulon modulates adaptive immunity and is essential for *Mycobacterium tuberculosis* persistence. American Journal of Respiratory and Critical Care Medicine. 2015;**191**(10):1185-1196

[65] Reed MB, Gagneux S, DeRiemer K, Small PM, Barry CE. The W-Beijing lineage of *Mycobacterium tuberculosis* overproduces triglycerides and has the DosR dormancy regulon constitutively upregulated. Journal of Bacteriology. 2007;**189**(7):2583-2589

[66] Diel R. Long-term effect of Bacille Calmette-Guérin vaccination in tuberculin skin testing: A new reality for TB prevention. Chest. 2017;**152**:235-236

[67] Rivas-Santiago CE, Sarkar S, Cantarella P, Osornio-Vargas Á, Quintana-Belmares R, Meng Q, et al. Air pollution particulate matter alters antimycobacterial respiratory epithelium innate immunity. Infection and Immunity. 2015;**83**(6):2507-2517

[68] Wang L, Turner MO, Elwood RK. A Meta-Analysis of the Effect of Bacille Calmette Guérin Vaccination on Tuberculin Skin Test Measurements [Internet]. 2002. Available from: www.thoraxjnl.com

[69] Schito M, Hanna D, Zumla A. Tuberculosis eradication versus control. International Journal of Infectious Diseases. 2017;**56**:10-13

[70] Maglione PJ, Xu J, Casadevall A, Chan J. Fcγ receptors regulate immune activation and susceptibility during *Mycobacterium tuberculosis* infection. The Journal of Immunology. 2008;**180**(5):3329-3338

[71] Martinez-Pomares L. The mannose receptor. Journal of Leukocyte Biology. 2012;**92**(6):1177-1186

[72] Kumar V. Macrophages: The Potent Immunoregulatory Innate Immune Cells. London, UK: IntechOpen; 2019. Available from: www.intechopen.com

[73] Nouailles G, Dorhoi A, Koch M, Zerrahn J, Weiner J, Faé KC, et al. CXCL5-secreting pulmonary epithelial cells drive destructive neutrophilic inflammation in tuberculosis. Journal of Clinical Investigation. 2014;**124**(3):1268-1282

[74] Mehra S, Pahar B, Dutta NK, Conerly CN, Philippi-Falkenstein K, Alvarez X, et al. Transcriptional reprogramming in nonhuman primate (*Rhesus macaque*) tuberculosis

granulomas. PLoS ONE. 2010;**5**(8):e12266. Available from: http://www.ncbi.nlm.nih.gov/pubmed/20824205

[75] Lin Y, Zhang M, Barnes PF. Chemokine production by a human alveolar epithelial cell line in response to *Mycobacterium tuberculosis*. Infection and Immunity. 1998 Mar 1;**66**(3):1121-1126

[76] Rohani MG, Beyer RP, Hacker BM, Dommisch H, Dale BA, Chung WO. Modulation of expression of innate immunity markers CXCL5/ENA-78 and CCL20/MIP3α by protease-activated receptors (PARs) in human gingival epithelial cells. Innate Immunity. 2010 Apr;**16**(2):104-114

[77] Cohen SB, Gern BH, Delahaye JL, Adams KN, Plumlee CR, Winkler JK, et al. Alveolar macrophages provide an early *Mycobacterium tuberculosis* niche and initiate dissemination. Cell Host and Microbe. 2018;**24**(3):439-446.e4

[78] Martinon F, Burns K, Tschopp J. The Inflammasome: A molecular platform triggering activation of inflammatory caspases and processing of proIL-β. Molecular Cell. 2002;**10**(2):417-426

[79] Apostolopoulos V, McKenzie IF. Role of the mannose receptor in the immune response. Current Molecular Medicine. 2001 Sep 1;**1**(4):469-474

[80] Queval CJ, Brosch R, Simeone R. The macrophage: A disputed fortress in the battle against *Mycobacterium tuberculosis*. Frontiers in Microbiology. 2017;**8**:2284

[81] Faridgohar M, Nikoueinejad H. New findings of Toll-like receptors involved in *Mycobacterium tuberculosis* infection. Pathogens and Global Health. 2017;**111**:256-264

[82] Schweizer A, Stahl PD, Rohrer J. A di-aromatic motif in the cytosolic tail of the mannose receptor mediates endosomal sorting. Journal of Biological Chemistry [Internet]. 2000;**275**(38):29694-29700. Available from: http://www.ncbi.nlm.nih.gov/pubmed/10896932

[83] Azad AK, Rajaram MV, Schlesinger LS. Exploitation of the macrophage mannose receptor (CD206) in infectious disease diagnostics and therapeutics. Journal of Cytology & Molecular Biology. 2014 Jan 10;**1**(1)

[84] Gazi U, Martinez-Pomares L. Influence of the mannose receptor in host immune responses. Immunobiology. 2009;**214**:554-561. Available from: http://www.ncbi.nlm.nih.gov/pubmed/19162368

[85] Martinez FO, Sica A, Mantovani A, Locati M. Macrophage activation and polarization. Frontiers in Bioscience. 2008;**13**:453-461

[86] Stahl PD, Ezekowitz RAB. The mannose receptor is a pattern recognition receptor involved in host defense. Current Opinion in Immunology. 1998;**10**(1):50-55

[87] Kang BK, Schlesinger LS. Characterization of mannose receptor-dependent phagocytosis mediated by Mycobacterium tuberculosis lipoarabinomannan. Infection and immunity. 1998;**66**(6):2769-2777. Available from: http://www.ncbi.nlm.nih.gov/pubmed/9596746

[88] Lowell CA. Src-family and Syk kinases in activating and inhibitory pathways in innate immune cells: Signaling cross talk. Cold Spring Harbor Perspectives in Biology. 2011;**3**:1-16

[89] May RC, Machesky LM. Phagocytosis and the actin cytoskeleton. Journal of Cell Science. 2001;**114**:1061-1077

[90] Bekale RB, Du Plessis SM, Hsu NJ, Sharma JR, Sampson SL, Jacobs M, et al. *Mycobacterium tuberculosis* and interactions with the host immune system: Opportunities for nanoparticle based immunotherapeutics and vaccines. Pharmaceutical Research. 2019 Jan;**36**(1):1-5

[91] Vergne I, Chua J, Deretic V. Tuberculosis toxin blocking phagosome maturation inhibits a novel Ca 2+/ calmodulin-PI3K hVPS34 cascade. Journal of Experimental Medicine. 2003;**198**(4):653-659

[92] Turner J, Torrelles JB. Mannose-capped lipoarabinomannan in Mycobacterium tuberculosis pathogenesis. Pathogens and Disease. 2018 Jun;**76**(4):fty026

[93] Correia-Neves M, Sundling C, Cooper A, Källenius G. Lipoarabinomannan in active and passive protection against tuberculosis. Frontiers in Immunology. 2019:1968

[94] Yuan C, Qu ZL, Tang XL, Liu Q, Luo W, Huang C, et al. *Mycobacterium tuberculosis* mannose-capped lipoarabinomannan induces IL-10-producing B cells and hinders CD4+Th1 immunity. iScience. 2019;**11**:13-30

[95] Cardona P, Cardona PJ. Regulatory T cells in *Mycobacterium tuberculosis* infection. Frontiers in Immunology. 2019:2139

[96] Liu PT, Stenger S, Li H, Wenzel L, Tan BH, Krutzik SR, et al. Toll-like receptor triggering of a vitamin D-mediated human antimicrobial response. Science. 2006;**311**(5768):1770-1773

[97] Gopalakrishnan A, Salgame P. Toll-like receptor 2 in host defense against *Mycobacterium tuberculosis*: To be or not to be-that is the question. Current Opinion in Immunology. 2016;**42**:76. Available from: /pmc/articles/ PMC5086274/

[98] Gehring AJ, Dobos KM, Belisle JT, Harding CV, Boom WH. *Mycobacterium tuberculosis* LprG (Rv1411c): A novel TLR-2 ligand that inhibits human macrophage class II MHC antigen processing. Journal of Immunology (Baltimore, Md: 1950). 2004;**173**(4):2660-2668. Available from: https://pubmed.ncbi.nlm.nih.gov/15294983/

[99] Taha RA, Kotsimbos TC, Song YL, Menzies D, Hamid Q. IFN-gamma and IL-12 are increased in active compared with inactive tuberculosis. American journal of Respiratory and Critical Care Medicine. 1997 Mar;**155**(3):1135-1139

[100] Leopold Wager CM, Hole CR, Campuzano A, Castro-Lopez N, Cai H, Caballero Van Dyke MC, et al. IFN-γ immune priming of macrophages in vivo induces prolonged STAT1 binding and protection against Cryptococcus neoformans. PLoS Pathogens. 2018 Oct 10;**14**(10):e1007358

[101] Alemán M. Neutrophil apoptosis in the context of tuberculosis infection. Tuberculosis. 2015;**95**:359-363

[102] Esin S, Counoupas C, Aulicino A, Brancatisano FL, Maisetta G, Bottai D, et al. Interaction of mycobacterium tuberculosis cell wall components with the human natural killer cell receptors NKp44 and toll-like receptor 2. Scandinavian Journal of Immunology. 2013;**77**(6):460-469. Available from: http://www.ncbi.nlm.nih.gov/ pubmed/23578092

[103] Ferwerda G, Girardin SE, Kullberg BJ, le Bourhis L, de Jong DJ, Langenberg DML, et al. NOD2 and toll-like receptors are nonredundant

recognition systems of mycobacterium tuberculosis. PLoS Pathogens. 2005;**1**(3):0279-0285

[104] Medzhitov R. Toll-like receptors and innate immunity. Nature Reviews Immunology. 2001;**1**:135-145

[105] Bafica A, Scanga CA, Feng CG, Leifer C, Cheever A, Sher A. TLR9 regulates Th1 responses and cooperates with TLR2 in mediating optimal resistance to *Mycobacterium tuberculosis*. Journal of Experimental Medicine. 2005;**202**(12):1715-1724

[106] Bartek IL, Rutherford R, Gruppo V, Morton RA, Morris RP, Klein MR, et al. The DosR regulon of *M. tuberculosis* and antibacterial tolerance. Tuberculosis. 2009;**89**(4):310-316

[107] Black GF, Thiel BA, Ota MO, Parida SK, Adegbola R, Boom WH, et al. Immunogenicity of novel DosR regulon-encoded candidate antigens of *Mycobacterium tuberculosis* in three high-burden populations in Africa. Clinical and Vaccine Immunology. 2009;**16**(8):1203-1212

[108] Kim J-S, Kim WS, Choi H-G, Jang B, Lee K, Park J-H, et al. *Mycobacterium tuberculosis* RpfB drives Th1-type T cell immunity via a TLR4-dependent activation of dendritic cells. Journal of Leukocyte Biology. 2013;**94**(4):733-749

[109] Guillerey C, Mourieś J, Polo G, Doyen N, HKW L, Chan S, et al. Pivotal role of plasmacytoid dendritic cells in inflammation and NK-cell responses after TLR9 triggering in mice. Blood. 2012;**120**(1):90-99

[110] Sun Z, Ren W, Xu Y, Zhang H, Li C. Preliminary study on the virulence of XDR-TB: Low virulence owing to less cytokine expression through the TLR 2 and TLR4 pathways in BLAB/C mice. Bio-Medical Materials and Engineering. 2014 Jan 1;24(6):3873-3882

[111] Commandeur S, van den Eeden SJF, Dijkman K, Clark SO, van Meijgaarden KE, Wilson L, et al. The in vivo expressed *Mycobacterium tuberculosis* (IVE-TB) antigen Rv2034 induces CD4+ T-cells that protect against pulmonary infection in HLA-DR transgenic mice and Guinea pigs. Vaccine. 2014;**32**(29):3580-3588. Available from: http://www.ncbi.nlm.nih.gov/pubmed/24837764

[112] Schön T, Juréen P, Giske CG, Chryssanthou E, Sturegård E, Werngren J, et al. Evaluation of wild-type MIC distributions as a tool for determination of clinical breakpoints for *Mycobacterium tuberculosis*. The Journal of Antimicrobial Chemotherapy. 2009;**64**(4):786-793. Available from: http://www.ncbi.nlm.nih.gov/pubmed/19633001

[113] Salie M, Daya M, Lucas LA, Warren RM, van der Spuy GD, van Helden PD, et al. Association of toll-like receptors with susceptibility to tuberculosis suggests sex-specific effects of TLR8 polymorphisms. Infection, Genetics and Evolution. 2015;**34**:221-229

[114] Bukhari M, Aslam MA, Khan A, Iram Q, Akbar A, Naz AG, et al. TLR8 gene polymorphism and association in bacterial load in southern Punjab of Pakistan: An association study with pulmonary tuberculosis. International Journal of Immunogenetics [Internet]. 2015;**42**(1):46-51. Available from: http://www.ncbi.nlm.nih.gov/pubmed/25572425

[115] Padhi A, Pattnaik K, Biswas M, Jagadeb M, Behera A, Sonawane A. *Mycobacteriumtuberculosis* LprEsuppresses TLR2-dependent cathelicidin and autophagy expression to enhance bacterial survival in macrophages.

The Journal of Immunology. 2019;**203**(10):2665-2678. Available from: https://www.jimmunol.org/content/203/10/2665

[116] Pecora ND, Gehring AJ, Canaday DH, Boom WH, Harding CV. *Mycobacterium tuberculosis* LprA is a lipoprotein agonist of TLR2 that regulates innate immunity and APC function. Journal of Immunology (Baltimore, Md: 1950). 2006;**177**(1):422-429. Available from: https://pubmed.ncbi.nlm.nih.gov/16785538/

[117] Heldwein KA, Liang MD, Andresen TK, Thomas KE, Marty AM, Cuesta N, et al. TLR2 and TLR4 serve distinct roles in the host immune response against *Mycobacterium bovis* BCG. Journal of Leukocyte Biology. 2003;**74**(2):277-286. Available from: https://pubmed.ncbi.nlm.nih.gov/12885945/

[118] Sepehri Z, Kiani Z, Kohan F, Ghavami S. Toll-like receptor 4 as an immune receptor against *Mycobacterium tuberculosis*: A systematic review. Laboratory Medicine. 2019;**50**(2):117-129. Available from: https://pubmed.ncbi.nlm.nih.gov/30124945/

[119] Stamm CE, Collins AC, Shiloh MU. Sensing of *Mycobacterium tuberculosis* and consequences to both host and bacillus. Immunological Reviews [Internet]. 2015;**264**(1):204. Available from: /pmc/articles/PMC4339209/

[120] Donovan ML, Schultz TE, Duke TJ, Blumenthal A. Type I interferons in the pathogenesis of tuberculosis: Molecular drivers and immunological consequences. Frontiers in Immunology. 2017;**8**(NOV):1633

[121] Kiemer AK, Senaratne RH, Hoppstädter J, Diesel B, Riley LW, Tabeta K, et al. Attenuated activation of macrophage TLR9 by DNA from virulent mycobacteria. Journal of Innate Immunity. 2009;**1**(1):29-45. Available from: https://pubmed.ncbi.nlm.nih.gov/20375564/

[122] Orme IM, Basaraba RJ. The formation of the granuloma in tuberculosis infection. Seminars in Immunology [Internet]. 2014;**26**(6):601-609. Available from: https://pubmed.ncbi.nlm.nih.gov/25453231/

[123] Korb VC, Chuturgoon AA, Moodley D. *Mycobacterium tuberculosis*: manipulator of protective immunity. International journal of Molecular Sciences. 2016 Mar;**17**(3):131

[124] Stockmann C, Schadendorf D, Klose R, Helfrich I. The impact of the immune system on tumor: Angiogenesis and vascular remodeling. Frontiers in Oncology. 2014;**4**(Apr):69

[125] Tezera LB, Bielecka MK, Chancellor A, Reichmann MT, Al Shammari B, Brace P, et al. Dissection of the host-pathogen interaction in human tuberculosis using a bioengineered 3-dimensional model. Elife. 2017 Jan 7;**6**:e21283

[126] Datta M, Via LE, Kamoun WS, Liu C, Chen W, Seano G, et al. Anti-vascular endothelial growth factor treatment normalizes tuberculosis granuloma vasculature and improves small molecule delivery. Proceedings of the National Academy of Sciences of the United States of America [Internet]. 2015;**112**(6):1827-1832. Available from: https://pubmed.ncbi.nlm.nih.gov/25624495/

[127] Jee B. Understanding the early host immune response against *Mycobacterium tuberculosis*. Central-European Journal of

Immunology. 2020;**45**(1):99. Available from: /labs/pmc/articles/PMC7226546/

[128] Flynn JL, Chan J. Immunology of tuberculosis. Annual Review of Immunology. 2001;**19**:93-129. Available from: https://pubmed.ncbi.nlm.nih.gov/11244032/

[129] Rohde K, Yates RM, Purdy GE, Russell DG. *Mycobacterium tuberculosis* and the environment within the phagosome. Immunological Reviews. 2007;**219**(1):37-54. Available from: https://pubmed.ncbi.nlm.nih.gov/17850480/

[130] Lee J, Hartman M, Kornfeld H. Macrophage apoptosis in tuberculosis. Yonsei Medical Journal [Internet]. 2009;**50**(1):1-11. Available from: https://pubmed.ncbi.nlm.nih.gov/19259342/

[131] Upadhyay S, Mittal E, Philips JA. Tuberculosis and the art of macrophage manipulation. Pathogens and Disease. 2018;**76**(4):37. Available from: https://academic.oup.com/femspd/article/76/4/fty037/4970761

[132] Flynn JL, Chan J, Lin PL. Macrophages and control of granulomatous inflammation in tuberculosis. Mucosal Immunology [Internet]. 2011;**4**(3):271-278. Available from: https://pubmed.ncbi.nlm.nih.gov/21430653/

[133] Wong KW. The role of ESX-1 in *Mycobacterium tuberculosis* pathogenesis. Microbiology Spectrum. 2017 May 19;**5**(3):5-3

[134] Manzanillo PS, Shiloh MU, Portnoy DA, Cox JS. *Mycobacterium tuberculosis* activates the DNA-dependent cytosolic surveillance pathway within macrophages. Cell Host & Microbe. 2012;**11**(5):469. Available from: /labs/pmc/articles/PMC3662372/

[135] Cambier CJ, O'Leary SM, O'Sullivan MP, Keane J, Ramakrishnan L. Phenolic glycolipid facilitates mycobacterial escape from microbicidal tissue-resident macrophages. Immunity. 2017;**47**(3):552. Available from: /labs/pmc/articles/PMC5610147/

Chapter 13

Role of CD14+ CD16+ Monocytes in the Pathogenesis of Periodontitis Associated Systemic Diseases

Raghunathan Jagannathan, Balaji Thodur Madapusi, Cakku Jalliah Venkatakrishnan, Lakshmipriya Sridhar, Saranya Varadarajan and Swaminathan Rajendran

Abstract

Monocytes are immune cells that form an important bridge between the innate and adaptive immune response. These cells exist in various phenotypes based on cell surface marker expression and participate in the pathobiology of many systemic diseases. Periodontitis is an inflammatory condition of the tooth attachment apparatus caused by microbial assault from the dental plaque biofilm. It is noteworthy that monocytes play a key role in mediating tissue destruction in periodontitis. The CD14+ CD16+ monocytes that bear both the surface markers are especially involved and upregulated in periodontitis and produce increased amounts of proinflammatory cytokines following microbial challenge. In this context and exploring the available literature, the present chapter aims to unravel the role of CD14+ CD16+ monocytes in periodontitis and systemic disease and also aims to elucidate the possible pathways by which periodontitis could be a key risk factor for systemic disease based on monocyte selection and participation.

Keywords: monocytes, periodontitis, antigens CD14, receptors IgG, periodontal diseases

1. Introduction

Periodontitis is a currently recognized as an inflammatory disease affecting the supporting structures of teeth, having its origin in microbiome of the oral cavity, influenced by plethora of local and systemic factors. Many evidences regarding periodontal disease are accumulated over a century now. It is consistently shown that the disease is initiated by bacteria, progressing at various stages, leading to tooth loss. However, over and above the loss of tooth, its immense contribution to systemic inflammatory level and load of cytokines is what affords high importance to this disease [1]. Evidence also supports that the sequel of complex interactions amongst the dysbiotic bacterial biofilm and the immune response of the host leads to disruption of homeostasis, setting a vicious cycle in to motion [2]. Therefore, the host immune system is unable to restore the homeostasis leading to the characteristic pathogenesis of periodontitis. In addition, this is also modified by various risk factors such as diabetes mellitus and smoking habits. They complicate the existing complex relationship between the host and the flora.

In this inflammatory process, monocytes and macrophages are considered to be the major cellular components of the innate immunity. Macrophages are seen as the primary host defense mechanism to neutralize the threat from microbes. They are derived from monocytes from blood and hence can migrate to the site of inflammation quickly [3]. The monocytes leave the blood stream in case of inflammation and differentiate into macrophages. In this process, various cellular subtypes have been identified in monocytes. Of the three monocytes- *viz.* classical, non-classical, or intermediate monocytes, the classical monocytes are the ones that become macrophages at the site of inflammation [4]. While non-classical monocytes take care of vasculature surveillance, the intermediate monocytes participate in the inflammatory cascade. Monocyte life is short and non-classical monocytes live longer than classical monocytes [4].

With regard to the subtypes, monocytes are also seen to express Cluster of differentiation molecules leading to the classification into various immunophenotypes. These molecules act as receptors or ligands mediating various functions of the cell. These molecules are designated by unique numbers and CD14 and CD16 are considered to be of importance in periodontal inflammation.CD14 cells are involved in recognition of microbial cell wall components and clearance of apoptotic cells [5]. CD16 monocytes induce IL-1beta production and leukocyte recruitment under non-infectious conditions [6].

In the past decades relation between increased presence of these CD14/16 monocytes in blood has been related to periodontal disease [7]. Further, these cells acquire macrophage like features while in circulation in blood [8]. The evidences for implicating them are on the rise. If well understood, these can have immense clinical implications, leading to clues to solve complex clinical conditions. Therefore, a these cells can be channels by which systemic inflammation is increased during periodontal disease. Therefore, it is necessary to understand their role in periodontal disease, based on the existing evidence.

2. Immune system in relation to periodontal disease

The immunology of periodontal disease deals with the interaction of host and the microorganisms in the micro-anatomical regions around the tooth. While the area of concern is small in size, it has complex local and systemic interactions. The science begins with the microbiological aspect. In this sense, the microbial population was initially identified and cultured. The implication of a pathogen to a disease requires satisfying the Socransky's criteria. According to this theory, the relative severity of disease was related to various groups of pathogens like the red, orange, green, orange-associated and *Aggregatibacter actinomycetemcomitans* complexes [9].

Subsequent to this stage of understanding, research took a different track to identify the molecular pathways involved in the host-bacterial interactions, which occur as a result of host responding to the microbial attack. It was also seen that response of the host is frequently detrimental to the host itself. In current scenario, the molecular pathways are being constantly studied in addition to identification and characterization of unculturable bacteria by metagenomics.

In current understanding, rather than implicating a single or group of microbes in periodontitis, the focus has shifted to characterizing the so called "dysbiosis" of the oral cavity. It is said that the shift of concentrations of various bacterial species are known to cause disease. Here the shift happens by reducing the symbiotic microbes and increasing the pathogenic ones. Further, what was not a pathogen earlier may become a virulent pathogen when the dysbiosis happens. For the host to be in the state of homeostasis, immune system helps to control the microbial colonization. It may be constituted by the salivary, the systemic and the gingival tissue immune systems.

This discussion pertains to local factors and hence salivary and gingival components take the major role. Gingival crevicular fluid (GCF), derived from gingival capillary beds has both resident and emigrating inflammatory cellular components and a wide range of innate, inflammatory and adaptive immune molecules. Saliva is known to contain enzymes and other defense molecules that act synergistically with GCF components [10, 11]. Therefore, due to interaction with pathogens the transudate of GCF becomes inflammatory exudate, kick starting the classical periodontal pathogenesis.

With respect to the cell mediated component of immunity, both T and B lymphocytes are observed. Further, there is an observation of unique subsets of helper and cytotoxic T-cells were involved in: modulating immune response, co-operating with B-cells in the induction of antibody synthesis, stimulating the release of cytokines for cellular communication to activate phagocytic cells; and aiding in the elimination of many intracellular and viral pathogens. Most circulating T-cells express a combination of cluster determinant (CD) markers, including CD2, CD3, CD4 (helper T-cells) or CD8 (cytotoxic T-cells), and a T-cell antigen receptor [12]. In addition to T-lymphocytes, the second primary cell type involved in activating the adaptive immune response is the monocyte/macrophage, which is responsible for antigen recognition, immune stimulation and the tissue consequences that follow immune stimulation.

Therefore, gingival health at the immune-histological level is the delicate balance between the subgingival microbiota and host resistance. Therefore, even under normal conditions, there exists a minimal inflammation with some inflammatory cells in the tissues. This seems to be crucial in maintaining the local homeostasis [13].

3. Monocytes as an integral part of the immune system

Monocytes are one of the major cellular elements of the innate immune system and have crucial roles to play in the tissue homeostasis. Monocytes are called the largest leucocyte, with their diameter between 12 to 20 μm [14]. These cells are easily identified in the blood due to their relatively large size and convoluted bilobed or kidney shaped nuclei [14]. Macrophages are derived from the monocytes and serves as a phagocyte that gulps the microbes in their vicinity. They can reach the site of inflammation in a very short time [15].

A monocyte can differentiate into various populations of macrophages and dendritic cells in order to regulate cellular homeostasis during infection and inflammation [16]. Monocytes are known to perform two distinct roles as follows:

1. They are the patrolling cells and identify microbial cells to orchestrate an immune response.

2. They express different pattern recognition receptors (PRRs), including toll-like receptors on their surfaces which interacts with pathogen-associated molecular

patterns present on the invading microbial cells [17]. It is in response to this stimuli, monocytes exit the bone marrow into the circulating blood to reach and infiltrate the tissues with infection within 12 to 24 hours [18].

Subsequent to their arrival at the affected site, the monocytes attach themselves to the endothelium and roll along the vascular surface. Subsequently, they extravasate and perform diapedesis to reach the area of inflammation. This is regulated by monocyte related, endothelial related and chemotaxis related factors. Monocytes from here on function as phagocytes, which present antigens from the foreign cells, to facilitate ingestion and removal of microbes, foreign materials, and necrotic cells. Further, antigen-presenting cells may also include macrophages, dendritic cells, B lymphocytes, and activated endothelial cells [19].

The role of monocytes is in the immune system is very versatile and is crucially related to various types of disorders of infectious and inflammatory origin. Monocytosis is a characteristic feature of numerous inflammatory and immune disorders such as rheumatoid arthritis, systemic lupus erythematous, and sarcoidosis. Hence, monocytes in periodontal inflammation and systemic circulation has been related in the recent days. Monocytes mediate inflammatory reaction by producing both cytokines mounting an substantial immune response and promoting healing by secreting anti-inflammatory cytokines [20].

Macrophages, present in all tissues are formed by differentiation of circulating peripheral-blood mononuclear cells. Monocytes form the blood stream, migrate into the tissue to old tissue-specific macrophages of the tissue. They become tissue specific as they perform their function. These macrophages can further differentiate into various specialized macrophages based on their location. Examples of this may include histiocytes in the connective tissue and osteoclasts in the bone [21].

4. Monocyte subpopulations

While monocytes are characterized for various functions, it is inevitable to classify it according to the function. Generally, they are classified as classical, non-classical, or intermediate monocytes [22]. Classical monocytes are those that can turn into macrophages at the site of injury. While, non-classical monocytes are mainly involved in vasculature surveillance, the Intermediate monocytes, called hyperinflammatory monocytes have major role in the inflammatory cascade [23]. The non-classical monocytes group accumulate at the sites of chronic bacterial infection, producing low levels of pro-inflammatory, but high levels of anti-inflammatory cytokines. Hence, this is more relevant to periodontal infections.

Recently, macrophages are designated pro-inflammatory macrophages (M1) and anti-inflammatory or resolution macrophages (M2) [24]. M1 macrophages are linked with the inflammatory mediators - interleukin (IL)-12 and IL-8. Hence they activate type 1 T helper cells. On the other hand, M2 macrophages are related with transforming growth factor-beta, vascular endothelial growth factor and epidermal growth factor, activating type 2 T helper cells. Therefore, there is a distinct difference in the roles of various subpopulations. During inflammation, subsequent to diapedesis for reaching the site of action, activation of M1 macrophage occurs, leading to production of tumor necrosis factor -α and IL-12. However, during the resolution of inflammation, M2 macrophages are activated inducing VEGF etc., leading to neo-angiogenesis and healing [25].

In this connection, description of monocytes in relation to CD factors is crucial for the critical understanding about its role. CD14 is known as monocyte/macrophage differentiation antigen on the surface of myeloid lineage. This protein has a major role in immune recognition and reactivation. However, recently CD14 is shown to be associated with the phagocytic clearance of apoptotic cells. The CD14 protein acts as a receptor for binding the lipopolysaccharides [26].

CD16− monocytes are known to produce both pro- and anti-inflammatory cytokines production in addition to leukocyte recruitment during infections, while CD16+ monocytes induce IL-1beta synthesis and leukocyte recruitment under non-infectious conditions [26].

It has been reported that various systemic diseases are associated with change in these proportions of monocyte subpopulations. This lower percentage of CD14+/CD16+ monocytes was found in rheumatoid arthritis [27]. Chronic kidney disease patients also show change in these monocytes [28]. With relevance to the original discussion, CD14 and CD16 were increased in chronic and aggressive periodontitis patients respectively [29]. The CD14+/CD16+ cells occur as about 10% of all blood monocytes. They have allow level expression of the CD14 molecule and a high level expression of the CD16 (Fc gamma R III) molecule. Specifically, phenotypic markers of the CD14+/CD16+ blood monocytes resemble tissue macrophages [30]. In this regard, it is worthwhile to note that these monocytes acquire phagocyte like properties even when they are in the blood stream. Therefore, increased production of these cells due to any reason may raise the systemic phagocyte load leading to unexpected mounting of immune response at a location unrelated to the site of production of these cells. In this regard, periodontal inflammation can play a major role in increasing the systemic inflammatory load, both on the basis of humoral and cell mediated pathways.

5. Periodontitis as an oral disorder with immune system role

Periodontitis as generally known, is characterized by a chronic inflammation of periodontal tissue associated with pathogens and modified by various local and systemic factors [13]. Therefore, the pathogenesis is complicated and slow process. In this regard, various imbalances of the immune system precipitated by the oral floral dysbiosis considered as an important factor in the etiopathogenesis of periodontitis [13]. Numerous works have focused on the external pathogenic factors and the clinical treatment of periodontitis. However there is limited documentation of changes in the molecular aspects of the immune system in such cases [13]. In the recent literature, the importance of the imbalance of the periodontal immune system is being focused. The abnormality of cytokines in the host immune response can have a far reaching impact on the human body [13].

6. Role of monocytes in pathogenesis of periodontitis

In a healthy or normobiotic gingival environment, Gram-positive cocci and rods predominate the system. As the plaque matures, there is a gradual transition in to a complex community that is predominated by gram-negative rods, filaments and the fusiforms [31]. This is one of the first steps towards progression to periodontal inflammation. Previous studies have demonstrated high prevalence of *prevotella* and *fusobacteria* in early periodontitis [31]. *P. intermedia* was found to be the predominant anaerobic species that predisposes to periodontitis [31]. Major periodontal pathogens are *Porphyromonas gingivalis*, *Tannerella forsythia* and *Treponema denticola*. When there is a shift in the microbiome, the host response is stimulated and inflammatory reaction sets in. The reaction may be modified by the composition of the flora. It is also known that this dysbiosis may facilitate a non-pathogenic organism to become a pathogen and express virulence. Therefore, this composition may be important to identify the stage of periodontal disease.

In this line of thinking, the CD14 molecule is recognized as primary factor for the innate recognition of bacteria. This CD14 is a 55-kDa glycoprotein that exist in both soluble and membrane bound form, represented as sCD14 and mCD14 respectively. The membrane bound form is immobilized by glycosylphosphatidylinositol tail and is found mainly on mature monocytes, macrophages, and activated neutrophils. Further, the soluble formin circulation is attributed to protease-mediated shedding/ cleavage of mCD14. The main role of sCD14 is to provide non-CD14 cells, sensitivity to bacterial products. These cells may be epithelium, fibroblast and so on. Therefore, it should be recognized that all forms of CD14 function as a receptor for byproducts of bacterial cell wall [32].

With regard to periodontium derived mesenchymal stromal cells, soluble CD14 causes radical increase in inflammatory response to bacterial products. Therefore, CD14 acts as a major factor for mounting an inflammatory response. On the other hand, CD16, a type III Fcγ receptor, is involved in antibody-dependent cell-mediated cytotoxicity. In the absence of CD16, this immunological activity is absent in cells. Further, treatment of CD16- monocytes with inflammatory mediators, would result in expression of CD16 in the cell membrane making them CD16+. Hence production of inflammatory mediators by CD14+ monocytes may result in up-regulation of CD16 in monocytes. This CD16+ monocytes require cell-cell contact by integrin for killing the target, by releasing cytotoxic granules [33].

While mechanisms of the host response to periodontal infection have been extensively studied, CD14 still remains an interesting molecule as its role to periodontitis still remains unclear. Reports have associated increased CD14 and CD16 monocytes in the vicinity of periodontitis [34]. Further, CD14+ monocytes are related to osteoclast development leading to influence on bone homeostasis [35]. Some reports have said that the expression of mCD14 in peripheral monocytes decreased in periodontitis, while some authors report no difference. However, majority of the reports show a positive association of sCD14 levels with periodontal disease. Therefore, an increase in production of sCD14 in moderate-to-severe and generalized periodontal breakdown cases may be expected. As a corollary, local levels of sCD14 can be observed in saliva and GCF. As an additional finding, scaling and root planning reduced salivary sCD14 levels.

Further, soluble CD14 can stimulate inflammation even in the absence of bacterial by products, thereby increasing the secretion of pro-inflammatory cytokines, chemokines, and mediators in the local and systemic cells [35].

An important finding is that *P. gingivalis* outer membrane vesicles can inactivate the CD14 receptor, cleaving the mCD14 from monocytes, resulting in decreased phagocytosis and pathogen elimination [36]. Therefore, Gingipains of *P. gingivalis* bypass the CD14 based immunity and invade the tissues. Therefore, resultant sCD14 may sensitize adjacent tissues and may enter blood stream leading to sensitization of somatic cells to bacterial byproducts. While host tries to produce more CD14 cells at the inflammatory site, bacteria cleave the CD14 locally, destroying tissues for its nourishment. In this pathway, it also leads to systemic complication.

In interesting phenomenon here is the vicious cycle of monocyte production by body and inactivation by pathogens, leading to flooding of location with cell debris and inflammatory mediators leading to progress of the disease. Other cells of the immune system contribute substantially to this process, thereby contributing to tissue destruction. Other cells of the immune system lead to secretion of various cytokines that directly and indirectly destroy the pathogens. In this nexus of interaction, if the intervention is successful, the periodontium restored to healthy state.

7. Periodontitis as a risk factor for systemic disease

Periodontal inflammation and systemic inflammation appear to be a two way traffic and is demonstrated in many instances. Several authors have reported the association between systemic diseases and periodontal diseases. Periodontium acts as a constant reservoir of infection due to periodontal flora that enters the blood stream, causing stimulation of systemic immunity. This stimulation leads to production of inflammatory mediators that adversely affects various systems of the body (**Figure 1**) [37].

Aspiration of oral flora can lead to respiratory infections. Constantly high levels of periodontal inflammation leads to increase of systemic C-reactive protein and interleukin (IL)-6 levels and consequent changes in atherosclerotic lesions. This would give rise to various cardiac or cerebrovascular events [38]. It is also reported that rheumatoid arthritis and periodontitis share common immunological processes [39]. In this line, well known bidirectional link exists between Diabetes mellitus

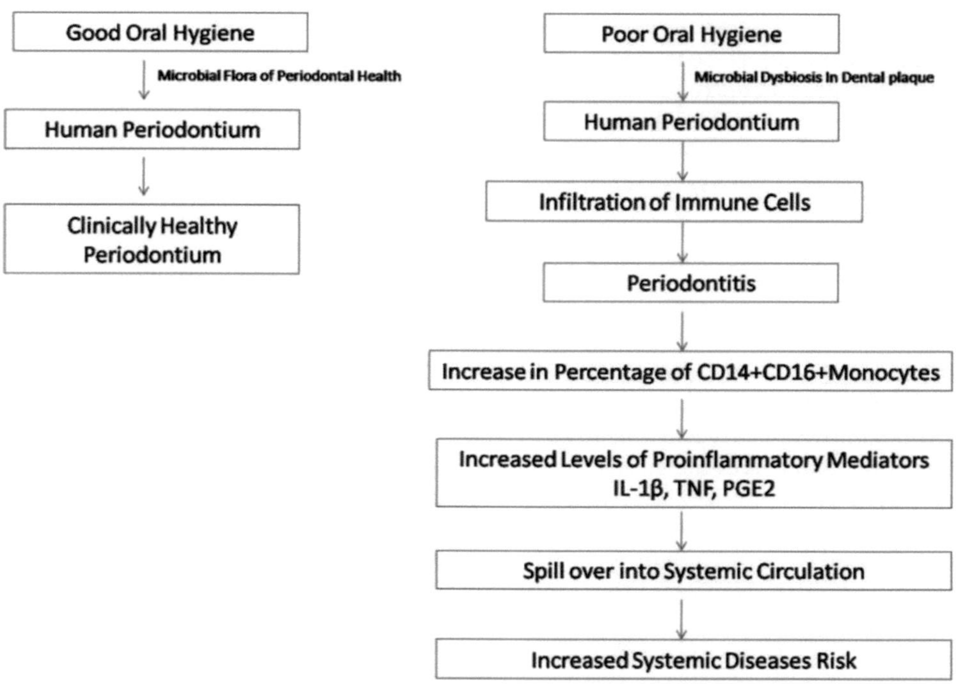

Figure 1.
Schematic representation of the role of non-classical monocytes.

and periodontitis [40]. It is also observed that periodontal flora can also worsen Alzheimer's disease by two mechanisms, viz. increased inflammatory cytokines and invasion of brain by microbes from periodontium. Other systems like renal, skin, reproductive and so on are affected by rise in systemic inflammation [38].

As discussed above, the relation between periodontal inflammation and systemic diseases is well established. The mechanism widely proposed is through increase in systemic inflammation. It is sensible to relate this with other systemic inflammatory diseases like rheumatoid arthritis, lupus erythematous, etc. This rise in systemic inflammation stimulates various organ systems to secrete their specific inflammatory mediators leading to inflammation in that organ. Like the well-known concept of "focus of infection", this may be called "focus of inflammation" for the purpose of understanding. Every bite or masticatory process would pump the periodontal inflammatory products into blood stream. In the initial stages the stimulus would be well below the threshold of other organs. With continuous and repeated stimulation of tissues by chemical messengers of inflammation, this would cause multiple pathways to be activated. As every organ system responds uniquely to inflammation, the manifestation may bring the patient to a clinician, who may not have any clue of the origin of inflammation. In the recent general medical practice, awareness of clinicians to this focus of inflammation has increased, and they regularly refer patients for clearance from dentist prior to any procedure or devising a treatment plan. The inflammatory condition most commonly manifests as a non-communicable disease like arthritis, cardiovascular disorders and so on, but indeed it is a product of infection.

Management of such infections systemically frequently includes anti-inflammatory drugs and seldom antibiotics. As periodontal infection is identified as a culprit in systemic disorders of wide range, proper administration of antibiotic is needed to solve the problem completely. Further, rise in periodontal inflammation can also be a byproduct of rise in systemic inflammation. For instance increased blood sugar level can bring about increase in systemic inflammation and its influence of periodontal inflammation. Uncontrolled diabetes is well known to increase periodontal inflammation. Hence therapeutics of periodontal inflammation is well intertwined with systemic inflammatory processes. Therefore, dentist must have opinion from a physician to completely assess and address the condition, to afford a proper and complete treatment.

8. Monocytes role in periodontitis systemic disease link

Monocytes are trafficked during chronic inflammation in a slow and well-orchestrated way. Increased monocytes in a location contributes significantly to the pool of monocytes available in circulation. Monocytosis could be initiated by the infection and it drives the monocyte precursor proliferation. As we have discussed amount of monocyte can be proportional to the size of inflammation. Further, removal of monocytes from circulation would leads to reduction in macrophage in the inflamed tissues. Therefore, periodontally stimulated monocytes can reach the systemic circulation and lead to recruitment of macrophages elsewhere in the body. As with inflammatory mediators stimulating inflammation in various far off organs, monocytes can do the same effect, driving cell based inflammation in the visceral and other organs, presenting clinically with a disease of unknown etiology. In this context, when monocytes reach other organs, the interaction of monocyte with that organ entirely be different and specific [41].

Further, monocytes recruited in chronic inflammatory condition can lead to increase in inflammation while those recruited in acute phase can heal the inflammation. This is due to change in subpopulation and difference in release of mediators of inflammation.

In this regard, many questions remain unanswered with respect to monocytes in chronic inflammation. We know that monocyte recruitment increases inflammation in chronic diseases, however, specific subpopulation that works in every organ is not yet found out. To elaborate, the questions to be answered are:

- What is the phenotype of monocyte that is released in to blood stream from periodontal inflammations?
- What are the systemic organs that are affected by released monocyte subpopulations?
- Does every organ get equally stimulated by released monocyte subpopulation or certain organs are resistant to periodontal inflammation induced monocytes?
- Do CD14+ and CD16+ monocyte alone drive the systemic inflammation? If not, what are the modifying factors?
- Will systemic suppression of monocyte lead to lesser recruitment of macrophage in periodontal inflammation?
- Will subpopulations interact in such a way as to stimulate each other destructively leading to destruction of periodontium?

As previously stated, monocytes appear to be a key factor in periodontal inflammation in this situation. Their CD14 and CD16 play an active involvement in periodontal inflammation that is "yet to be fully investigated." The role of CD14 and CD16 monocytes in systemic immunity, on the other hand, has been thoroughly investigated. As a result of the spillage of monocytes and their by-products into the bloodstream, somatic cells are stimulated, and inflammation increases brutally. By increasing inflammation, this rise in systemic inflammation would have a vicious effect on periodontal tissues.

9. Clinical implications

Though the complete knowledge of monocytes is yet to be achieved, its clinical implications are profound and need attention by not just dentists but also by physicians and other specialists. As explained in the previous section, every system in the body can be potentially affected by this pathologic process.

With respect to the cardiovascular system, chronic periodontitis is well associated with coronary heart disease (CHD) and increases the risk with other contributory factors. The link may be through direct infection or due to increase in systemic inflammation, coupled with genetic factors. Elevated inflammatory markers reaching the atherosclerotic lesions may increase the risk for cardiac or cerebrovascular events [42]. Further, monocyte increase is associated with cardiac diseases [43].

With respect to respiratory system, in addition to flora directly contributing to various diseases, it is important to note that there is an association of monocyte increase in fibrotic diseases [44]. Hence periodontitis may contribute to poor outcome in such cases.

With regard to muscular system, macrophages are needed to repair the injured skeletal muscles [45]. Circulating monocytes contribute to this process. However, with increase in systemic inflammation due to periodontitis, this healing may be delayed. Nevertheless, evidence to this statement is not clearly available. With regard to skeletal system, it has been well discussed about rheumatic arthritis and periodontitis have similar pathophysiology. Therefore, monocytes from periodontal inflammation can increase the arthritis and lead to poor outcome.

As a major observation, CD16+ and CD14+ monocytes are associated with preterm labor. It has been suggested that CD16 can be a marker of preterm labor [46]. In addition, low birth weight and other adverse pregnancy outcomes have been reported to be associated with periodontitis. However, the contributory role of monocytes, especially CD14+ and CD16+ have not been reported. However, even subclinical periodontal infections can trigger adverse pregnancy outcomes as reported by Raj et al. [47].

Diabetes mellitus and periodontal infection is previously discussed. In addition, role of monocytes in diabetes is well explained recently by Kantar et al. [48]. According to them, monocytes and macrophages may be considered as "protagonists" in the inflammatory pathways of Diabetes mellitus and actually mediate all complications in various organs. However, they do not instigate the process, but only do role play of destruction. Previous authors have also associated obesity with increases CD14+ and CD16+ monocytes [49]. It has been said that periodontal inflammation is associated with malignancy [50]. However, role of monocytes in this mediation is yet to be reported in the literature.

In connection with nervous system disorders, Alzheimer's disease has been associated with periodontal disorders. Monocytes are useful in clearing the amyloid plaque deposited, but it also increases the pre-existing inflammation in the central nervous system [51]. However, specific role of CD14+ and CD16+ monocytes from periodontal origin is yet unexplored.

With this information, it is to be understood that periodontitis is associated with all these disorders. Immune system of the body is involved with all other systems for defense. However, periodontitis interferes with this system through various pathways including monocytes. Therefore, periodontitis assumes phenomenal importance in all disciplines of medicine and dentistry. The awareness should be spread to all medical and paramedical experts to aid in proper management of patients who come with pain and suffering.

10. Conclusion

With the previous collection of evidence discussed in this chapter, apparently monocytes have large number of roles in the immune system. It has various subpopulations catering to specific needs in specific tissues. In this discussion, CD14 and CD16 cells are focused upon. However, the evidence from literature is scanty in several aspects. It is necessary to study the immunological pathways that involve the said monocytes from periodontal origin. This lacuna should be addressed to improve the standard of care provided to patients. Systemic manifestations of periodontitis may present as a disorder of specific system and the patient may seek advice either from a physician or a specialist of that organ system. In the absence of this background knowledge, the therapy may not be successful, as origin of the disorder is not addressed. Furthering the research in this direction can solve a lot of puzzles in both medicine and dentistry.

In the other direction, role of systemically originated monocytes in periodontium should also be further explored. This bidirectional approach is the key to breaking this vicious cycle. Very few diseases have been thoroughly explored in this regard like Diabetes Mellitus. However, potential role of other inflammatory disorders should be explored. An important fact here is that, in a vicious cycle involving periodontium and other organs, periodontium is easily accessible for therapy that breaks the said cycle compared to other visceral organs. Hence physicians should advice patients to consult dental clinicians to get their periodontitis under good control so that other organs may be prevented from damage. If periodontal therapy can stop a lot of disorders, then the burden of care and expenditure for health would reduce considerably in the global level.

Conflict of interest

The authors declare no conflict of interest.

Author details

Raghunathan Jagannathan[1*], Balaji Thodur Madapusi[1], Cakku Jalliah Venkatakrishnan[1], Lakshmipriya Sridhar[2], Saranya Varadarajan[3] and Swaminathan Rajendran[3]

1 Tagore Dental College and Hospital, Chennai, Tamilnadu, India

2 Chettinad Dental College and Research Institute, Chennai, Tamilnadu, India

3 Sri Venkateswara Dental College and Hospital, Chennai, Tamilnadu, India

*Address all correspondence to: doctorraghunathan@gmail.com

References

[1] Papapanou PN. Periodontitis: Consensus report of workgroup 2 of the 2017 world workshop on the classification of periodontal and peri-implant diseases and conditions. Journal of Periodontology. 2018;**89**(Suppl. 1):S173-S182

[2] Cekici A. Inflammatory and immune pathways in the pathogenesis of periodontal disease. Periodontology. 2000;**2014**(64):57-80. DOI: 10.1111/prd.12002

[3] Almubarak A, Tanagala KKK, Papapanou PN, Lalla E, Momen-Heravi F. Disruption of monocyte and macrophage homeostasis in periodontitis. Frontiers in Immunology. 2020;**11**:330. DOI: 10.3389/fimmu.2020.00330

[4] Carlin LM, Stamatiades EG, Auffray C, Hanna RN, Glover L, Vizcay-Barrena G. Nr4a1-dependent Ly6C(low) monocytes monitor endothelial cells and orchestrate their disposal. Cell. 2013;**153**:362-375. DOI: 10.1016/j.cell.2013.03.010

[5] Zamani F, ZareShahneh F, Aghebati-Maleki L, Baradaran B. Induction of CD14 expression and differentiation to monocytes or mature macrophages in Promyelocytic cell lines: New approach. Advanced Pharmaceutical Bulletin. 2013;**3**(2):329-332. DOI: 10.5681/apb.2013.053

[6] Balboa L, Barrios-Payan J, Gonzalez-Dominguez E, Lastrucci C, Lugo-Villarino G, Mata-Espinoza D, et al. Diverging biological roles among human monocyte subsets in the context of tuberculosis infection. Clinical Science (London). 2015;**129**(4):319-330. DOI: 10.1042/CS20150021

[7] Nagasawa T, Kobayashi H, Aramaki M, Kiji M, Oda S, Izumi Y. Expression of CD14, CD16 and CD45RA on monocytes from periodontitis patients. Journal of Periodontal Research. 2004;**39**(1):72-78. DOI: 10.1111/j.1600-0765.2004.00713.x

[8] Ziegler-Heitbrock HW, Fingerle G, Ströbel M, Schraut W, Stelter F, Schütt C, et al. The novel subset of CD14+/CD16+ blood monocytes exhibits features of tissue macrophages. European Journal of Immunology. 1993;**23**(9):2053-2058. DOI: 10.1002/eji.1830230902

[9] Teles RP, Teles FRF, Loesche WJ, et al. Rediscovering Sig Socransky, the genius and his legacy. Journal of Dental Research. 2012;**91**(5):433-439. DOI: 10.1177/0022034512443689

[10] Ebersole JL. Humoral immune responses in gingival crevice fluid: Local and systemic implications. Periodontology. 2000;**2003**(31):135-166. DOI: 10.1034/j.1600-0757.2003.03109.x

[11] Fábián TK, Hermann P, Beck A, Fejérdy P, Fábián G. Salivary defense proteins: Their network and role in innate and acquired oral immunity. International Journal of Molecular Sciences. 2012;**13**(4):4295-4320. DOI: 10.3390/ijms13044295

[12] Singh A, Mehdi AA, Srivastava RN, Verma NS. Immunoregulation of bone remodelling. International Journal of Critical Illness & Injury Science. 2012;**2**:75-81

[13] Ebersole JL. Immune responses in periodontal diseases. In: Wilson TG Jr, Kornman KS, editors. Fundamentals of Periodontics. 2nd ed. Chicago, IL: Quintessence Publishing Co., Inc.; 2003. pp. 111-143

[14] Wang SY, Mak KL, Chen LY, Chou MP, Ho CK. Heterogeneity of human blood monocyte: Two subpopulations with different sizes, phenotypes and functions. Immunology. 1992;**77**(2):298-303

[15] Mills CD, Ley K. M1 and M2 macrophages: The chicken and the egg of immunity. Journal of Innate Immunity. 2014;**6**:716-726. DOI: 10.1159/000364945

[16] Yáñez A, Coetzee SG, Olsson A, Muench DE, Berman BP, Hazelett DJ, et al. Granulocyte-monocyte progenitors and monocyte-dendritic cell progenitors independently produce functionally distinct monocytes. Immunity. 2017;**47**(5):890-902.e4

[17] Santoni G, Cardinali C, Morelli MB, Santoni M, Nabissi M, Amantini C. Danger- and pathogen-associated molecular patterns recognition by pattern-recognition receptors and ion channels of the transient receptor potential family triggers the inflammasome activation in immune cells and sensory neurons. Journal of Neuroinflammation. 2015;**12**:21

[18] Issekutz AC, Issekutz TB. Quantitation and kinetics of blood monocyte migration to acute inflammatory reactions, and IL-1 alpha, tumor necrosis factor-alpha, and IFN-gamma. Journal of Immunology. 1993;**151**(4):2105-2115

[19] Jakubzick CV, Randolph GJ, Henson PM. Monocyte differentiation and antigen-presenting functions. Nature Reviews. Immunology. 2017;**17**(6):349-362

[20] Yang J, Zhang L, Yu C, Yang XF, Wang H. Monocyte and macrophage differentiation: Circulation inflammatory monocyte as biomarker for inflammatory diseases. Biomarker Research. 2014;**2**(1):1

[21] Gordon S, Taylor PR. Monocyte and macrophage heterogeneity. Nature Reviews Immunology. 2005;**5**:953-964

[22] Thomas G, Tacke R, Hedrick CC, Hanna RN. Nonclassical patrolling monocyte function in the vasculature. Arteriosclerosis, Thrombosis, and Vascular Biology. 2015;**35**:1306-1316. DOI: 10.1161/ATVBAHA.114.304650

[23] Geissmann F, Jung S, Littman DR. Blood monocytes consist of two principal subsets with distinct migratory properties. Immunity. 2003;**19**:71-82. DOI: 10.1016/s1074-7613(03)00174-2

[24] Stout RD, Suttles J. Functional plasticity of macrophages: Reversible adaptation to changing microenvironments. Journal of Leukocyte Biology. 2004;**76**:509-513

[25] Das A, Sinha M, Datta S, Abas M, Chaffee S, Sen CK. Monocyte and macrophage plasticity in tissue repair and regeneration. The American Journal of Pathology. 2015;**185**:2596-2606. DOI: 10.1016/j.ajpath.2015.06.001

[26] Balboa L, Barrios-Payan J, Gonzalez-Dominguez E, Lastrucci C, Lugo-Villarino G, Mata-Espinoza D, et al. Diverging biological roles among human monocyte subsets in the context of tuberculosis infection. Clinical Science (London). 2015;**129**(4):319-330. DOI: 10.1042/CS20150021

[27] Cairns AP, Crockard AD, Bell AL. The CD14+ CD16+ monocyte subset in rheumatoid arthritis and systemic lupus erythematosus. Rheumatology International. 2002;**21**(5):189-192. DOI: 10.1007/s00296-001-0165-8

[28] Ramírez R, Carracedo J, Merino A, Soriano S, Ojeda R, Alvarez-Lara MA,

et al. CD14+CD16+ monocytes from chronic kidney disease patients exhibit increased adhesion ability to endothelial cells. Contributions to Nephrology. 2011;**171**:57-61. DOI: 10.1159/000327134

[29] Nagasawa T, Kobayashi H, Aramaki M, Kiji M, Oda S, Izumi Y. Expression of CD14, CD16 and CD45RA on monocytes from periodontitis patients. Journal of Periodontal Research. 2004;**39**(1):72-78. DOI: 10.1111/j.1600-0765.2004.00713.x

[30] Ziegler-Heitbrock HW, Fingerle G, Ströbel M, Schraut W, Stelter F, Schütt C, et al. The novel subset of CD14+/CD16+ blood monocytes exhibits features of tissue macrophages. European Journal of Immunology. 1993;**23**(9):2053-2058. DOI: 10.1002/eji.1830230902

[31] Salako NO, Rotimi VO, Preeta R, Khodakhast F. The bacteriology of the supragingival plaque of child dental patients in Kuwait. Medical Principles and Practice. 2004;**13**(4):191-195. DOI: 10.1159/000078314

[32] Hirsch V, Blufstein A, Behm C, Andrukhov O. The alterations in CD14 expression in periodontitis: A systematic review. Applied Sciences. 2021;**11**(5):2444. DOI: 10.3390/app11052444

[33] Yeap WH, Wong KL, Shimasaki N, Teo EC, Quek JK, Yong HX, et al. CD16 is indispensable for antibody-dependent cellular cytotoxicity by human monocytes. Scientific Reports. 2016;**6**:34310. DOI: 10.1038/srep34310

[34] Jagannathan R, Lavu V, Rao SR. Comparison of the proportion of non-classic (CD14+CD16+) monocytes/macrophages in peripheral blood and gingiva of healthy individuals and patients with chronic periodontitis. Journal of Periodontology. 2014;**85**(6):852-858. DOI: 10.1902/jop.2013.120658

[35] Ichise Y, Saegusa J, Tanaka-Natsui S, Naka I, Hayashi S, Kuroda R, et al. Soluble CD14 induces pro-inflammatory cytokines in rheumatoid arthritis fibroblast-like synovial cells via toll-like receptor 4. Cell. 2020;**9**(7):1689. DOI: 10.3390/cells9071689

[36] Wilensky A, Tzach-Nahman R, Potempa J, Shapira L, Nussbaum G. Porphyromonasgingivalisgingipains selectively reduce CD14 expression, leading to macrophage hyporesponsiveness to bacterial infection. Journal of Innate Immunity. 2015;**7**(2):127-135. DOI: 10.1159/000365970

[37] Arigbede AO, Babatope BO, Bamidele MK. Periodontitis and systemic diseases: A literature review. Journal of Indian Society Periodontology. 2012;**16**(4):487-491. DOI: 10.4103/0972-124X.106878

[38] Bui FQ, Almeida-da-Silva CLC, Huynh B, Trinh A, Liu J, Woodward J, et al. Association between periodontal pathogens and systemic disease. Biomedical Journal. 2019;**42**(1):27-35. DOI: 10.1016/j.bj.2018.12.001

[39] Yu S, Nakashima N, Xu BH, Matsuda T, Izumihara A, Sunahara N, et al. Pathological significance of elevated soluble CD14 production in rheumatoid arthritis: in the presence of soluble CD14, lipopolysaccharides at low concentrations activate RA synovial fibroblasts. Rheumatology International. 1998;**17**(6):237-243. DOI: 10.1007/s002960050041

[40] Preshaw PM, Alba AL, Herrera D, Jepsen S, Konstantinidis A, Makrilakis K, et al. Periodontitis and diabetes: A two-way relationship.

Diabetologia. 2012;**55**(1):21-31. DOI: 10.1007/s00125-011-2342-y

[41] Ingersoll MA, Platt AM, Potteaux S, Randolph GJ. Monocyte trafficking in acute and chronic inflammation. Trends in Immunology. 2011;**32**(10):470-477. DOI: 10.1016/j.it.2011.05.001

[42] Genco R, Offenbecker S, Beck J. Periodontal disease and cardiovascular disease: Epidemiology and possible mechanisms. Journal of the American Dental Association (1939). 2002;**133**:145-125

[43] Olivares R, Ducimetière P, Claude JR. Monocyte count: A risk factor for coronary heart disease? American Journal of Epidemiology. 1993;**137**(1):49-53. DOI: 10.1093/oxfordjournals.aje.a116601

[44] Scott M, Quinn K, Li Q, Carroll R, Warsinske H, Vallania F, et al. Increased monocyte count as a cellular biomarker for poor outcomes in fibrotic diseases: A retrospective, multicentre cohort study. The Lancet Respiratory Medicine. 2019;**7**:497-508. DOI: 10.1016/S2213-2600(18)30508-3

[45] Côté CH, Bouchard P, van Rooijen N, et al. Monocyte depletion increases local proliferation of macrophage subsets after skeletal muscle injury. BMC Musculoskeletal Disorders. 2013;**14**:359. DOI: 10.1186/1471-2474-14-359

[46] Kim J, Ko Y, Kwon K, Koo S, Rhee Y, Kang B, et al. Analysis of monocyte subsets and toll-like receptor 4 expression in peripheral blood monocytes of women in preterm labor. Journal of Reproductive Immunology. 2012;**94**(2):190-195. DOI: 10.1016/j.jri.2012.02.002

[47] Rai B, Kaur J, Kharb S. Pregnancy gingivitis and periodontitis and its systemic effect. The Internet Journal of Dental Science [Internet]. 2009;**6**. Available from: http://www.ispub.com/journal/the_internet_journal_of_dental_science/volume_6_number_2_25/article/pregnancy_gingivitis_and_periodontitis_and_its_systemic_effect.html

[48] Kanter JE, Hsu CC, Bornfeldt KE. Monocytes and macrophages as protagonists in vascular complications of diabetes. Frontiers in Cardiovascular Medicine. 2020;**7**:10. DOI: 10.3389/fcvm.2020.00010

[49] Krinninger P, Ensenauer R, Ehlers K, Rauh K, Stoll J, Krauss-Etschmann S, et al. Peripheral monocytes of obese women display increased chemokine receptor expression and migration capacity. The Journal of Clinical Endocrinology & Metabolism. 2014;**99**(7):2500-2509. DOI: 10.1210/jc.2013-2611

[50] Meyer MS, Joshipura K, Giovannuci E, MichandiDS. Periodontal disease and cancer. Cancer Causes & Control. 2008;**19**:895-807

[51] Feng Y, Li L, Sun XH. Monocytes and Alzheimer's disease. Neuroscience Bulletin. 2011;**27**(2):115-122. DOI: 10.1007/s12264-011-1205-3

Section 5

Macrophages in Viral Infections

Chapter 14

Interaction of Ebola Virus with the Innate Immune System

Parastoo Yousefi and Alireza Tabibzadeh

Abstract

The Ebola viruses (EBOVs) are known as one the most lethal viruses. EBOV systemic infection can cause damage to vital organs and lead to death. The immune responses of the innate immune system and inflammatory cascade are critical elements in the EBOV pathogenesis and mortality. The primary innate immune system response can shape the adaptive immune responses. The innate immune response, due to the pattern-recognition receptors (PRRs), can induce interferons (IFN). IFN is a critical element in the antiviral response. The EBOV can evade the IFN and innate immunity using different mechanisms, whereas a well-controlled and sufficient innate immune response is vital for limiting the EBOV infection. In this regard, a hyperactive inflammation response may lead to cytokine storms and death. In this chapter, we have tried to provide a perspective on the pathogenesis and molecular mechanisms of the innate immune system and its interaction with EBOV infection.

Keywords: Ebola virus, immunity, innate immune responses, macrophages, VP35

1. Introduction

The Ebola virus (EBOV) genus and Marburg viruses are classified in the *Filoviridae* family and *Mononegavirales* order [1]. The EBOV contains a linear single-stranded RNA genome of 18.9-kilobase length and a membrane glycoprotein [2, 3]. Over the past 40 years, there have been 34 episodes of EBOV outbreaks in 11 different Sub-Saharan African countries. The first outbreaks occurred in 1971 in the Democratic Republic of the Congo (DRC) and Sudan [3]. These outbreaks amassed a total of more than 34000 cases and led to 14000 deaths [3]. EBOV Sudan, Bundibugyo, Zaire, and Reston are important species of the EBOV infection in humans [4]. The basic reproductive number (R0) of the EBOV is estimated to be in the range of 1.51–2.53 [4].

Some therapeutic and vaccination strategies have been introduced against the EBOV so far. The remdesivir, monoclonal antibodies [5], and rVSV-ZEBOV (vesicular stomatitis virus-based vaccine which is expressing the glycoprotein of a Zaire Ebola virus) [6] are considered ongoing advances in this area for EBOV treatment and transmission control.

Innate immunity and interferons (IFN) production are one of the most important immune responses to viral infections. Interaction between the Ebola virus and innate immunity with a well-regulated inflammation response can be life-saving in

IntechOpen

patients with the Ebola virus disease (EBD) [7]. The interaction of the EBOV with the innate immune system is a multifactorial condition, and it is largely associated with cytokines, chemokines, inflammation mediators, the NK cell receptors, and pathogen-associated molecular patterns (PAMPs), such as killer immunoglobulin-like receptor (KIR) and Toll-like receptors (TLRs) [8, 9]. The signaling pathways in the innate immune system are triggered after PAMPs detected by pattern-recognition receptors (PRRs) [10]. Based on protein domain homology, the PRRs are classified into six groups TLRs, a retinoic acid-inducible gene I (RIG-I)-like receptors (RLRs), nucleotide oligomerization domain (NOD)-like receptors (NLRs), C-type lectin receptors (CLRs), absent in melanoma-2 (AIM2)-like receptors (ALRs), and cyclic GMP-AMP synthase and stimulator of interferon genes (cGAS-STING pathway) [11, 12]. PRRs are also able to recognize molecules released by damaged cells (The damage-associated molecular pattern-DAMPs) and activate natural immunity [13, 14]. The detection of PAMPs or DAMPs by PRRs increases the transcription of genes encoding cytokine and chemokine, IFN type 1, and antimicrobial proteins (AMPs) [15]. Furthermore, most of the TLRs recognize double-stranded RNA (dsRNA) whereas TLR7 and TLR8 bind single-stranded RNA (ssRNA) in endosomes [16]. After recognition, TLRs recruit several adaptor proteins, including Myeloid Differentiation primary response 88 (MyD88), TIR-domain-containing adaptor protein (TIRAP), TIR-domain-containing adapter-inducing interferon-β (TRIF), and TRIF-related adapter molecule (TRAM) [17]. This initiates downstream signaling cascades that lead to the activation of transcription factors, such as transcription factors NF-κB, interferon regulatory factor 3/7 (IRF3/7), and activator protein-1 (AP-1). These factors stimulate the transcription of genes in the cell nucleus and increase the secretion of pro-inflammatory cytokines and IFN [15, 18]. RIG-1 and melanoma differentiation-associated gene 5 (MDA5), recognize viral ss/dsRNA molecule leads to the translocation of NF-kB, mitogen-activated protein kinases (MAPKs), as well as interferon regulatory factors IRF3, IRF7 [19]. RIG-1 signaling pathway plays a crucial role in the antiviral innate immune response. Activated RIG-1 can interact with signaling adaptor protein mitochondrial antiviral signaling protein (MAVS), also known as IFN-β promoter stimulator 1 (IPS-1), to induction of NF-κB signaling or interferon pathways. It was revealed that upon viral infection, MAVs form high-molecular-weight aggregates downstream of RIG-1 and MDA5 signaling [20]. Activated MAVS–RIG-I signaling ultimately results in the activation of the antiviral IFN-I pathway [21]. The binding of type I and III IFNs to their receptors activates the Jak–STAT pathway, which is responsible for enhancing IFN-stimulated gene expression, which includes antiviral genes, such as Viperin, MxA, MxB, IFITMs, OAS, and PKR [22, 23]. One of the most important complexes, which participate in host defense by sensing viral infection and promoting innate immune system response, is the inflammasome, first described by Martinon in 2002 [24]. The best-studied inflammasome sensor is NOD-like receptor pyrin domain-containing protein 3 (NLRP3), which consists of a sensor molecule (NLRP3), the adaptor protein ASC, also called PYCARD, and an effector pro-caspase-1 [25]. Activated caspase is required for the cleavage of the inactivated interleukin-1 family (IL-1), such as pro-IL-18 and pro-IL-1β to the mature forms to initiate inflammasome [26].

Dendritic cells (DCs) and macrophages are one of the main axes for filoviruses infections due to the activation of the adaptive immune [27, 28]. In addition, the macrophage's infection and attachment by EBOV result in downstream signaling for alteration of the expression profile in these cells. This alteration leads to the pro-inflammatory cytokine release and virus spreading, which both are important elements in the disease progression and outcome [29, 30]. In this regard, in the current chapter, we tried to provide a perspective on the pathophysiology and molecular mechanisms of the innate immune system and its interaction with EBOV infection.

2. Ebola virus: history and epidemiology

Over the past 40 years, there are 34 episodes of the EBOV outbreak in more than 10 different Sub-Saharan African countries leading to numerous cases and deaths [31]. Different species of the EBOV have been reported thus far. Three important species are known as Sudan, Bundibugyo, and Reston [32]. The responsible species for the 2014 outbreak of EBOV was identified as the Zaire ebolavirus [32]. The EBOV disease is a zoonotic disease in nature and the major route for transmission is contact with the infected animal especially chimpanzees, fruit bats, and antelope [2, 33]. The virus genome could be detectable for 10 weeks postmortem [34]. Any contact with bodily fluids is a major route for transmission of EBOV [35]. Even after the survival from the disease the viral genome can be detected in semen for 179 days and leads to sexual transmission in some cases [36]. Fever, fatigue, diarrhea, and tachycardia are the most common symptoms and based on the infected strain and the patient's age, 43% of mortality is reported over the 8 days following the infection [37]. In convalesce or a long time after the remission, some rare complications and long-term sequels, such as uveitis or blurred vision, sleeping problems, and meningoencephalitis are reported [38–40].

3. EBOVE virology and pathogenicity

3.1 Virology and classification

The Ebola virus (EBOV) genus in *Filoviridae* is a member of the great order of *Mononegavirales* [1]. There are seven important genes in EBOV. The nucleoprotein (NP) is curial for replication and virus formation. Also, viral protein 35 (VP35) is important in the IFN synthesis blocking and virus replication while VP40 acts as an element in virus formation and intracellular trafficking. The glycoprotein (GP) is a major element for viral entry and induces lymphocyte apoptosis by soluble GPs. EBOV VP30 has been assumed to function as a transcription activation factor, which is essential for viral replication. VP24 is necessary for the formation of nucleocapsids (NC) and nucleocapsid-like structures, and Ebola virus L proteins act as subunits of RNA-dependent RNA polymerase, which along with VP35, is necessary for viral replication and transcription [41–43]. A summary of the function of genes is provided in **Table 1**.

The VP35 is a key viral protein in the EBOV virulence. This unique protein inhibits the induction of IFN type I in the infected cell. The IFN type I has long been declared a key element in the host's innate antiviral response [45]. In this regard, the VP35 is considered the most important for virus immune evasion [46]. The IFN blocking strategy in EBOV is not limited to VP35. Other EBOV protein VP24 can actively bind to the karyopherin alpha (KPNA) and interfere with the IFN STAT1 downstream signaling [47]. Furthermore, VP24 seems to be essential for the EBOV replication in macrophages of the guinea pig as an animal model [48].

Viral gene name	Important functions
VP24	formation of nucleocapsids (NC) and nucleocapsid-like structures, inhibit IFN signaling
L	RNA-dependent RNA polymerase
glycoprotein (GP)	viral entry induces lymphocyte apoptosis and reduces neutralizing antibodies by soluble GPs
NP	Nucleoprotein formation
VP40	Virus assembly
VP35	inhibits the induction of IFN type I
VP30	transcription activation factor

Table 1.
A summary of the important functions of the Ebola virus genes [41, 44].

3.2 Pathogenicity and treatment

The EBOV represents an affinity to a wide range of the cellular receptors for virus attachment to the cells. Following the systemic virus infection, viral cytopathology and immune-mediated cell damage are two essential steps of the EBOV pathogenesis and tissue damage [49]. One of the suggested pathogenic mechanisms of the EBOV is the antibody-dependent augmentation of the infection through the attachment of the antibodies to the virus and the C1q-C1q receptor of the complement in the cell surfaces [50].

One of the most important therapeutic agents for EBOV is the remdesivir. The remdesivir acts as an inhibitor of the virus RNA polymerase and leads to chain termination [51]. Efforts for the treatment of the EBOV also lead to some monoclonal antibodies against this virus; for instance, old and newer versions of these monoclonal antibodies are ZMapp, MAb114, and REGN-EB3 [5].

4. Innate immune system and EBOV

4.1 Primary innate immune response and inflammation

Interaction between the Ebola virus and innate immunity suggested that a fast and well-regulated inflammation response could be life-saving in patients with the Ebola virus disease (EBD). While a massive monocyte/macrophage activation could be lethal [7]. The mononuclear phagocytes are import element in the EBD pathology [52].

Biomarkers are suggestive elements for disease prognosis and pathogenesis. Some markers such as apoptosis antigen-Fas, IFN-β, IL-29, IL-5, TNFR-II, and FAS ligand levels are associated with the moderate disease while the D-dimer, Granzyme B, IL-10, IL-6, IL-8, TNFR-I, vWF (von Willebrand factor), monocyte chemoattractant proteins and thrombomodulin are associate with severe disease [53]. Furthermore, up-regulation of the IL-1β and IL-6 can suggest a non-fatal infection while the increase in TNF-α, IFN-ϒ, IL-10, IL-1 receptor antagonist, neopterin, IL-8, IL-15, and IL-16 is associated with the lethal outcome [7, 54–56]. By considering all these markers, it has been suggested that in a general view an increase in cytokines and cytokine storm, which it is, represents a hyperactive of the innate immune responses and in the other way, suppression of the adaptive immune responses and lymphocyte apoptosis is the main pathogenesis feature of the EBD and lethal infections [55].

The lymphocyte apoptosis leads to lymphocyte depletion. This apoptotic feature is not due to the replication and infection of the lymphocytes but it mediates through viral and immune system stimulations [57]. sGP, a viral protein produced during EBOV infection and accumulates at high concentrations in the serum, serves as a decoy to prevent the immune system from fighting the infection by binding EBOV-neutralizing antibodies [58]. It is assumed that glycosylation of transmembrane GP may affect neutralizing antibody binding [59]. Virally infected cells, release inflammation mediators that induce Fas and TNF-associated apoptosis-inducing ligands (TRAIL) pathways that can result in lymphocyte apoptosis and lack of an effective adaptive immune response [60–62]. In EBOV infection, lymphocytes are not directly infected, but apoptosis of lymphocytes is a pathological feature of infection. It is hypothesized that the factors (such as TRAIL, TNF-a, and Fas ligand) secreted by macrophages and dendritic cells infected in EBOV, cause lymphocyte apoptosis [52, 60].

Investigation of the EBOV infection in asymptomatic people suggested strong activation of the innate immune system and inflammation, which leads to adaptive immune activation and cytotoxic T cell responses. The strong activation of the innate immune system, inflammation and adaptive immune activation are considered as the optimum immune response to EBOV [63]. The main concept of the current section is summarized in **Figure 1**. The figure represents the EBOV infection in lethal and non-lethal scenarios and the role of the innate immune and inflammation in this process. In addition, some important interactions of the EBOV proteins are noted, for instance, the role of the VP35 and VP24 in type I interferon blocking or the role of the soluble glycoproteins in lymphocyte apoptosis.

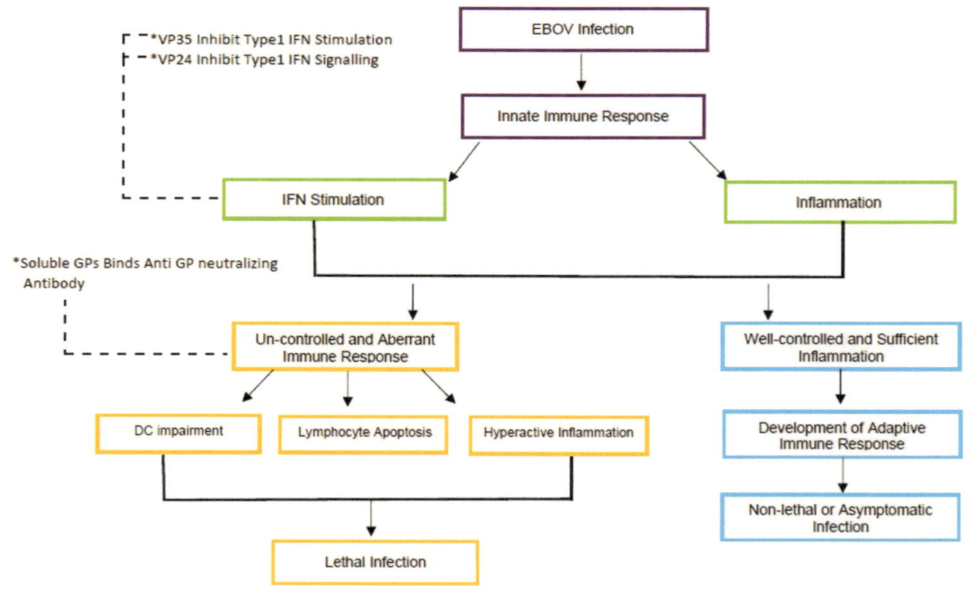

Figure 1.
A summary of the EBOV infection in lethal and non-lethal scenarios and the role of the innate immune and inflammation. After the EBOV, infection such as any other viral infection innate immunity induces inflammation and IFN. The VP35 and VP24 of the EBOV block the IFN production. A well-controlled and sufficient innate immune response, while it leads to the adaptive immune response, is assumed main cause of asymptomatic or non-lethal infections.

4.2 Innate immunity receptors and EBOV

The interaction of the EBOV and the innate immune system is not only limited to the cytokines, chemokines, or inflammation mediators. In this regard, the NK cell and T cell receptors, which are known as killer immunoglobulin-like receptors (KIR), are critical. The role of the NK cells in response to the EBOV viral-like particles highlighted the importance of these cells in the innate immune response to the EBOV [64]. The KIRs are important elements in the host response to infectious diseases. KIR2DS1 and KIR2DS3 of repertoire genotypes of the KIR represent more susceptibility to fatal EBOV [8].

In the EBOV infection, the interaction of the innate and adaptive immune responses is critical for the disease outcome. The Toll-like receptor 4 (TLR4) is a vital element in response to the EBOV glycoprotein and activation of the antigen-presenting cells and T cells. By considering this, TLR4 responses represent a vital role in the regulation of innate and adaptive immunity [9]. The interaction of the TLR4 and monocytes (as antigen-presenting cells) highlighted the importance of the monocytes in the regulation of the immune response. The evidence supports the alteration of the transcriptional patterns in monocytes in EBD [65]. Furthermore, one of the major elements in inflammation and IFN stimulation is NLRP3 [66]. The EBOV infection could increase the IL-1β and IL-18 by the NLRP3 inflammasome activation [67]. This factor highlights the importance of the NLRP3 in pro-inflammatory cytokine production and innate immune system responses.

5. Macrophages and other important innate immune cells in Ebola virus innate immune responses

The DCs and macrophages infection with the EBOV is critical for adaptive immune activation. The EBOV infection leads to macrophage activation (by increasing the CD163 marker) and decreases T cell activation (by reducing in CD25 marker) in severe cases [68]. The macrophage's infection leads to reductions in the co-stimulatory molecules in these cells, which are known as the main adaptive immune activation and the axis of the antigen presentation [27, 28]. The macrophage infection also leads to alteration in pro-inflammatory cytokine releases, such as IL-1β, TNF-α, and IL-6, which could dysregulate the inflammation [69]. Furthermore, monocytes infection with EBOV is a toll on the virus spreading all around the body [69]. The EBOV uses a mimicking of the apoptosis process for attachment and entry macrophages due to the TAM receptor tyrosine kinases and integrin αV [70]. However, it seems that other cell surface receptors such as DC-SIGN and DC-SIGNR or macrophage galactose-type calcium-type lectin (MGL) are critical for the EBOV infection in DC and macrophages [71, 72]. The attachment of the virus to macrophages regardless of the virus entry or macrophage infection affects the macrophage's expression profile. This alteration is led macrophages to produce high levels of pro-inflammatory and pro-apoptotic signals [30].

Macrophages and dendritic cells are important cell targets of EBOV and the main innate immune cells that secrete cytokines, and chemokines following infection [29, 69]. Although macrophages and DCs are still able to initiate coagulation and inflammation, they are not able to stop the spreading of the Ebola virus systemically due to their impaired ability [28, 73]. These dysfunctions have a major impact on the innate and adaptive immune systems [74]. Macrophages and DCs are the essential cells of innate immunity and provide a bridge between innate and adaptive immunity [75]. It will highlight the importance of these cells in the disease outcome (**Figure 1**). Furthermore, VP24 and VP35 block latent lymphocyte stimulation through the IFN response [73]. All these clues are critical to combine and work as chains for limiting the infection through sufficient and well-controlled innate immune response activation, which leads to adaptive immune responses.

6. Conclusions

In this chapter, we tried to provide a perspective on the EBOV infection and innate immune responses. In a glimpse, it is worth mentioning that innate immune responses are critical in the EBOV infection. Sufficient and well-controlled innate immune responses may lead to optimum cytokine release and adaptive immune activation. In contrast, an overreacted innate immunity could affect and hyper-inflammation response.

The macrophages and DCs are also key elements in EBOV infection due to pro-inflammatory response and virus spreading. The EBOV uses different strategies to dysregulate and evade innate immune responses.

VP35 and VP24 of the virus inhibit the IFN type I stimulation in infected cells. Furthermore, the soluble GPs of the EBOV can induce apoptosis in T cells. The interaction of the EBOV with innate immunity is the most fundamental feature of the infection and determines the disease outcome.

Acknowledgements

We sincerely acknowledge the IntechOpen publication editorial office and Jelena Vrdoljak the Author Service Manager in IntechOpen for her incredible efforts.

Conflict of interest

The authors declare no conflict of interest.

Author details

Parastoo Yousefi* and Alireza Tabibzadeh*
Department of Virology, School of Medicine, Iran University of Medical Sciences, Tehran, Iran

*Address all correspondence to: parastoo_y@yahoo.com
and alireza.tabibzadeh@outlook.com; tabibzadeh.a@iums.ac.ir

References

[1] ICTV. https://talk.ictvonline.org/taxonomy/. visit 2 March 2022

[2] Pourrut X et al. The natural history of Ebola virus in Africa. Microbes and Infection. 2005;7(7-8):1005-1014

[3] Li Y, Chen S. Evolutionary history of Ebola virus. Epidemiology & Infection. 2014;**142**(6):1138-1145

[4] Althaus CL. Estimating the reproduction number of Ebola virus (EBOV) during the 2014 outbreak in West Africa. PLoS Currents. 2014;**2014**:6

[5] Mulangu S et al. A randomized, controlled trial of Ebola virus disease therapeutics. New England Journal of Medicine. 2019;**381**(24):2293-2303

[6] Lévy Y et al. Prevention of Ebola virus disease through vaccination: Where we are in 2018. The Lancet. 2018;**392**(10149):787-790

[7] Baize S et al. Inflammatory responses in Ebola virus-infected patients. Clinical & Experimental Immunology. 2002;**128**(1):163-168

[8] Wauquier N et al. Association of KIR2DS1 and KIR2DS3 with fatal outcome in Ebola virus infection. Immunogenetics. 2010;**62**(11):767-771

[9] Lai C-Y et al. Ebola virus glycoprotein induces an innate immune response in vivo via TLR4. Frontiers in Microbiology. 2017;**8**:1571

[10] Iwasaki A, Medzhitov R. Toll-like receptor control of the adaptive immune responses. Nature Immunology. 2004;**5**(10):987-995

[11] Abe T, Marutani Y, Shoji I. Cytosolic DNA-sensing immune response and viral infection. Microbiology and Immunology. 2019;**63**(2):51-64

[12] He S et al. Research advancement of innate immunity and pattern recognition receptors. Chinese Journal of Animal Nutrition. 2017;**29**(11):3844-3851

[13] Amarante-Mendes GP et al. Pattern recognition receptors and the host cell death molecular machinery. Frontiers in Immunology. 2018:2379

[14] Akira S, Uematsu S, Takeuchi O. Pathogen recognition and innate immunity. Cell. 2006;**124**(4):783-801

[15] Takeuchi O, Akira S. Pattern recognition receptors and inflammation. Cell. 2010;**140**(6):805-820

[16] Dalpke AH, Helm M. RNA mediated Toll-like receptor stimulation in health and disease. RNA Biology. 2012;**9**(6):828-842

[17] Jang T-h, Park HH. Crystal structure of TIR domain of TLR6 reveals novel dimeric interface of TIR–TIR interaction for toll-like receptor signaling pathway. Journal of Molecular Biology. 2014;**426**(19):3305-3313

[18] Kawai T, Akira S. The role of pattern-recognition receptors in innate immunity: Update on Toll-like receptors. Nature Immunology. 2010;**11**(5):373-384

[19] Jensen S, Thomsen AR. Sensing of RNA viruses: A review of innate immune receptors involved in recognizing RNA virus invasion. Journal of Virology. 2012;**86**(6):2900-2910

[20] Hou F et al. MAVS forms functional prion-like aggregates to activate and

propagate antiviral innate immune response. Cell. 2011;**146**(3):448-461

[21] Servant MJ, Grandvaux N, Hiscott J. Multiple signaling pathways leading to the activation of interferon regulatory factor 3. Biochemical Pharmacology. 2002;**64**(5-6):985-992

[22] Schoggins JW. Interferon-stimulated genes: Roles in viral pathogenesis. Current Opinion in Virology. 2014;**6**:40-46

[23] He F et al. Filovirus VP24 proteins differentially regulate RIG-I and MDA5-dependent Type I and III interferon promoter activation. Frontiers in Immunology. Jan 5, 2022;**12**:694105

[24] Martinon F, Burns K, Tschopp J. The inflammasome: A molecular platform triggering activation of inflammatory caspases and processing of proIL-β. Molecular Cell. 2002;**10**(2):417-426

[25] Menu P, Vince J. The NLRP3 inflammasome in health and disease: The good, the bad and the ugly. Clinical & Experimental Immunology. 2011;**166**(1):1-15

[26] Lamkanfi M, Dixit VM. Mechanisms and functions of inflammasomes. Cell. 2014;**157**(5):1013-1022

[27] Mahanty S et al. Cutting edge: Impairment of dendritic cells and adaptive immunity by Ebola and Lassa viruses. The Journal of Immunology. 2003;**170**(6):2797-2801

[28] Bosio CM et al. Ebola and Marburg viruses replicate in monocyte-derived dendritic cells without inducing the production of cytokines and full maturation. The Journal of Infectious Diseases. 2003;**188**(11):1630-1638

[29] Gupta M et al. Monocyte-derived human macrophages and peripheral blood mononuclear cells infected with Ebola virus secrete MIP-1α and TNF-α and inhibit poly-IC-induced IFN-α in vitro. Virology. 2001;**284**(1):20-25

[30] Wahl-Jensen V et al. Ebola virion attachment and entry into human macrophages profoundly effects early cellular gene expression. PLoS Neglected Tropical Diseases. 2011;**5**(10):e1359

[31] Rugarabamu S et al. Forty-two years of responding to Ebola virus outbreaks in Sub-Saharan Africa: A review. BMJ Global Health. 2020;**5**(3):e001955

[32] Baize S et al. Emergence of Zaire Ebola virus disease in Guinea. New England Journal of Medicine. 2014;**371**(15):1418-1425

[33] Rewar S, Mirdha D. Transmission of Ebola virus disease: An overview. Annals of Global Health. 2014;**80**(6):444-451

[34] Prescott J et al. Postmortem stability of Ebola virus. Emerging Infectious Diseases. 2015;**21**(5):856

[35] Judson S, Prescott J, Munster V. Understanding ebola virus transmission. Viruses. 2015;**7**(2):511-521

[36] Mate SE et al. Molecular evidence of sexual transmission of Ebola virus. New England Journal of Medicine. 2015;**373**(25):2448-2454

[37] Bah EI et al. Clinical presentation of patients with Ebola virus disease in Conakry, Guinea. New England Journal of Medicine. 2015;**372**(1):40-47

[38] Varkey JB et al. Persistence of Ebola virus in ocular fluid during convalescence. New England Journal of Medicine. 2015;**372**(25):2423-2427

[39] Jacobs M et al. Late Ebola virus relapse causing meningoencephalitis:

A case report. The Lancet. 2016; **388**(10043):498-503

[40] Clark DV et al. Long-term sequelae after Ebola virus disease in Bundibugyo, Uganda: A retrospective cohort study. The Lancet Infectious Diseases. 2015;**15**(8):905-912

[41] Jain S et al. Structural and functional aspects of Ebola virus proteins. Pathogens. 2021;**10**(10):1330

[42] Watt A et al. A novel life cycle modeling system for Ebola virus shows a genome length-dependent role of VP24 in virus infectivity. Journal of Virology. 2014;**88**(18):10511-10524

[43] Boehmann Y et al. A reconstituted replication and transcription system for Ebola virus Reston and comparison with Ebola virus Zaire. Virology. 2005;**332**(1):406-417

[44] He FB, Melén K, Kakkola L, Julkunen I. Interaction of ebola virus with the innate immune system. In: Okware SI, editor. Emerging Challenges in Filovirus Infections [Internet]. London: IntechOpen; 2019 [cited 2022 May 02]. Available from: https://www.intechopen.com/chapters/67614. DOI: 10.5772/intechopen.86749

[45] Basler CF et al. The Ebola virus VP35 protein functions as a type I IFN antagonist. Proceedings of the National Academy of Sciences. 2000;**97**(22):12289-12294

[46] Woolsey C et al. A VP35 mutant Ebola virus lacks virulence but can elicit protective immunity to wild-type virus challenge. Cell Reports. 2019;**28**(12):3032-3046

[47] Xu W et al. Ebola virus VP24 targets a unique NLS binding site on karyopherin alpha 5 to selectively compete with nuclear import of phosphorylated STAT1. Cell Host & Microbe. 2014;**16**(2):187-200

[48] Mateo M et al. VP24 is a molecular determinant of Ebola virus virulence in guinea pigs. The Journal of Infectious Diseases. 2011;**204**(suppl_3):S1011-S1020

[49] Baseler L et al. The pathogenesis of Ebola virus disease. Annual Review of Pathology: Mechanisms of Disease. 2017;**12**:387-418

[50] Takada A et al. Antibody-dependent enhancement of Ebola virus infection. Journal of Virology. 2003;**77**(13):7539-7544

[51] Tchesnokov EP et al. Mechanism of inhibition of Ebola virus RNA-dependent RNA polymerase by remdesivir. Viruses. 2019;**11**(4):326

[52] Hensley LE et al. Proinflammatory response during Ebola virus infection of primate models: Possible involvement of the tumor necrosis factor receptor superfamily. Immunology Letters. 2002;**80**(3):169-179

[53] McElroy AK et al. Kinetic analysis of biomarkers in a cohort of US patients with Ebola virus disease. Reviews of Infectious Diseases. 2016;**63**(4): 460-467

[54] Villinger F et al. Markedly elevated levels of interferon (IFN)-γ, IFN-α, interleukin (IL)-2, IL-10, and tumor necrosis factor-α associated with fatal Ebola virus infection. The Journal of Infectious Diseases. 1999;**179**(Suppl_1):S188-S191

[55] Wauquier N et al. Human fatal zaire ebola virus infection is associated with an aberrant innate immunity and with massive lymphocyte apoptosis. PLoS Neglected Tropical Diseases. 2010;**4**(10):e837

[56] Hutchinson KL, Rollin PE. Cytokine and chemokine expression in humans infected with Sudan Ebola virus. The Journal of Infectious Diseases. 2007;**196**(Suppl_2):S357-S363

[57] Geisbert TW et al. Apoptosis induced in vitro and in vivo during infection by Ebola and Marburg viruses. Laboratory Investigation. 2000;**80**(2):171-186

[58] Ito H et al. Ebola virus glycoprotein: Proteolytic processing, acylation, cell tropism, and detection of neutralizing antibodies. Journal of Virology. 2001;**75**(3):1576-1580

[59] Francica JR et al. Steric shielding of surface epitopes and impaired immune recognition induced by the ebola virus glycoprotein. PLoS Pathogens. 2010;**6**(9):e1001098

[60] Bradfute SB et al. Mechanisms and consequences of ebolavirus-induced lymphocyte apoptosis. The Journal of Immunology. 2010;**184**(1):327-335

[61] Zaki S, Goldsmith C. Pathologic features of filovirus infections in humans. Current Topics in Microbiology and Immunology. 1999;**235**:97-116

[62] Prescott JB et al. Immunobiology of Ebola and Lassa virus infections. Nature Reviews Immunology. 2017;**17**(3):195-207

[63] Leroy E et al. Early immune responses accompanying human asymptomatic Ebola infections. Clinical & Experimental Immunology. 2001;**124**(3):453-460

[64] Warfield KL et al. Role of natural killer cells in innate protection against lethal ebola virus infection. The Journal of Experimental Medicine. 2004;**200**(2):169-179

[65] Menicucci AR et al. Transcriptome analysis of circulating immune cell subsets highlight the role of monocytes in Zaire Ebola virus Makona pathogenesis. Frontiers in Immunology. 2017;**8**:1372

[66] Chong WC et al. The complex interplay between endoplasmic reticulum stress and the NLRP3 inflammasome: A potential therapeutic target for inflammatory disorders. Clinical & Translational Immunology. 2021;**10**(2):e1247

[67] Halfmann P, Hill-Batorski L, Kawaoka Y. The induction of IL-1β secretion through the NLRP3 inflammasome during Ebola virus infection. The Journal of Infectious Diseases. 2018;**218**(suppl_5): S504-S507

[68] McElroy AK et al. Macrophage activation marker soluble CD163 associated with fatal and severe Ebola virus disease in humans. Emerging Infectious Diseases. 2019;**25**(2):290

[69] Ströher U et al. Infection and activation of monocytes by Marburg and Ebola viruses. Journal of Virology. 2001;**75**(22):11025-11033

[70] Dahlmann F et al. Analysis of Ebola virus entry into macrophages. The Journal of Infectious Diseases. 2015;**212**(suppl_2):S247-S257

[71] Simmons G et al. DC-SIGN and DC-SIGNR bind ebola glycoproteins and enhance infection of macrophages and endothelial cells. Virology. 2003;**305**(1):115-123

[72] Usami K et al. Involvement of viral envelope GP2 in Ebola virus entry into cells expressing the macrophage galactose-type C-type lectin. Biochemical and Biophysical Research Communications. 2011;**407**(1):74-78

[73] Bray M, Geisbert TW. Ebola virus: The role of macrophages and dendritic cells in the pathogenesis of Ebola hemorrhagic fever. The International Journal of Biochemistry & Cell Biology. 2005;**37**(8):1560-1566

[74] Mohamadzadeh M, Chen L, Schmaljohn AL. How Ebola and Marburg viruses battle the immune system. Nature Reviews Immunology. 2007;**7**(7):556-567

[75] Olukitibi TA et al. Dendritic cells/macrophages-targeting feature of Ebola glycoprotein and its potential as immunological facilitator for antiviral vaccine approach. Microorganisms. 2019;**7**(10):402

Chapter 15

Macrophage Polarization in Viral Infectious Diseases: Confrontation with the Reality

Perla Abou Atmeh, Soraya Mezouar and Jean-Louis Mège

Abstract

The role of macrophages in viral infections is well documented. Their activation status also called macrophage polarization categorized by the dichotomy of M1 and M2 phenotype remained poorly investigated. Recent studies have shown the complexity of macrophage polarization in response to viral infection and the limits of its use in infected individuals. The aim of this chapter is to reappraise the concept of macrophage polarization in viral infectious diseases, which are more complicated than the models of macrophage-virus interaction. If this concept has been largely used to describe activation status of myeloid cells in experimental conditions, it has to be assessed in light of high-throughput technologies at molecular and phenotypic levels. We update knowledge on macrophage polarization in viral infectious diseases with a special attention for severe acute respiratory syndrome coronavirus-2 (SARS-CoV-2) infection leading to coronavirus disease (COVID-19). Hence, we propose an overview of the concept of macrophages as targets for therapeutic intervention in viral infectious disease. Finally, we tempted to focus our approach on patient investigation restricting the use of *in vitro* experiments and animal models to mechanistic questions.

Keywords: macrophages, myeloid cells, polarization, viral diseases

1. Introduction

First described in 1882 by Ilya Mechnikov, macrophages or "phagocytes" are distributed widely in the body where they acquire specific tissue identities and functions [1]. Macrophages are key effectors of tissue homeostasis contributing to wound healing and tissue repair. When tissue homeostasis is altered, monocytes are recruited from blood to tissues where they differentiate into macrophages. These latter are critical components of innate and adaptive immunity and contribute to inflammation and host defense.

During infection, macrophages represent the first cells on the battle front. They can act as scavengers by engulfing and destroying pathogens or altered host cells, alert the immune system through the secretion of lipid mediators, cytokines, and chemokine; or present antigens to T lymphocytes [2]. The expression of lectins, scavenger receptors, and immunoglobulin receptors enables macrophage phagocytosis, antibody-dependent cell phagocytosis (ADCP) and cytotoxicity (ADCC) [3].

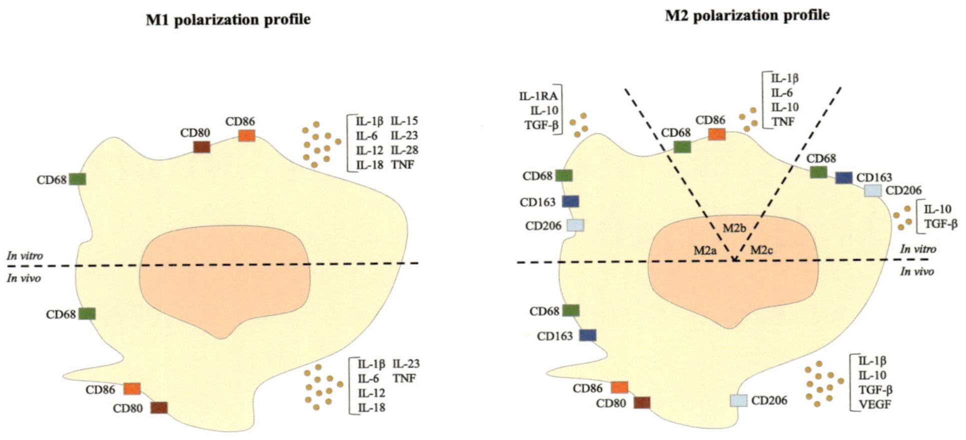

Figure 1.
In vitro and in vivo macrophage polarization markers and protein secretion.

They are also equipped with pattern recognition receptors (PRRs) that following their stimulation lead to the activation of transcription factors, the release of toxic mediators (reactive oxygen intermediates, proteases, inflammatory molecules) [3]. Because of their ability to promote adaptive immune response to virus via antibody release and CD8 T cell activation, macrophages can contribute to the cure of viral infections.

According to their function in pathological conditions, macrophages are considered as activated or alternatively activated also referred to as M1 and M2 polarization phenotype, respectively. The polarization of macrophages is a concept introduced to describe the features of myeloid cell activation and to classify them in functional categories (**Figure 1**), according to initially reported polarization of immune response into Th1 and Th2 types [4–6]. The M1 macrophages are induced by Th1 cytokines such as interferon (IFN)-γ and/or lipopolysaccharide (LPS) and present a pro-inflammatory phenotype. They are characterized by the secretion of inflammatory cytokines including tumor necrosis factor (TNF), interleukin (IL)-1α, IL-1β, IL-6, IL-12, IL-23, and also the expression of several markers including CD80, CD86, and CD68. The M2 macrophages are likely more heterogeneous: they have been classified into four categories, M2a, M2b, M2c, and M2d, depending on the stimulus [7, 8]. As described in **Table 1**, macrophages stimulated by IL-4 or IL-13 lead to an M2a profile associating the expression of CD206, IL-1 receptor type 2 (IL1-R2) and arginase and the secretion of transforming growth factor (TGF)-β and IL-10. M2b macrophages are induced by immune complexes, Toll-like receptor (TLR) ligands, or IL-1β. This profile is associated with the secretion of inflammatory cytokines (TNF, IL-1β, IL-6), IL-10, and the chemokine CCL1. M2c macrophages are induced by IL-10, TGF-β, or glucocorticoids; they expressed CD163 and CD206 and exhibit anti-inflammatory activity through the secretion of IL-10 and TGF-β. Finally, M2d polarization is initiated by TLRs (TLR2, TLR4, TLR7, and TLR9) or adenosine receptor ligands (A2A) with the secretion of vascular endothelial growth factor (VEGF) supporting pro-angiogenic and pro-tumoral functions [9–11]. It is becoming evident that these categories of activation states are an over-simplification of the diversity of macrophage activation modes. We have tried to reappraise the concept of macrophage polarization by associating the type of polarization with the agonist [12]. This approach allows to propose several activation profiles with LPS, IFN-γ, or their combination instead

	Stimuli	Marker expression	Cytokine production	Chemokine production	Functions
M1	IFN-γ, LPS, GM-CSF, TNF	CD68, CD86, CD80, MHC-II, IL1R, TLR2, TLR4, iNOS, SOCS3, IL-12^{high}/ IL-10^{low}, IL-6, TNF	TNF, IL-1β, IL-6, IL-12, IL-23	CCL10, CCL11, CCL5, CCl8, CCL9, CCL2, CCL3, CCL4	• Pro-inflammation • Microbicidal • Tumor resistance
M2a	IL-4, IL-13	CD163, CD206, MHC-II, TGM2, IL-1R II, scavenger receptors, Arg-1	IL-10, TGF-β, IL-1ra	CCL17, CCL22, CCL24	• Anti-inflammatory • Wound healing
M2b	LPS + immune complexe, IL-1 β, immune complexes, TLRs	CCL1, CD86, IL-6, IL-10^{high}/ IL-12^{low}, TNF, MHC-II	IL-1β, IL-6, IL-10, TNF	CCL1	• Immunoregulation • Tumor progression • Promoting infection
M2c	Glucocorticoids, IL-10, TGF-β	CD163, TLR8, TLR1, CD206	IL-10, TGF-β	CCR2	• Phagocytosis • Immunosuppression • Tissue remodeling
M2d	IL-6, adenosine, leukocyte inhibitory factor, TLRs	VEGF	IL-10, TGF-β, TNF, IL-12	CCL5, CXCL10, CXCL16	• Angiogenesis • Tumor progression

IFN: interferon, LPS: polysaccharide; GM-CSF: granulocyte macrophage colony stimulating factor; TLR: Toll like receptor; MHC: major histocompatibility complex; iNOS: inducible nitric oxide; Arg: arginase; TNF: tumor necrosis factor; IL: interleukin; TGF: transforming growth factor; VEGF: vascular endothelial growth factor.

Table 1.
In vitro macrophages polarization sub-types.

of a unique M1 activation state [13, 14]. In clinical situations, it has been shown that tumor-associated macrophages (TAMs) are clearly specialized cell populations in which polarization and functions are related: M1-like and M2-like TAMs have anti-tumoral and pro-tumoral activities, respectively [15]. In other clinical situations including infectious diseases, such functional dichotomy is rarely observed [7], and the functional role of macrophage polarization remains an exception.

The mechanisms of macrophage polarization have been the object of a broad literature. It appears now that the metabolism of macrophages is different according to their polarization. Hence, M1 macrophages exhibit increased glycolysis and broken tricarboxylic acid (TCA) cycle, leading to the accumulation of succinate and citrate. In contrast, M2 macrophages have intact TCA cycle leading to the generation of adenosine triphosphate (ATP) [16, 17]. It is becoming evident that the polarization of macrophages is determined by transcriptional changes, as shown by using new technologies [4]. In aortic macrophages studied *in vivo* by scRNA-seq, Chang et al. identified three classes of macrophages: resident-like, inflammatory, and a final group with strong expression of triggering receptor expressed on myeloid cells 2 (TREM2) [18]. Interestingly, M2 markers are found in the inflammatory macrophage population, suggesting that the traditional classification of macrophage polarization does not fully reflect the diversity of the *in vivo* macrophage populations (**Figure 1**). Quantitative mass spectrometry imaging has also been proposed to investigate macrophage polarization *in situ*. It enabled the cartography of functional macrophage population and the visualization of their distribution in normal and pathological tissues [19–22]. In addition, macrophage polarization requires dynamic and reversible epigenomic marks at enhancers and promoters of signal responsive genes [4]. The epigenetic mechanisms of M2 polarization reveal the role of histone methylation and acetylation. Hence, the overexpression of DNA methyltransferase 3B or the loss of histone deacetylase-3 (HDAC3) promotes M2 phenotype. The histone demethylase JMJD3 (lysine demethylase 6B, KDM6B) is activated by IL-4 and binds M2 genes, leading to repress M1 inflammatory program. In contrast, IFN-γ increases chromatin accessibility [4, 23]. Finally, polarization and functional responses of macrophages are influenced by differential expression of microRNAs: the literature has reported miRs specialized in M1 polarization and miRs increasing M2-like responses [24].

Is the specialization of M1/M2-like macrophages evolutionary conserved? Two ancient molecular mechanisms, inducible nitric oxide synthase 2 (iNOS2) and arginase (Arg), characterize macrophage polarization. If the ability to produce large amounts of nitric oxide in response to microbial agonists, a hallmark of M1 macrophages, has emerged with vertebrates, the Arg pathway is described in both prokaryotes and eukaryotes [25]. The cytosolic and mitochondrial Args are encoded by two genes, and it has been shown that the duplication of Arg gene occurred after the separation of vertebrates and invertebrates [26]. Hence, it is likely that macrophage polarization occurs during early vertebrate evolution [27].

The aim of this chapter is to update the knowledge about macrophage polarization in viral infections with a special focus on severe acute respiratory syndrome coronavirus-2 (SARS-CoV-2) infection. We are deciding to analyze papers reporting infections in humans and to restrict animal models for specific questions. The analysis of the literature reveals the heterogeneous definition of macrophage polarization and the frequently inappropriate use of this concept. It is the reason why the final paragraph will describe how macrophage polarization can be studied in patients (**Table 2**) and to propose some recommendations for investigating infected patients.

	M1 macrophage	M2 macrophage
Marker expression	CD68, CD86, CD80	CD68, CD86, CD80, CD163, CD206
Cytokine	TNF, IL-1β, IL-6, IL-12, IL-23, IL-18	IL-10, TGF-β, TNF, VEGF, IL-1β
Functions	Pro-inflammatory and anti-tumoral	Pro- and/or anti-inflammatory

TNF: tumor necrosis factor; IL: interleukin; TGF: transforming growth factor; VEGF: vascular endothelial growth factor.

Table 2.
In vivo polarization of macrophage sub-types.

2. Viral infectious diseases in humans

As obligate intracellular pathogens, viruses require host cells to replicate. Innate defenses are essentials to block or inhibit cell infection, to eliminate virus from infected cells, and to alert cells the adaptive immunity. This crucial stage is regulated by myeloid cells including, dendritic cells, and mainly by macrophages. The early response is based on [1] the recognition of pathogen-associated molecular patterns (PAMPs) by PRRs, [2] the elimination of foreign agents [3] and the activation of type I and II IFNs, and interferon-stimulated gene (ISG), which have broad-spectrum antiviral activity [28, 29]. Although this defense is effective, a complete cure of the infection requires mounting adaptive immune response that is controlled to prevent immune pathogenicity. Macrophage-mediated immune response can be circumvented or hijacked by the virus to allow its replication and persistence in the host.

The first studies highlighting the interaction between myeloid cells and viruses date back to the end of 1970s [30, 31]. In a general point of view, macrophages polarize into M1 following a contact with viruses, which induces a pro-inflammatory response while the phenotype M2 is often found at late stages of infection [32]. It has been reported that virulent strains of viruses will "bias" the M1 polarization profile of macrophages into M2. In contrast, attenuated viruses lead to an M2 polarization profile M2 [33]. M1-activated macrophages play a key role in the elimination of viruses through several strategies, including the secretion of reactive species [34], secretion of antiviral cytokines [35], or activation of other immune cells such as T cells and natural killers [36, 37]. Hence, some viruses are able to counteract M1 macrophages in order to obtain an environment favorable to their replication. Indeed, some viruses are able to inhibit production of nitric oxide [38–41] or pro-inflammatory cytokines [42–44], suppress antigen presentation [45–48], or simply modulate the signaling pathways associated with polarization by inducing M2 phenotype [8, 49–51]. We previously addressed the role of macrophage polarization in bacterial infections [7, 52]; the aim of the present talk is to assess the role of macrophage polarization in viral infections by selecting typical viral infections.

2.1 Hepatitis viruses

Five viruses, known as hepatitis A, B (HBV), C (HCV), D, and E, are responsible for the majority of acute and chronic hepatitis. HBV infection is responsible of acute self-resolving disease in adults but not in early life. Hepatic macrophages whatever their origin are involved in host response to HBV. HBV antigen and nucleic acids are detected in monocytes and macrophages from patients with hepatitis. The interaction of HBV with macrophages including hepatic macrophages may affect macrophage polarization by suppressing M1 polarization and promoting M2 polarization [53]. M1-associated cytokines are likely protective as shown by higher risk of HBV reactivation and hepatotoxicity in patients with anti-TNF treatment given for inflammatory diseases [54]. During the progression of HBV-related disease (from mild chronic hepatitis B to decompensated cirrhosis), M2-type monocytes expressing CD163 and CD206 are increased, whereas the frequency of cells expressing M1 markers decreases. Monocytes and Kupffer cells expressing an M2 profile are predicting a poor clinical outcome [55]. The non-protective effect of M2-type polarization is illustrated by the observation that IL-10 gene promoter polymorphisms are associated with HBV progression [44]. The measurement of soluble CD163 and soluble mannose receptor may be a pertinent approach of follow-up of patients with chronic hepatitis. Both markers are released during liver damage and are associated with M2 polarization and fibrosis; their levels are reduced after antiviral treatment [56]. The relationship between chronic evolution of hepatitis B, fibrosis, and infiltration of liver by M2-like macrophages has been demonstrated in a humanized mouse model of infection [57].

HCV is transmitted between adults and is responsible for a high percentage of chronic infections with a major risk of liver cirrhosis and hepatocellular carcinoma [58]. The co-culture of monocyte-derived macrophages with HCV-infected hepatocytes induces M2 surface markers. TGF-β produced by these polarized macrophages activates hepatic stellate cells, leading to fibrosis. However, monocytes and macrophages do not seem completely polarized at the cytokine level [59]. Cell-free virus or exosome-packaged HCV induces the differentiation of monocytes into macrophages with M2 phenotype and non-polarized cytokine production under the control of TLR7/8. Interestingly, TLR7/8 is overexpressed in pro-fibrotic monocytes from chronic HCV-infected patients [60]. It has been also shown that HCV core protein inhibits phagocytosis activity of M1 and M2 macrophages and $CD4^+$ T cell activation induced by M1 macrophages but promotes that induced by M2 macrophages [61]. M1 and M2 macrophages generated from chronic HCV patients lose their phenotypic characteristics, suggesting that chronic HCV infection is rather associated with an impaired polarization than a reprogramming of macrophages [62]. Finally, in biopsies of HCV-infected patients, it has been shown that non-infected cells such as Kupffer cells are a source of IFNs, demonstrating the interplay between hepatic cells [63]. Taken together, these data suggest that HBV and HCV share the ability to interfere with M1-type macrophage polarization, thus accounting for viral persistence, hepatic fibrosis, and evolution to carcinoma.

2.2 Human immunodeficiency virus (HIV)

The permissivity of monocytes and macrophages to HIV depends on their differentiation stage, polarization status, and tissue location [64]. The M1/M2 polarization of macrophages impacts the steps of viral cycle including entry, reverse transcription, transcription, and posttranscription. As the level of inflammatory cytokines is high in the early stage of HIV-1 infection [65, 66], it is likely that M1-like macrophages play a role in HIV infection. The entry of R5 and R5/X4 HIV in M1-like macrophages is decreased because of cytokine-mediated downregulation of CD4 and CCR5. In contrast, M1 cytokines such as TNF increase viral transcription. In M2 macrophages elicited by IL-4/IL-13 and/or IL-10-mediated deactivated macrophages, both entry and replication of HIV-1 are decreased [64]. The implication of TNF in M1 polarization of HIV-infected macrophages is debated [67]. Hence, it is likely that M1 macrophages enable the formation of viral reservoirs early in the disease. At later stages, an M2 shift of macrophages is observed. At the onset of acquired immunodeficiency syndrome (AIDS), deactivated macrophages predominate via enhanced clearance of apoptotic cells, which is known to promote M2-like macrophages [68]. Severe evolution of HIV infection is associated with elevated IL-10 levels, but not IL-4 levels, suggesting that AIDS is characterized by IL-10-mediated M2-like phenotype [69]. These findings have been confirmed in acute and chronic HIV and SIV infections. Hence, at the beginning of the infection, the central nervous system, heart, and blood vessels exhibit M1-like macrophages, whereas M2-like macrophages are observed in later responses [32]. It is likely that $CD163^+$ M2 macrophages play a protective role in SIV-infected macaques through their anti-inflammatory functions [70]. It has been proposed that the persistence of initial activation in patients with chronic infection and successful antiviral therapy is correlated to non-AIDS complications such neurocognitive disorder and cardiovascular dysfunctions [71]. Unfortunately, few markers have been investigated in these studies, and it is likely that more precise data will be necessary to reanalyze the polarization of macrophages in HIV infection [71, 72].

2.3 Flavivirus

Flavivirus is responsible for infections essentially dominated by dengue virus (DENV) and Zika virus (ZIKV). First, DENV infection presents a large spectrum of clinical presentations from moderate symptoms to classical dengue and hemorrhagic dengue. Monocytes and macrophages are involved in the infection pathogenesis. Macrophage-colony-stimulating factor (M-CSF)-differentiated macrophages (M2-like macrophages) are poorly sensitive to DENV infection. In contrast, granulocyte macrophage CSF (GM-CSF)-differentiated macrophages (M1-like macrophages) are highly susceptible to DENV infection with high release of cytokines and activation of NLRP3 inflammasome [73]. Nevertheless, some biomarkers such as soluble CD163, known to be associated with M2 polarization of macrophages, seem predictive of severe dengue [74]. In pediatric dengue patients compared with healthy individuals, the number of M2-like macrophages is increased with decreased number of M1-like macrophages. In dengue patients with bleeding trend, both macrophage subsets are decreased and are associated with decreased platelet count [48]. Second, ZIKV is associated with numerous cases of microcephaly and/or central nervous system malformations. ZIKV infects myeloid cells and has a tropism for placenta including maternal and fetal tissues. It has been shown that ZIKV replicates in both placenta macrophages, also named Hofbauer cells, and trophoblasts [75]. Two lineages of ZIKV, African and Asian, have been described, and it has been shown that they exhibit differences in pathogenicity despite close sequence homology [76, 77]. While the Asian strain of ZIKV elicits an expansion of non-classical monocytes from healthy donors and M2-skewed immunosuppressive program, African strain promotes a M1 program [78].

2.4 Cytomegalovirus (CMV)

Human CMV (hCMV) uses TLR2 and intracytosoplasmic sensors to invade monocytes and macrophages [79]. In monocytes, hCMV stimulates a transcriptomic program in which M1 genes are enriched [80]. On the other hand, a product of hCMV genome, *UL111A* gene, encodes functional homologs of human IL-10 during both productive and latent phases of CMV infection [81]. In $CD14^+$ monocytes, the viral IL-10 induces M2c phenotype associating increased expression of CD163 and CD14 and downregulation of HLA-DR. The viral IL-10 also upregulates heme oxygenase 1 (HO-1), a driver of phenotype shift to M2 macrophages [82] known to also down-modulate M1-associated cytokines and poorly stimulate $CD4^+$ T cells [83]. We hypothesize that CMV triggers an M1 program in monocytes and that the release of viral or human IL-10 leads bystander monocytes to be reprogrammed toward an M2 phenotype. The polarization of monocytes in response to hCMV is likely necessary for their differentiation into macrophages. Recently, it has been shown that hCMV stimulates the expression of M1 and M2 markers in monocytes and activates PI3K-Akt axis, leading to caspase 3 activation [84]. CMV susceptibility is dependent on polarization of myeloid cells. M1-like macrophages are more resistant to CMV than M2-like macrophages, and it is likely that this resistance is related to the ability of M1-like macrophages to induce IFN-γ production by natural killer (NK) cells [85]. This hypothesis is supported by two other studies. Although hCMV susceptibility is higher in M2-like macrophages, productive and persistent viral infection is observed in both M1- and M2-like macrophages. Infected M1- and M2-like macrophages are efficient in stimulating proliferation of autologous T cells from hCMV-seropositive donors [86]. The susceptibility of M2 macrophages is optimal in the early phase of hCMV infection, whereas, in the late phase, macrophage activation necessary for viral replication is dependent on the activation of mammalian target of rapamycin (mTORC)1 complex, as confirmed with experiments including rapamycin [87].

2.5 Influenza virus

Four *influenza* virus genera (A, B, C, and D) belonging to *orthomyxoviridae* are responsible for flu, a seasonal respiratory epidemics, or pandemics, such as the "Great Influenza" pandemics of 1918 [88]. The severity of influenza pneumonia depends on host susceptibility and strain diversity and can lead to acute respiratory distress syndrome and lethality. These latter complications are associated with uncontrolled inflammatory response. Numerous evidences show that macrophages including alveolar macrophages are involved in the pathophysiology of influenza virus infections via a direct viral infection or the overproduction of cytokines. This is emphasized by the observation that over-pathogenic strains of *influenza* virus productively infect monocytes [89]. Animal models demonstrate that macrophage reprogramming is critical in outcome of influenza virus infections. Hence, GM-CSF protects from mortality and morbidity and redirects responses of alveolar macrophages from M1-like to M-2-like activation. This finding was unexpected because GM-CSF is known as an M1 inducer and depresses arginase, a canonical marker of M2-like status [90]. The inactivation of NOS (nitric oxide synthase) 2 and IFN-γ favors M2 reprogramming and improves outcome of viral infection [91]. In contrast, the treatment of macrophages with baicalin that possesses antiviral properties stimulated an M1 phenotype shift associated with activation of IFN pathway and inhibition of influenza virus replication [92].

The evidences of macrophage polarization in humans infected with influenza virus are scarce. In one study of patients from the 2009 to 2010 pandemics, monocytes have been reported as a marker of severity independently of viral load [93]. Monocytes from patients with severe infection exhibit increased expression of M1 markers and TNF production and a down-modulation of CD163, an M2 marker. Murine models of influenza virus infection also show high proportion of recruited M1 monocytes and decreased number of resident M2 alveolar macrophages, confirming that the severity of influenza virus infection is associated with macrophage reprogramming toward an M1 phenotype [93].

2.6 Severe acute respiratory syndrome coronavirus 2 (SARS-CoV-2)

SARS-CoV-2, a strain of the coronavirus family, causes coronavirus disease-2019 (COVID-19) characterized in the most severe cases by an increased production of cytokines including IL-1α, IL-1β, IL-6, IL-7, TNF, type I and II IFN, CCL2, CCL3, and CXCL10 [94, 95]. This cytokine storm was initially observed in influenza syndrome that occurs after systemic infection and immunotherapy [96] before it was extended to describe immune response in COVID-19 patients [97]. To better understand the pathophysiology of this emergent disease, the researchers focused on the response of myeloid cells such as macrophages or dendritic cells. Macrophages are permissive to SARS-CoV-2 infection but no viral replication is observed *in vitro* [98, 99]. Interestingly, the production of inflammatory cytokines and chemokines is observed after SARS-CoV-2 infection of macrophages but not after infection of monocyte-derived dendritic cells [98, 100]. The release of TNF, IL-1β, IL-10, IFN-α/β, and IL-6 by infected-macrophages leads to type I IFN-immune response, suggesting a protective role against viral infection [100].

The polarization of macrophages in COVID-19 has also been investigated. Alveolar macrophages respond differently to infection depending on their polarization status. After SARS-CoV-2 infection, M1 macrophages are associated with viral spreading, whereas M2 polarization induces virus degradation and infection limitation. Indeed, macrophages from human ACE2 transgenic mice present an increased infection rate after *in vitro* treatment by IFN-γ or LPS compared with IL-4 treatment [101]. These results are controversial because the SARS-CoV-2 infection of M1 and M2 macrophages from the THP-1 cell line is similar [99]. The gene expression study of lung alveoli from COVID-19 patients reveals different macrophage patterns depending on their polarization profile. The gene expression study of lung alveoli from COVID-19 patients shows that highly inflammatory macrophages are mostly found in patients with severe COVID-19 [102, 103]. Thus, the polarization of macrophages during infection by SARS-CoV-2 is suggested as determining the severity of the disease, even if involved molecular mechanisms remain unexplored to date.

3. Macrophage polarization and treatment of viral infections

The role of deregulated immune response in pathogenesis of viral infections such as COVID-19 pandemics justifies the use of drugs that target host response and exhibit anti-infective properties. Hence, chloroquine and hydroxychloroquine are known for their antiviral and immunomodulatory effects, which lead to propose these molecules in the treatment of SARS-Cov2 infection [104]. Beyond the debate about the efficiency of chloroquine and hydroxychloroquine, their immunomodulatory properties affect the macrophage polarization. It is established that treatment with chloroquine can reverse the polarization of TAMs from M2 to M1 phenotype in tumor models [105]. Similarly, chloroquine and hydroxychloroquine interfere with LPS-mediated M1 polarization of macrophages [106]. The combination of hydroxychloroquine and azithromycin is interesting since this latter molecule is known to induce M2 macrophage polarization [106, 107]. Ivermectin, a macrocyclic lactone known for its antiparasitic effect, has an anti-inflammatory effect promoting M2 polarization of macrophages without effect on viral load; it has been proposed to limit the inflammation of respiratory tract and to improve COVID-19 outcome [108]. Remdesivir, an adenosine analog, reduces inflammatory gene expression and has been largely used in COVID-19 treatment [109].

As mentioned above, M1 polarization of macrophages is a determining phenotype against viral infections. The artificial induction of macrophage M1 polarization may be an interesting adjuvant to antiviral treatment for non-COVID19 infectious diseases. Baicaline has been proposed to limit influenza virus infection via the M1 polarization of macrophages, thus activating their antiviral function via the IFN signaling pathway [92, 110]. It is important to note that viral infections can lead to hyperactivation of macrophages, leading to an excessive inflammatory response known as macrophage activation syndrome. In this context, anti-inflammatory molecules such as tofacitinib, anti-IL1R, or IL-6R have been clinically tested, particularly for COVID-19 [111, 112].

4. Conclusion and perspectives

As the first line of defense, macrophages represent key immune cells against viral infections. In general, the antiviral response is mediated by a pro-inflammatory response of polarized M1 macrophages. Some viruses are able to counteract the antiviral response of macrophages by modulating their polarization by switching the M1 phenotype to M2 phenotype. It should also be noted that viruses such as influenza and SARS-CoV-2 are capable of modulating an M1 over-polarization of macrophages responsible for severe diseases. Interestingly, modulation of macrophage polarization has been investigated as a therapeutic strategy. However, the *in vivo* polarization profile remains more intricate compared with *in vitro* situations. This can be explained by the techniques classically used for investigating macrophage polarization (gene or protein expression) whose limitation is that the observed signals result from a mixture of diverse cells. Hopes for quantitative mass spectrometry imaging as a tissue-level investigative tool remain unanswered to date. Thus, clarifying the tools for investigating macrophage polarization in clinical settings and the associated molecular mechanisms are key steps in the development of therapies in viral infections.

Acknowledgements

Soraya Mezouar was supported by a "Fondation pour la Recherche Médicale" postdoctoral fellowship (reference: SPF20151234951). This work was supported by the French Government under the "Investissements d'avenir" (Investments for the future) program managed by the "Agence Nationale de la Recherche" (reference: 10-IAHU-03).

Author contributions

P.A.A, S.M., and J.L.M. conceived and wrote the manuscript.

Declaration of interest

The authors declare no competing interests.

Author details

Perla Abou Atmeh[1,2†], Soraya Mezouar[1,2†] and Jean-Louis Mège[1,2,3*†]

1 Aix-Marseille Univ, IRD, APHM, MEPHI, Marseille, France

2 IHU-Méditerranée Infection, Marseille, France

3 Aix-Marseille Univ, APHM, Hôpital de la Conception, Laboratoire d'Immunologie, Marseille, France

*Address all correspondence to: jean-louis.mege@univ-amu.fr

† Contributed equally.

References

[1] Lavin Y, Mortha A, Rahman A, Merad M. Regulation of macrophage development and function in peripheral tissues. Nature Reviews. Immunology. 2015;**15**(12):731-744

[2] Murray PJ, Wynn TA. Protective and pathogenic functions of macrophage subsets. Nature Reviews. Immunology. 2011;**11**(11):723-737

[3] Kumar V. Phagocytosis: Phenotypically simple yet a mechanistically complex process: Phagocytosis is a very complex but crucial process playing a pivotal role in embryonic development and host defense to maintain immune homeostasis. International Reviews of Immunology. 2020;**39**(3):118-150

[4] Locati M, Curtale G, Mantovani A. Diversity, mechanisms, and significance of macrophage plasticity. Annual Review of Pathology. 2020;**15**:123-147

[5] Martinez FO, Gordon S. The M1 and M2 paradigm of macrophage activation: Time for reassessment. F1000prime Reports. 2014;**6**:13

[6] Mills CD, Ley K. M1 and M2 macrophages: The chicken and the egg of immunity. Journal of Innate Immunity. 2014;**6**(6):716-726

[7] Benoit M, Desnues B, Mege JL. Macrophage polarization in bacterial infections. Journal of Immunology. 2008;**181**(6):3733-3739

[8] Wang L, Zhang S, Wu H, Rong X, Guo J. M2b macrophage polarization and its roles in diseases. Journal of Leukocyte Biology. 2019;**106**(2):345-358

[9] Nikovics K, Favier AL. Macrophage identification in situ. Biomedicines. 2021;**9**(10):1393

[10] Pinhal-Enfield G, Ramanathan M, Hasko G, Vogel SN, Salzman AL, Boons GJ, et al. An Angiogenic switch in macrophages involving synergy between toll-like receptors 2, 4, 7, and 9 and adenosine A2A receptors. The American Journal of Pathology. 2003;**163**(2):711-721

[11] Ferrante CJ, Pinhal-Enfield G, Elson G, Cronstein BN, Hasko G, Outram S, et al. The adenosine-dependent angiogenic switch of macrophages to an M2-like phenotype is independent of interleukin-4 receptor alpha (IL-4Rα) signaling. Inflammation. 2013;**36**(4):921-931

[12] Murray PJ, Allen JE, Biswas SK, Fisher EA, Gilroy DW, Goerdt S, et al. Macrophage activation and polarization: Nomenclature and experimental guidelines. Immunity. 2014;**41**(1):14-20

[13] Murray PJ. Macrophage polarization. Annual Review of Physiology. 2017;**79**(1):541-566

[14] Ouedraogo R, Daumas A, Capo C, Mege JL, Textoris J. Whole-cell MALDI-TOF mass spectrometry is an accurate and rapid method to analyze different modes of macrophage activation. Journal of Visualized Experiments. 2013;**82**:50926

[15] Wu K, Lin K, Li X, Yuan X, Xu P, Ni P, et al. Redefining tumor-associated macrophage subpopulations and functions in the tumor microenvironment. Frontiers in Immunology. 2020;**11**:1731

[16] O'Neill LAJ. A broken Krebs cycle in macrophages. Immunity. 2015;**42**(3):393-394

[17] O'Neill LAJ, Kishton RJ, Rathmell J. A guide to

immunometabolism for immunologists. Nature Reviews. Immunology. 2016;**16**(9):553-565

[18] Chang Z, Wang Y, Liu C, Smith W, Kong L. Natural products for regulating macrophages M2 polarization. Current Stem Cell Research & Therapy. 2020;**15**(7):559-569

[19] Unsihuay D, Mesa Sanchez D, Laskin J. Quantitative mass spectrometry imaging of biological systems. Annual Review of Physical Chemistry. 2021;**72**:307-329

[20] Holzlechner M, Strasser K, Zareva E, Steinhäuser L, Birnleitner H, Beer A, et al. In situ characterization of tissue-resident immune cells by MALDI mass spectrometry imaging. Journal of Proteome Research. 2017;**16**(1):65-76

[21] Roussel M, Bartkowiak T, Irish JM. Picturing polarized myeloid phagocytes and regulatory cells by mass cytometry. Methods in Molecular Biology (Clifton, N.J.). 2019; **1989**:217-226

[22] Porta Siegel T, Hamm G, Bunch J, Cappell J, Fletcher JS, Schwamborn K. Mass spectrometry imaging and integration with other imaging modalities for greater molecular understanding of biological tissues. Molecular Imaging and Biology. 2018;**20**(6):888-901

[23] Foster SL, Hargreaves DC, Medzhitov R. Gene-specific control of inflammation by TLR-induced chromatin modifications. Nature. 2007;**447**(7147):972-978

[24] Zhong Y, Yi C. MicroRNA-720 suppresses M2 macrophage polarization by targeting GATA3. Bioscience Reports. 2016;**36**(4):e00363

[25] Edholm ES, Rhoo KH, Robert J. Evolutionary aspects of macrophages polarization. Results and Problems in Cell Differentiation. 2017;**62**:3-22

[26] Dzik JM. Evolutionary roots of arginase expression and regulation. Frontiers in Immunology. 2014;**5**:544

[27] Hodgkinson J, Grayfer L, Belosevic M. Biology of bony fish macrophages. Biology. 2015;**4**(4):881-906

[28] Thompson MR, Kaminski JJ, Kurt-Jones EA, Fitzgerald KA. Pattern recognition receptors and the innate immune response to viral infection. Viruses. 2011;**3**(6):920-940

[29] Feng J, Wickenhagen A, Turnbull ML, Rezelj VV, Kreher F, Tilston-Lunel NL, et al. Interferon-stimulated gene (ISG)-expression screening reveals the specific antibunyaviral activity of ISG20. Jung JU, editor. Journal of Virology. 2018;**92**(13):e02140-e02117

[30] Wardley RC, Wilkinson PJ. The growth of virulent African swine fever virus in pig monocytes and macrophages. The Journal of General Virology. 1978;**38**(1):183-186

[31] Gazzolo L, Moscovici C, Moscovici MG. Persistence of avian oncoviruses in chicken macrophages. Infection and Immunity. 1979;**23**(2):294-297

[32] Burdo TH, Walker J, Williams KC. Macrophage polarization in AIDS: Dynamic Interface between anti-viral and anti-inflammatory macrophages during acute and chronic infection. Journal of Clinical and Cellular Immunology. 2015;**6**(3):333

[33] Ferrer MF, Thomas P, López Ortiz AO, Errasti AE, Charo N, Romanowski V, et al.

Junin virus triggers macrophage activation and modulates polarization according to viral strain pathogenicity. Frontiers in Immunology. 2019;**10**:2499

[34] Camini FC, da Silva Caetano CC, Almeida LT, de Brito Magalhães CL. Implications of oxidative stress on viral pathogenesis. Archives of Virology. 2017;**162**(4):907-917

[35] Arango Duque G, Descoteaux A. Macrophage cytokines: Involvement in immunity and infectious diseases. Frontiers in Immunology. 2014;**5**(491):491. Available from: http://journal.frontiersin.org/article/10.3389/fimmu.2014.00491/abstract

[36] Guerriero JL. Macrophages. In: International Review of Cell and Molecular Biology [Internet]. Elsevier; 2019. pp. 73-93. Available from: https://linkinghub.elsevier.com/retrieve/pii/S1937644818300698

[37] Zwirner NW, Domaica CI, Fuertes MB. Regulatory functions of NK cells during infections and cancer. Journal of Leukocyte Biology. 2021;**109**(1):185-194

[38] Kao YJ, Piedra PA, Larsen GL, Colasurdo GN. Induction and regulation of nitric oxide synthase in airway epithelial cells by respiratory syncytial virus. American Journal of Respiratory and Critical Care Medicine. 2001;**163**(2):532-539

[39] Santiago-Olivares C, Rivera-Toledo E, Gómez B. Nitric oxide production is downregulated during respiratory syncytial virus persistence by constitutive expression of arginase 1. Archives of Virology. 2019;**164**(9):2231-2241

[40] Granja AG, Sabina P, Salas ML, Fresno M, Revilla Y. Regulation of inducible nitric oxide synthase expression by viral A238L-mediated inhibition of p65/RelA acetylation and p300 transactivation. Journal of Virology. 2006;**80**(21):10487-10496

[41] Odkhuu E, Komatsu T, Naiki Y, Koide N, Yokochi T. Sendai virus C protein inhibits lipopolysaccharide-induced nitric oxide production through impairing interferon-β signaling. International Immunopharmacology. 2014;**23**(1):267-272

[42] Bradley JH, Harrison A, Corey A, Gentry N, Gregg RK. Ebola virus secreted glycoprotein decreases the anti-viral immunity of macrophages in early inflammatory responses. Cellular Immunology. 2018;**324**:24-32

[43] Zhu W, Banadyga L, Emeterio K, Wong G, Qiu X. The roles of Ebola virus soluble glycoprotein in replication, pathogenesis, and countermeasure development. Viruses. 2019;**11**(11):999

[44] McElroy AK, Nichol ST. Rift Valley fever virus inhibits a pro-inflammatory response in experimentally infected human monocyte derived macrophages and a pro-inflammatory cytokine response may be associated with patient survival during natural infection. Virology. 2012;**422**(1):6-12

[45] Hurtado C, Bustos MJ, Granja AG, de León P, Sabina P, López-Viñas E, et al. The African swine fever virus lectin EP153R modulates the surface membrane expression of MHC class I antigens. Archives of Virology. 2011;**156**(2):219-234

[46] Rehm KE, Connor RF, Jones GJB, Yimbu K, Roper RL. Vaccinia virus A35R inhibits MHC class II antigen presentation. Virology. 2010;**397**(1):176-186

[47] Rehm KE, Connor RF, Jones GJB, Yimbu K, Mannie MD, Roper RL. Vaccinia virus decreases major histocompatibility complex (MHC) class II antigen presentation, T-cell priming, and peptide association with MHC class II. Immunology. 2009;**128**(3):381-392

[48] Schaefer MR, Wonderlich ER, Roeth JF, Leonard JA, Collins KL. HIV-1 Nef targets MHC-I and CD4 for degradation via a final common β-COP–dependent pathway in T cells. Hope TJ, editor. PLoS Pathogens. 2008;**4**(8):e1000131

[49] Wilson HM. SOCS proteins in macrophage polarization and function. Frontiers in Immunology. 2014;**5**:357. Available from: http://journal.frontiersin.org/article/10.3389/fimmu.2014.00357/abstract

[50] Kwon Y, Meyer K, Peng G, Chatterjee S, Hoft DF, Ray R. Hepatitis C virus E2 envelope glycoprotein induces an Immunoregulatory phenotype in macrophages. Hepatology. 2019;**69**(5):1873-1884

[51] Ouyang P, Rakus K, van Beurden SJ, Westphal AH, Davison AJ, Gatherer D, et al. IL-10 encoded by viruses: A remarkable example of independent acquisition of a cellular gene by viruses and its subsequent evolution in the viral genome. The Journal of General Virology. 2014;**95**(2):245-262

[52] Mezouar S, Mege JL. New tools for studying macrophage polarization: Application to bacterial infections. In: Prakash H, editor. Macrophages [Internet]. London, UK: IntechOpen; 2021. Available from: https://www.intechopen.com/books/macrophages/new-tools-for-studying-macrophage-polarization-application-to-bacterial-infections

[53] Faure-Dupuy S, Delphin M, Aillot L, Dimier L, Lebossé F, Fresquet J, et al. Hepatitis B virus-induced modulation of liver macrophage function promotes hepatocyte infection. Journal of Hepatology. 2019;**71**(6):1086-1098

[54] Temel T, Cansu DÜ, Korkmaz C, Kaşifoğlu T, Özakyol A. The long-term effects of anti-TNF-α agents on patients with chronic viral hepatitis C and B infections. International Journal of Rheumatic Diseases. 2015;**18**(1):40-45

[55] Liang J, Long Z, Zhang Y, Wang J, Chen X, Liu X, et al. Chloride intercellular channel 3 (CLIC-3) suppression-mediated macrophage polarization: A potential indicator of poor prognosis of hepatitis B virus-related acute-on-chronic liver failure. Immunology and Cell Biology. 2022:imcb.12542

[56] Laursen TL, Wong GLH, Kazankov K, Sandahl T, Møller HJ, Hamilton-Dutoit S, et al. Soluble CD163 and mannose receptor associate with chronic hepatitis B activity and fibrosis and decline with treatment: sCD163 and sMR in chronic hepatitis B. Journal of Gastroenterology and Hepatology. 2018;**33**(2):484-491

[57] Bility MT, Cheng L, Zhang Z, Luan Y, Li F, Chi L, et al. Hepatitis B virus infection and immunopathogenesis in a humanized mouse model: Induction of human-specific liver fibrosis and M2-like macrophages. Walker CM, editor. PLoS Pathogens. 2014;**10**(3):e1004032

[58] Scheel TKH, Rice CM. Understanding the hepatitis C virus life cycle paves the way for highly effective therapies. Nature Medicine. 2013;**19**(7):837-849

[59] Saha B, Kodys K, Szabo G. Hepatitis C virus-induced monocyte

differentiation into polarized M2 macrophages promotes stellate cell activation via TGF-β. Cellular and Molecular Gastroenterology and Hepatology. 2016;**2**(3):302-316.e8

[60] Saha B, Kodys K, Adejumo A, Szabo G. Circulating and exosome-packaged hepatitis C single-stranded RNA induce monocyte differentiation via TLR7/8 to polarized macrophages and fibrocytes. Journal of immunology (Baltimore, Md. : 1950). 2017;**198**(5):1974-1984

[61] Hou Z, Zhang J, Han Q, Su C, Qu J, Xu D, et al. Hepatitis B virus inhibits intrinsic RIG-I and RIG-G immune signaling via inducing miR146a. Scientific Reports. 2016;**6**(1):26150

[62] Ahmed F, Ibrahim A, Cooper CL, Kumar A, Crawley AM. Chronic hepatitis C virus infection impairs M1 macrophage differentiation and contributes to CD8+ T-cell dysfunction. Cell. 2019;**8**(4):E374

[63] Park SH, Rehermann B. Immune responses to HCV and other hepatitis viruses. Immunity. 2014;**40**(1):13-24

[64] Herbein G, Varin A. The macrophage in HIV-1 infection: From activation to deactivation? Retrovirology. 2010;**7**(1):33

[65] Lafeuillade A, Tamalet C, Pellegrino P, Tourres C, Yahi N, Vignoli C, et al. High viral burden in lymph nodes during early stages of HIV-1 infection. AIDS (London, England). 1993;**7**(11):1527-1528

[66] Emilie D, Peuchmaur M, Maillot MC, Crevon MC, Brousse N, Delfraissy JF, et al. Production of interleukins in human immunodeficiency virus-1-replicating lymph nodes. The Journal of Clinical Investigation. 1990;**86**(1):148-159

[67] Porcheray F, Samah B, Léone C, Dereuddre-Bosquet N, Gras G. Macrophage activation and human immunodeficiency virus infection: HIV replication directs macrophages towards a pro-inflammatory phenotype while previous activation modulates macrophage susceptibility to infection and viral production. Virology. 2006;**349**(1):112-120

[68] Ogden CA, Pound JD, Batth BK, Owens S, Johannessen I, Wood K, et al. Enhanced apoptotic cell clearance capacity and B cell survival factor production by IL-10-activated macrophages: Implications for Burkitt's lymphoma. Journal of Immunology (Baltimore, Md.: 1950). 2005;**174**(5):3015-3023

[69] Sandanger Ø, Ryan L, Bohnhorst J, Iversen AC, Husebye H, Halaas Ø, et al. IL-10 enhances MD-2 and CD14 expression in monocytes and the proteins are increased and correlated in HIV-infected patients. Journal of Immunology (Baltimore, Md.: 1950). 2009;**182**(1):588-595

[70] Yearley JH, Pearson C, Shannon RP, Mansfield KG. Phenotypic variation in myocardial macrophage populations suggests a role for macrophage activation in SIV-associated cardiac disease. AIDS Research and Human Retroviruses. 2007;**23**(4):515-524

[71] Akiyama H, Jalloh S, Park S, Lei M, Mostoslavsky G, Gummuluru S. Expression of HIV-1 intron-containing RNA in microglia induces inflammatory responses. Journal of Virology. 2020;**95**(5):e01386-20

[72] Lv T, Cao W, Li T. HIV-related immune activation and inflammation: Current understanding and strategies. Journal of Immunology Research. 2021;**2021**:7316456

[73] Wu MF, Chen ST, Yang AH, Lin WW, Lin YL, Chen NJ, et al. CLEC5A is critical for dengue virus-induced inflammasome activation in human macrophages. Blood. 2013;**121**(1):95-106

[74] Rahman K, Desai C, Iyer SS, Thorn NE, Kumar P, Liu Y, et al. Loss of junctional adhesion molecule a promotes severe steatohepatitis in mice on a diet high in saturated fat, fructose, and cholesterol. Gastroenterology. 2016;**151**(4):733-746.e12

[75] Quicke KM, Bowen JR, Johnson EL, McDonald CE, Ma H, O'Neal JT, et al. Zika virus infects human placental macrophages. Cell Host & Microbe. 2016;**20**(1):83-90

[76] Wang L, Valderramos SG, Wu A, Ouyang S, Li C, Brasil P, et al. From mosquitos to humans: Genetic evolution of Zika virus. Cell Host & Microbe. 2016;**19**(5):561-565

[77] Miner JJ, Diamond MS. Zika virus pathogenesis and tissue tropism. Cell Host & Microbe. 2017;**21**(2):134-142

[78] Foo SS, Chen W, Chan Y, Bowman JW, Chang LC, Choi Y, et al. Asian Zika virus strains target CD14+ blood monocytes and induce M2-skewed immunosuppression during pregnancy. Nature Microbiology. 2017;**2**(11):1558-1570

[79] Baasch S, Ruzsics Z, Henneke P. Cytomegaloviruses and macrophages-friends and foes from early on? Frontiers in Immunology. 2020;**11**:793

[80] Chan G, Bivins-Smith ER, Smith MS, Smith PM, Yurochko AD. Transcriptome analysis reveals human cytomegalovirus reprograms monocyte differentiation toward an M1 macrophage. Journal of Immunology (Baltimore, Md.: 1950). 2008;**181**(1):698-711

[81] Jenkins C, Abendroth A, Slobedman B. A novel viral transcript with homology to human interleukin-10 is expressed during latent human cytomegalovirus infection. Journal of Virology. 2004;**78**(3):1440-1447

[82] Naito Y, Takagi T, Higashimura Y. Heme oxygenase-1 and anti-inflammatory M2 macrophages. Archives of Biochemistry and Biophysics. 2014;**564**:83-88

[83] Avdic S, Cao JZ, McSharry BP, Clancy LE, Brown R, Steain M, et al. Human cytomegalovirus interleukin-10 polarizes monocytes toward a deactivated M2c phenotype to repress host immune responses. Journal of Virology. 2013;**87**(18):10273-10282

[84] Cojohari O, Mahmud J, Altman AM, Peppenelli MA, Miller MJ, Chan GC. Human cytomegalovirus mediates unique monocyte-to-macrophage differentiation through the PI3K/SHIP1/Akt signaling network. Viruses. 2020;**12**(6):E652

[85] Romo N, Magri G, Muntasell A, Heredia G, Baía D, Angulo A, et al. Natural killer cell-mediated response to human cytomegalovirus-infected macrophages is modulated by their functional polarization. Journal of Leukocyte Biology. 2011;**90**(4):717-726

[86] Bayer C, Varani S, Wang L, Walther P, Zhou S, Straschewski S, et al. Human cytomegalovirus infection of M1 and M2 macrophages triggers inflammation and autologous T-cell proliferation. Journal of Virology. 2013;**87**(1):67-79

[87] Poglitsch M, Weichhart T, Hecking M, Werzowa J, Katholnig K, Antlanger M, et al. CMV late phase-induced mTOR activation is essential for efficient virus replication in

polarized human macrophages. American Journal of Transplantation: Official Journal of the American Society of Transplantation and the American Society of Transplant Surgeons. 2012;**12**(6): 1458-1468

[88] Vemula S, Zhao J, Liu J, Wang X, Biswas S, Hewlett I. Current approaches for diagnosis of influenza virus infections in humans. Viruses. 2016;**8**(4):96

[89] Roberts JMK, Simbiken N, Dale C, Armstrong J, Anderson DL. Tolerance of honey bees to Varroa mite in the absence of deformed wing virus. Viruses. 2020;**12**(5):575

[90] Halstead ES, Umstead TM, Davies ML, Kawasawa YI, Silveyra P, Howyrlak J, et al. GM-CSF overexpression after influenza a virus infection prevents mortality and moderates M1-like airway monocyte/ macrophage polarization. Respiratory Research. 2018;**19**(1):3

[91] Sun K, Metzger DW. Inhibition of pulmonary antibacterial defense by interferon-γ during recovery from influenza infection. Nature Medicine. 2008;**14**(5):558-564

[92] Geng P, Zhu H, Zhou W, Su C, Chen M, Huang C, et al. Baicalin inhibits influenza a virus infection via promotion of M1 macrophage polarization. Frontiers in Pharmacology. 2020;**11**:01298

[93] Cole SL, Dunning J, Kok WL, Benam KH, Benlahrech A, Repapi E, et al. M1-like monocytes are a major immunological determinant of severity in previously healthy adults with life-threatening influenza. JCI Insight. 2017;**2**(7):e91868

[94] Lucas C, Wong P, Klein J, Castro TBR, Silva J, Sundaram M, et al. Longitudinal analyses reveal immunological misfiring in severe COVID-19. Nature. 2020;**584**(7821):463-469

[95] Arunachalam PS, Wimmers F, Mok CKP, Perera RAPM, Scott M, Hagan T, et al. Systems biological assessment of immunity to mild versus severe COVID-19 infection in humans. Science. 2020;**369**(6508):1210-1220

[96] Fajgenbaum DC, June CH. Cytokine Storm. The New England Journal of Medicine. 2020;**383**(23):2255-2273

[97] Mehta P, McAuley DF, Brown M, Sanchez E, Tattersall RS, Manson JJ, et al. COVID-19: Consider cytokine storm syndromes and immunosuppression. Lancet (London, England). 2020; **395**(10229):1033-1034

[98] Yang D, Chu H, Hou Y, Chai Y, Shuai H, Lee ACY, et al. Attenuated interferon and proinflammatory response in SARS-CoV-2-infected human dendritic cells is associated with viral antagonism of STAT1 phosphorylation. The Journal of Infectious Diseases. 2020;**222**(5):734-745

[99] Boumaza A, Gay L, Mezouar S, Bestion E, Diallo AB, Michel M, et al. Monocytes and macrophages, targets of severe acute respiratory syndrome coronavirus 2: The clue for coronavirus disease 2019 immunoparalysis. The Journal of Infectious Diseases. 2021;**224**(3):395-406

[100] Zheng J, Wang Y, Li K, Meyerholz DK, Allamargot C, Perlman S. Severe acute respiratory syndrome coronavirus 2-induced immune activation and death of monocyte-derived human macrophages and dendritic cells. The Journal of Infectious Diseases. 2021;**223**(5): 785-795

[101] Lv J, Wang Z, Qu Y, Zhu H, Zhu Q, Tong W, et al. Distinct uptake, amplification, and release of SARS-CoV-2 by M1 and M2 alveolar macrophages. Cell Discovery. 2021;**7**(1):24

[102] Liao M, Liu Y, Yuan J, Wen Y, Xu G, Zhao J, et al. Single-cell landscape of bronchoalveolar immune cells in patients with COVID-19. Nature Medicine. 2020;**26**(6):842-844

[103] Channappanavar R, Fehr AR, Vijay R, Mack M, Zhao J, Meyerholz DK, et al. Dysregulated type I interferon and inflammatory monocyte-macrophage responses cause lethal pneumonia in SARS-CoV-infected mice. Cell Host & Microbe. 2016;**19**(2):181-193

[104] Meyerowitz EA, Vannier AGL, Friesen MGN, Schoenfeld S, Gelfand JA, Callahan MV, et al. Rethinking the role of hydroxychloroquine in the treatment of COVID-19. The FASEB Journal. 2020;**34**(5):6027-6037

[105] Chen D, Xie J, Fiskesund R, Dong W, Liang X, Lv J, et al. Chloroquine modulates antitumor immune response by resetting tumor-associated macrophages toward M1 phenotype. Nature Communications. 2018;**9**(1):873

[106] Vitte J, Michel M, Mezouar S, Diallo AB, Boumaza A, Mege JL, et al. Immune modulation as a therapeutic option during the SARS-CoV-2 outbreak: The case for antimalarial aminoquinolines. Frontiers in Immunology. 2020;**11**:2159

[107] Haydar D, Cory TJ, Birket SE, Murphy BS, Pennypacker KR, Sinai AP, et al. Azithromycin polarizes macrophages to an M2 phenotype via inhibition of the STAT1 and NF-κB signaling pathways. Journal of Immunology. 2019;**203**(4):1021-1030

[108] Melo GD, Lazarini F, Larrous F, Feige L, Kornobis E, Levallois S, et al. Attenuation of clinical and immunological outcomes during SARS-CoV-2 infection by ivermectin. EMBO Molecular Medicine. 2021;**13**(8). Available from: https://onlinelibrary.wiley.com/doi/10.15252/emmm.202114122

[109] Yin L, Zhao H, Zhang H, Li Y, Dong Y, Ju H, et al. Remdesivir alleviates acute kidney injury by inhibiting the activation of NLRP3 inflammasome. Frontiers in Immunology. 2021;**12**:652446

[110] Li R, Wang L. Baicalin inhibits influenza virus a replication via activation of type-I IFN signaling by reducing miR-146a. Molecular Medicine Reports. 2019. Available from: http://www.spandidos-publications.com/10.3892/mmr.2019.10743

[111] Napoli C, Benincasa G, Criscuolo C, Faenza M, Liberato C, Rusciano M. Immune reactivity during COVID-19: Implications for treatment. Immunology Letters. 2021;**231**:28-34

[112] Mahmudpour M, Roozbeh J, Keshavarz M, Farrokhi S, Nabipour I. COVID-19 cytokine storm: The anger of inflammation. Cytokine. 2020;**133**:155151

Chapter 16

Macrophages and HIV/AIDS Pathogenesis: Lessons from the Rhesus Macaque Model

Elizabeth S. Didier and Marcelo J. Kuroda

Abstract

Destruction of $CD4^+$ T cells is a primary cause of immunodeficiency in Human Immunodeficiency Virus (HIV)-infected humans and Simian Immunodeficiency Virus (SIV)-infected rhesus macaques. Tissue macrophages, however, also contribute to AIDS pathogenesis. Studies on rhesus macaque lung revealed the presence of at least two types of macrophages comprising short-lived lung interstitial macrophages in the parenchyma that are not present in bronchoalveolar lavage (BAL), and the long-lived alveolar macrophages that predominate in BAL and rarely divide. Increased blood monocyte turnover was associated with death of infected short-lived tissue macrophages and terminal disease progression during AIDS. Antiretroviral therapy (ART) treatment of SIV-infected macaques effectively prevented active infection of short-lived macrophages in tissues and delayed disease progression. Interestingly however, longer-lived macrophages remained infected and survived despite ART. This suggests that the long-lived macrophages contribute to establishing a virus reservoir and that these infected persistent cells likely become dysregulated to promote chronic inflammation. Furthermore, macrophages are the predominant immunological cells in heart, adipose tissue, and lung, and these were primarily of the long-lived macrophage subset. Information about macrophages garnered from the SIV rhesus macaque model provides a basis to further develop intervention strategies that target macrophages for reducing chronic inflammatory co-morbidities and remove a contributing viral reservoir for achieving cure.

Keywords: Macrophage, HIV, SIV, pathogenesis, inflammation, rhesus macaque, virus reservoir

1. Introduction

Macrophages are immune cells located in tissues throughout the body that early in life, originate from the yolk sac during development and later from bone marrow-derived blood monocytes. Macrophages regulate inflammation and tissue repair to maintain or re-establish homeostasis in response to environmental exposures [1–4]. These cells exhibit tremendous plasticity and have been categorized in relation to their surface marker expression as well as pro- and anti-inflammatory responses [5–7].

Results from murine studies initially drove the categorization of polarized macrophage populations and origins. These contributed to better understanding monocyte and macrophage differentiation and plasticity in humans [5, 6]. Nonhuman primates that physiologically resemble humans, also contributed to the in vivo characterization of short-lived and long-lived macrophages using approaches that are difficult to perform in humans [8]. In addition, studies using the SIV-rhesus macaque infection model that simulates the disease pathogenesis observed in humans with HIV infection have afforded further characterization of macrophages in vivo [9–11].

Prior to the era of antiretroviral therapy (ART) application, HIV or SIV infection commonly led to AIDS resulting from a loss of $CD4^+$ T cells [12, 13]. We also learned that an increase in monocyte turnover apparently required to replace damaged tissue macrophages, also correlated with terminal disease progression [14, 15]. The loss in $CD4^+$ T cells and infected short-lived macrophages facilitated the development of opportunistic infections and cancers leading to death. HIV- or SIV infected hosts administered ART, however, survive with low-to-undetectable plasma viral levels, but typically develop HIV/SIV-associated non-AIDS conditions resembling chronic inflammatory diseases that occur in the elderly but at an earlier age than in non-HIV/SIV-infected individuals, a process sometimes considered accelerated or accentuated aging [16]. Chronic inflammation is likely a result of macrophage dysregulation which can be more readily evaluated in rhesus macaques infected with SIV and treated with ART. And, although, $CD4^+$ T lymphocytes serve as a primary target of infection, HIV and SIV are lentiviruses that also infect macrophages, especially as $CD4^+$ T cells decline in numbers leaving macrophages more available for infection [3, 17–23]. These macrophage subpopulations appear to exhibit distinct functions during progressing stages of HIV/SIV infection [22, 24–26]. Thus, studies on SIV in rhesus macaques are relevant for addressing macrophage subpopulations and their roles in pathogenesis in vivo.

2. Macrophages plasticity

Metchnikoff described macrophages as large (macro) cells that eat (phage) particles and phagocytize dead cells, debris, and pathogens as a first-line of innate immune responses, which remains a primary function of these cells [5, 6]. Macrophages also present antigen in the context of major histocompatibility complex antigens to promote adaptive immune responses by lymphocytes. To facilitate these functions, macrophages exhibit plasticity or polarized activation states that impact secretion of and responsiveness to a wide range of cytokines and chemokines to regulate inflammation, tissue repair, and (re)establishment of homeostasis [5, 6]. The activation of macrophages to perform these functions is multi-dimensional and impacted by intrinsic and extrinsic tissue environmental stimuli. Exposures to extrinsic stimuli including cell debris, pathogenic agents, or toxins trigger innate immune responses, recruitment of immune cells and secretion of a wide array of chemokines and cytokines. These extrinsic stimuli were further characterized using in vitro models of macrophage polarization. At one end of this spectrum, Th1 signals such as interferon stimulate M1 “classical” macrophages to promote acute inflammatory responses in response to intracellular pathogens. On the other end of the spectrum, Th2 factors such as IL4 stimulate M2 “alternative” macrophages to exhibit anti-inflammatory and anthelmintic responses as well as wound healing or tissue repair. These categorizations were further refined into a range of intermediate activation states and chronic or smoldering inflammation [6, 27]. Intrinsic factors impacting function consider macrophage origin via monocyte derivation versus resident embryonic progenitor status. Resident macrophages of embryonic yolk sac origin function in tissue remodeling and clearance of dead cells while monocyte-derived macrophages appear to function in microbial defense. It had long been believed that tissue macrophages are continually replaced by recruited blood monocytes that differentiate into tissue macrophages. More recently, studies in mice demonstrated that resident macrophages can undergo self-renewal [28]. In addition, monocyte-derived macrophages may acquire resident macrophage characteristics yet retain some epigenetic and transcriptional distinctions, suggesting that tissue environment may be more physiologically relevant than macrophage origin [6, 28, 29]. However, it is less clear and has been difficult to determine if embryonic-derived resident macrophages self-renew in nonhuman primates or humans throughout life [6, 28].

3. Tools to study macrophage populations in vivo in rhesus macaques

Rhesus macaque monocytes and macrophages express a wide range of biomarkers and cytokines / chemokines similar to those in humans, which can be identified via immune-detection and molecular biology methods. Surface biomarkers for CD14 and CD16 expression are commonly used to identify subpopulations of classical ($CD14^+$, $CD16^-$) pro-inflammatory, intermediate / transitional ($CD14^+$, $CD16^+$) and non-classical ($CD14^{+/-}$, $CD16^-$) anti-inflammatory monocytes that traffic to tissues where they differentiate into macrophages [6]. Among surface markers, tissue macrophages express scavenger receptors (e.g. CD163), Toll-like receptors (TLR), scavenger and lectin receptors (e.g. CD163, CD206), glycoproteins (e.g. lysosomal-associated membrane protein CD68) and MHC class II moieties for recognition of pathogens and antigen presentation.

In addition to analyzing surface biomarker expression, these cells have been characterized as short-lived macrophages having recently differentiated from trafficking monocytes or as longer-lived (i.e. resident) macrophages. An approach to identify shorter-lived macrophages in rhesus macaques is to monitor the incorporation of thymidine analogues such as 5-bromo-2′-deoxyuridine (BrdU). BrdU has a short half-life of a few hours in vivo and incorporates in cells dividing during this time, including monocyte precursors in bone marrow. Immunostaining then can be applied to detect the recently dividing monocytes and follow their trafficking patterns from bone marrow to blood to tissues, as well as their turnover rates [14, 22, 24–26, 30, 31]. To detect longer-lived macrophages, dextran, a branched polymer of anhydroglucose can be administered. Phagocytic cells take up fluorescein-labeled dextran, and long-lived macrophages containing the conjugated dextran can be identified weeks or months later whereas the shorter-lived cells with dextran die in a few days and are replaced with recently-recruited unlabeled cells [22, 32].

4. SIV infection in nonhuman primates

SIV infections in nonhuman primates have served as invaluable animal models for HIV infection and AIDS research [12, 13, 33]. Nonhuman primates are similar to humans physiologically and immunologically. Advantages to using nonhuman primates in SIV/HIV research is the ability to closely regulate parameters such as time, dose, and route of infection, as well as control for confounders such as smoking, diet, or illicit drug use. Experimental procedures for longitudinal tissue sampling, experimental vaccine testing, and therapeutic investigations also can be performed more readily in nonhuman primates. Naturally-infected nonhuman primate hosts such as African green monkeys and sooty mangabeys exhibit few clinical signs of disease from persistent or non-progressing SIV infection. Conversely, non-natural nonhuman primate hosts experimentally infected with SIV such as rhesus macaques, pigtail macaques, and cynomolgus macaques, exhibit a course of disease similar to that in humans with HIV infection. The differences between these non-pathogenic and pathogenic nonhuman primate models, respectively, provided opportunities to study comparative mechanisms of pathogenesis and immunity related to distinct outcomes of infection [34].

5. Increased monocyte turnover correlated to onset of terminal disease/AIDS in the absence of ART

Declining $CD4^+$ T cells is a key biomarker for immune-deficiency, morbidity, and mortality during HIV and SIV infections of rhesus macaques [13, 35]. However, in SIV-infected rhesus macaques, we observed exceptions whereby a few animals with relatively higher levels of $CD4^+$ T cells still developed AIDS while others exhibited low $CD4^+$ T cell numbers ($\leq$10% of baseline) with no obvious clinical signs of AIDS [14, 15, 36, 37] (Video 1: https://www.youtube.com/watch?v=g-RfAJyZsg0&t=23s and Video 2: https://www.youtube.com/watch?v=ynIom7fefxs&t=68s). Interestingly, while the number of monocytes in blood remained level, the percentage of recently dividing blood monocytes undergoing turnover, based on incorporation of BrdU administered 24 hours previously, drastically increased during terminal disease progression to AIDS in SIV-infected macaques [14, 25, 36–38]. To assess this observation further, machine learning algorithm modeling was applied to measure the relative contribution of covariates (singly or in combination) of monocyte turnover rate, percent $CD4^+$ T-cell loss, plasma viral levels, and viral strains to survival time or days until necropsy based on clinical AIDS criteria [15]. Matched time-point data sets were used (not imputed) and results from animals surviving to experimentally-timed endpoints were excluded. By Boosted Forest regression, monocyte turnover had the highest proportion of contribution to days until AIDS-associated necropsy (0.475 or 47.5%) followed by $CD4^+$ T-cell loss (0.216 or 21.6%), viral load (0.187 or 18.7%) or virus strain (below random) [15]. Classification categorization using decision tree algorithm modeling to analyze the flow chart-like proportion of the co-variates in predicting survival time in SIV-infected rhesus macaques further demonstrated that monocyte turnover (MTO) predicted a significantly shorter survival time among animals with $\geq$13.2% monocyte turnover rate followed by $CD4^+$ T cell decline. These results led to further investigations to delineate macrophage subpopulations and their roles in SIV/HIV infection pathogenesis.

6. Tissue macrophages in the pathogenesis of HIV/SIV infection

Increased monocyte turnover during terminal disease progression to AIDS suggested that monocytes and macrophages contribute to pathogenesis. While $CD4^+$ T cells are preferentially targeted by HIV/SIV, macrophages also become infected with HIV/SIV, especially if a tissue contains few T cells (i.e. brain) or after CD4⁺ T cell decline [19, 39, 40]. Infected macrophages are detected throughout the body [3, 4, 41–50]. Furthermore, resident macrophages infected with virus are resistant to apoptosis [17, 42, 51–53] and cytotoxic CD8 T cell lysis [54] thereby supporting their likely contribution to the virus reservoir.

a. **Lung.** In lung tissues and BAL fluids of rhesus macaques, two predominant populations of macrophages have been identified and characterized using in vivo administration of BrdU and dextran in conjunction with immunostaining methods to identify short-lived and long-lived macrophages, respectively [24]. Short-lived interstitial macrophages were relatively smaller in size, express CD163 (scavenger receptor) and primarily located in the lung interstitial tissue. Long-lived alveolar macrophages were relatively larger, double-positive (DP) for expressing both CD163 and CD206 (mannose receptor), and predominated in the alveolar spaces but also found in the interstitial tissue [24]. During terminal disease progression in SIV-infected rhesus macaques, the short-lived single-positive $CD163^{+}CD206^{-}$ macrophages in the interstitial lung tissues were readily infected and destroyed by SIV infection [25]. This loss in short-lived tissue macrophages may induce the increased production and turnover of monocytes to traffic and replace the damaged tissue macrophage that occurs during the transition from chronic to terminal disease progression after SIV infection. Furthermore, lung tissue lesions were progressively more severe with increasing monocyte turnover rates and macrophage accumulation (**Figure 1**) [25, 26]. Interestingly, resident long-lived double-positive $CD163^{+}CD206^{+}$ alveolar macrophages survived SIV infection despite efficacy in ART for reducing plasma viral loads to possibly become a virus reservoir [25]. In addition, while SIV-infected as well as uninfected $CD4^{+}$ T cells were killed in lungs of infected rhesus macaques, macrophages did

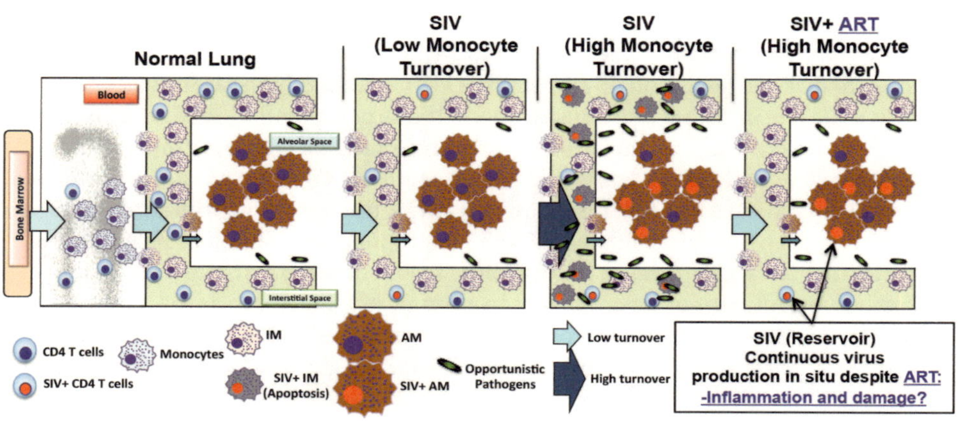

Figure 1.
Proposed mechanism of lung tissue damage in SIV-infected macaques undergoing ART. The lung contains at least two populations of macrophages; shorter-lived interstitial macrophages (IM) and longer-lived alveolar macrophages (AM). IM become massively infected with SIV and undergo a high rate of apoptosis that correlates with increased blood monocyte turnover. Conversely, SIV infection of the longer-lived AM does not lead to high rate of apoptosis compared to that of IM. ART appears to successfully block or inhibit SIV infection in IM but not in longer-lived AM. We thus expect that elimination of SIV-infected longer-lived AM, as well as SIV-infected $CD4^{+}$ T cells, is crucial to reduce inflammation and reverse pulmonary disease progression in SIV-infected aged macaques undergoing ART.

not decline and persisted, even if infected further indicating a population of long-lived macrophages that likely contribute to the virus reservoir [19].

b. **Brain**. Four populations of microglial, meningeal, choroid plexus, and peivascular macrophages exist in the brain [40, 55]. Resident microglial macrophages and macrophages of the meninges and choroid plexus exhibit low turnover rates and although infectable, are not major sites of HIV or SIV infection. Perivascular macrophages are located at the intersection between the central nervous system (CNS) and blood where systemic stimuli are encountered. These macrophages function in antigen presentation via MHC class II expression, exhibit a relatively higher turnover rate than parenchymal microglia during homeostasus, and are repopulated by peripheral monocytes that express $CD14^{high}CD16^{intermed}$ to then express CD206 and CD163 [56]. In SIV-infected macaques, perivascular macrophages that were replaced by trafficking infected monocytes establish CNS infection, whereas direct intrathecal injection with virus failed to produce brain infection [55, 57, 58]. The virus-infected perivascular macrophages were immunophenotypically similar to the trafficking activated ($CD16^{+}$) blood monocyte subsets and expressed CD163 [59]. Furthermore, increased monocyte turnover via BrdU kinetics, recruitment to brain, and accumulation of macrophages correlated with severity of encephalitis and neuronal injury in SIV-infected rhesus macaques. Encephalitic lesions were primarily comprised of myeloid cells including parenchymal macrophages, i.e. microglia, and perivascular macrophage cuffs, and macrophage accumulation better correlated with neurocognitive decline severity than did virus production [60, 61]. In addition, macrophage activation in relation to production of soluble CD163 (sCD163) in plasma and cerebral spinal fluid correlated with reduced neurocognition and virus levels further supporting macrophage contributions to SIV/HIV disease [38, 59, 61]. Macrophages of the brain could be reactivated to produce infectious virus using a virus outgrowth assay to also support their potential as a virus resevoir [41].

c. **Intestine**. The intestinal tract is a primary and early site of HIV/SIV infection that leads to massive depletion of intestinal $CD4^{+}$ T cells and high rate of viral replication [12]. The intestine also houses among the largest population of macrophages [62], and increased accumulation of intestinal macrophages was reported in HIV-positive patients [63] as well as in the ileum of SIV-infected rhesus macaques, especially during acute SIV infection and AIDS, but not during the chronic stage of infection [21]. The accumulated $CD163^{+}$ macrophages exhibited reduced phagocytic function that appeared to contribute to loss of intestinal integrity fueling further recruitment of macrophages in attempt to remove debris [64]. In rhesus macaques, two subsets of macrophages that comprised $CD163^{+}$ $CD206^{+}$ double-positive (DP) macrophages and $CD163^{+}$ $CD206^{-}$ single-positive (SP) macrophages were detected in the intestines using flow cytometry analyses [22]. In uninfected macaques, DP macrophages predominated over the SP macrophages. Forty-eight hours after BrdU administration, the majority of recently-dividing labeled cells were $CD163^{+}$ macrophages in the jejunum and colon in uninfected rhesus macaques that increased in SIV-infected animals [15]. Thus, monocytes appeared to migrate more rapidly from blood to intestine (lamina propria) during progression to AIDS.

DP macrophages predominated over SP macrophages in the lamina propria of uninfected rhesus macaques but SP macrophages were more common in the lamina propria of SIV-infected animals with increased monocyte turnover. Interestingly, in the submucosa and muscular mucosa, DP macrophages were more frequent than SP macrophages in both infected and uninfected animals and there was a statistically significantly higher mean DP:SP macrophage ratio in the lamina propria of uninfected macaques compared to infected animals exhibiting higher monocyte turnover. In contrast, there were no significant differences in the submucosa DP:SP macrophage ratios of uninfected versus SIV-infected macaques with intermediate-to-higher monocyte turnover. Similar trends were observed for the DP:SP macrophage ratios in the jejunum of uninfected compared to infected animals with higher monocyte turnover [22]. This suggested that during terminal stages of SIV infection in animals with higher monocyte turnover, there was a loss in DP macrophages with concurrent increases in SP macrophages in the lamina propria, whereas submucosal DP and SP macrophage levels remained steady even after SIV infection and disease progression.

DP macrophages appeared to localize and remain primarily in the submucosa regardless of SIV infection status and appeared to comprise a long-lived macrophage population. This is relevant because long-lived (vs short-lived) macrophages would more likely serve as a virus reservoir, become dysregulated, and thereby contribute to chronic inflammation and pathogenesis. To explore this, we analyzed the distribution of colon macrophages that incorporated and retained the dextran (i.e. long-lived macrophages) relative to those that were labeled with thymidine analogues, BrdU or EdU (i.e. recently-dividing short-lived macrophages) [22]. $BrdU^{+}CD163^{+}$ macrophages were only in the lamina propria but not in the submucosa. Conversely, two months after dextran injection, $dextran^{+}CD163^{+}$ macrophages exclusively localized in the submucosa where there were ~ 10 times more DP macrophages than SP macrophages. These findings suggested DP macrophages in the submucosa are long-lived cells and that short-lived macrophages migrate from blood to lamina propria where they remain for shorter periods of time [22]. The presence of HIV-infected macrophages in human intestine and SIV-infected macrophages in rhesus macaque intestine supports the contribution of macrophages to gut pathogenesis and another tissue site of the virus reservoir [22, 23, 39].

d. **Heart.** In an early study characterizing heart tissues of rhesus macaques, macrophages were uniformly distributed throughout the heart in animals of all age groups ranging from infants to elderly adults, and were more prevalent than $CD3^{+}$ T cells and $CD20^{+}$ B cells [32]. Macrophages comprised approximately 2% of heart tissue cells in the younger animals and increased to a mean of nearly 4% in the older adults. $CD163^{+}$ macrophages predominated over $HAM56^{+}$ and $CD206^{+}$ macrophages, and were detected at significantly higher percentage in the older animals between 13 and 24 years of age as well as in heart tissues exhibiting severe histopathology or inflammation in animals of all age groups. In vivo dextran labeling and retention indicated that at least half of the macrophages were longer-lived in healthy adult heart tissues and may comprise the tissue-resident population of macrophages.

In heart tissues of SIV-infected rhesus macaques, increased numbers of $CD163^{+}$ macrophages were associated with pathology and fibrosis, and macrophages infected with SIV expressed CD163 with some also expressing HAM56 [65, 66].

In our studies of rhesus macaques, the majority of heart tissue macrophages were $CD163^+$ and long-lived (i.e. retained dextran), regardless of whether animals were chronically infected with or without ART [32] and Petkov et al., submitted]. Short-lived macrophages were rarely detected in the hearts of SIV-infected macaques at low monocyte turnover stage and of uninfected macaques with low histopathology scores [32]. In uninfected animals with higher histopathology scores (i.e. cardiac disease) or in SIV-infected animals with increased monocyte turnover, higher percentages of $BrdU^+$ short-lived macrophages were detected in heart suggesting infiltration of monocyte-derived short-lived macrophages during disease progression. Reduction in monocyte traffic to the heart of SIV-infected rhesus macaques via anti-alpha-4 integrin antibody reduced lesion severity in the heart and decreased levels of $CD163^+CD68^+$ macrophages, implicating accumulation of short-lived macrophages as a promoter of SIV-associated heart disease [67]. Unpublished results from our lab suggested that the level of long-lived macrophage infection also influences the dynamics and recruitment of short-lived macrophages related to heart tissue damage during HIV infection. In addition, HIV and SIV infections appear to accelerate biological aging based on increased or earlier onset of chronic inflammatory diseases, including CVD [68–75]. Cellularity of heart tissues declined with age in rhesus macaques [32] and there also was a reduction in heart tissue cellularity in SIV-infected younger adult macaques similar to that in uninfected older animals. Thus an increase in macrophages relative to tissue cellularity may contribute to loss of tissue homeostasis during natural aging and SIV/HIV-associated accelerated aging.

e. **Adipose tissue.** Tissue macrophages also constitute a major portion of the immune cell population in adipose [76–78]. Macrophages in subcutaneous adipose tissue of rhesus macaques and humans expressed CD68 and predominated over T cells and B cells [79]. CD68 was heavily expressed on cells of the monocyte and macrophage lineage [80] along with CD163 and CD206 that appear to reflect 'anti-inflammatory' macrophages [81, 82]. In subcutaneous adipose tissue of rhesus macaques, there were at least two major macrophage subsets. $CD68^+CD163^+CD206^+$ macrophages were more common than the $CD68^+CD163^-CD206^-$ macrophages, suggesting the predominant population exhibited an 'anti-inflammatory' phenotype. While triple-positive adipose tissue macrophages were found throughout the tissue, $CD68^+CD163^-CD206^-$ were mainly detected inside crown-like structures and interstitial clusters, intimating these macrophages may be associated with pathology and inflammation [79]. As also observed in heart tissue macrophages, the vast majority of subcutaneous adipose tissue macrophages in rhesus macaques were longer-living (i.e. retained in vivo administered dextran) [32, 79]. These longer-lived subcutaneous adipose macrophages co-expressed CD68, CD163, and CD206. The $CD68^+$ macrophages that did not contain dextran were generally found in the crown-like structure and interstitial spaces, and also were negative for CD163 and CD206. A small but distinct subpopulation of these macrophages simultaneously expressed Ki67 in their nuclei, located to the crown-like structure and interstitial clusters, but also to the interstitial spaces, suggesting that they were self-renewing at the time of sampling. Though only a small proportion of macrophages were self-renewing at any one time, these observations provide evidence that, like in mice, adipose tissue macrophages from rhesus macaques are predominantly long-lived and may self-maintain in tissue via slow local proliferation.

Adipose tissue macrophages also have provided evidence that CD14$^+$ adipose tissue macrophages become infected with HIV and simian immunodeficiency virus (SIV) [45]. During SIV infection of cynomolgus macaques, subcutaneous macrophages also exhibited a pro-inflammatory phenotype expressing CD14 but not CD163 or CD206 [83] thereby contributing to the chronic inflammation often observed during SIV/HIV infection.

7. Future goals: targeting macrophages to reduce pathogenesis

Macrophages regulate inflammation and contribute to the SIV/HIV reservoir, thereby affecting pathogenesis of infection. Two general approaches have been applied experimentally to target macrophages in macaques that may benefit treatments for HIV. Bisphosphonates have been used for treating osteoporosis and other bone diseases, and target bone macrophages or osteoclasts to inhibit bone resorption [84]. In rhesus and cynomologus macaques, liposome-encapsulated alendronate administered intravenously reduced levels of CD14$^+$CD16$^-$ and CD14$^-$CD16$^+$ monocytes as well as CD163$^+$ tissue macrophages with relatively low or no toxicity [85]. Liposome-clodronate inoculated intracisternally selectively depleted CD206$^+$ perivascular macrophages of the brain as well as CD14$^+$ monocytes in SIV-infected rhesus macaques [56]. A second approach was to apply natalizumab, an antibody to α-4-integrin that inhibits monocyte/macrophage trafficking. This antibody reduced neuropathology and cardiac pathology in SIV-infected rhesus macaques [56, 67]. Increasing evidence for the presence of SIV/HIV-infected and persistent macrophage reservoirs supports further studies and approaches for modulating or targeting macrophages to achieve cure.

Acknowledgements

The authors gratefully acknowledge research funding from the National Institutes of Health (grants AI097059, AI110163, and MH108458, to M.J.K., AG052349 to E.S.D., HL139278 to E.S.D. and M.J.K., OD011104, OD010568, and OD024282 to the Tulane National Primate Research Center and OD011107 to the California National Primate Research Center).

Author contributions

E.S.D. and M.J.K. conceived and wrote the manuscript.

Declaration of interest

The authors declare no competing interests.

Author details

Elizabeth S. Didier[1,2] and Marcelo J. Kuroda[1,2]*

1 Center for Immunology and Infectious Diseases, University of California, Davis, CA, USA

2 California National Primate Research Center, University of California, Davis, CA, USA

*Address all correspondence to: mjkuroda@ucdavis.edu

References

[1] DiNapoli SR, Hirsch VM, Brenchley JM. Macrophages in progressive human immunodeficiency virus/Simian immunodeficiency virus infections. Journal of Virology. 2016;**90**(17):7596-7606

[2] Gordon S, Plüddemann A. The mononuclear phagocytic system. generation of diversity. Frontiers in Immunology. 2019;**10**(1893):1-10

[3] Kruize Z, Kootstra NA. The role of macrophages in HIV-1 persistence and pathogenesis. Front Microbiology. 2019;**10**:2828

[4] Khanal S, Schank M, El Gazzar M, Moorman JP, Yao ZQ. HIV-1 latency and viral reservoirs: Existing reversal approaches and potential technologies, targets, and pathways involved in HIV latency studies. Cells. 2021;**10**(2):1-23

[5] Mosser DM, Edwards JP. Exploring the full spectrum of macrophage activation. Natural Review Immunology. 2008;**8**(12):958-969

[6] Murray PJ. Macrophage polarization. Annual Review of Physiology. 2017;**79**:541-566

[7] Ross EA, Devitt A, Johnson JR. Macrophages: The good, the bad, and the gluttony. Frontiers in Immunology. 2021;**12**:708186

[8] Didier ES, MacLean AG, Mohan M, Didier PJ, Lackner AA, Kuroda MJ. Contributions of nonhuman primates to research on aging. Veterinary Pathology. 2016;**53**(2):277-290

[9] Goulder P, Deeks SG. HIV control: Is getting there the same as staying there? PLoS Pathogens. 2018;**14**(11):e1007222

[10] Martins MA, Watkins DI. What is the predictive value of animal models for vaccine efficacy in humans? Rigorous Simian immunodeficiency virus vaccine trials can be instructive. Cold Spring Harbor Perspectives in Biology. 2018;**10**(4):1-10

[11] Williams K, Lackner A, Mallard J. Non-human primate models of SIV infection and CNS neuropathology. Current Opinion in Virology. 2016;**19**:92-98

[12] Veazey RS, DeMaria M, Chalifoux LV, Shvetz DE, Pauley DR, Knight HL, et al. Gastrointestinal tract as a major site of $CD4^+$ T cell depletion and viral replication in SIV infection. Science (New York, NY). 1998;**280**(5362):427-431

[13] Evans DT, Silvestri G. Nonhuman primate models in AIDS research. Current Opinion in HIV and AIDS. 2013;**8**(4):255-261

[14] Hasegawa A, Liu H, Ling B, Borda JT, Alvarez X, Sugimoto C, et al. The level of monocyte turnover predicts disease progression in the macaque model of AIDS. Blood. 2009;**114**(14):2917-2925

[15] Takahashi N, Ardeshir A, Holder GE, Cai Y, Sugimoto C, Mori K, et al. Comparison of predictors for terminal disease progression in simian immunodeficiency virus/simian-HIV-infected rhesus macaques. AIDS (London, England). 2021;**35**(7):1021-1029

[16] Pathai S, Bajillan H, Landay AL, High KP. Is HIV a model of accelerated or accentuated aging? The Journals of Gerontology Series A, Biological Sciences and Medical Sciences. 2014;**69**(7):833-842

[17] Abbas W, Tariq M, Iqbal M, Kumar A, Herbein G. Eradication of HIV-1 from the macrophage reservoir: An uncertain goal? Viruses. 2015;7(4):1578-1598

[18] Clayton KL, Garcia JV, Clements JE, Walker BD. HIV infection of macrophages: Implications for pathogenesis and cure. Pathogens & Immunity. 2017;**2**(2):179-192

[19] Li Y, Kang G, Duan L, Lu W, Katze MG, Lewis MG, et al. SIV infection of lung macrophages. PloS One. 2015;**10**(5):e0125500

[20] Micci L, Alvarez X, Iriele RI, Ortiz AM, Ryan ES, McGary CS, et al. $CD4^+$ depletion in SIV-infected macaques results in macrophage and microglia infection with rapid turnover of infected cells. PLoS Pathogens. 2014;**10**(10):e1004467

[21] Swan ZD, Wonderlich ER, Barratt-Boyes SM. Macrophage accumulation in gut mucosa differentiates AIDS from chronic SIV infection in rhesus macaques. European Journal of Immunology. 2016;**46**(2):446-454

[22] Takahashi N, Sugimoto C, Allers C, Alvarez X, Kim WK, Didier ES, et al. Shifting dynamics of intestinal macrophages during Simian immunodeficiency virus infection in adult rhesus macaques. Journal of Immunology (Baltimore, Md : 1950). 2019;**202**(9):2682-2689

[23] Zalar A, Figueroa MI, Ruibal-Ares B, Baré P, Cahn P, de Bracco MM, et al. Macrophage HIV-1 infection in duodenal tissue of patients on long term HAART. Antiviral Research. 2010;**87**(2):269-271

[24] Cai Y, Sugimoto C, Arainga M, Alvarez X, Didier ES, Kuroda MJ. In vivo characterization of alveolar and interstitial lung macrophages in rhesus macaques: Implications for understanding lung disease in humans. Journal of Immunology (Baltimore, Md : 1950). 2014;**192**(6):2821-2829

[25] Cai Y, Sugimoto C, Arainga M, Midkiff CC, Liu DX, Alvarez X, et al. Preferential destruction of interstitial macrophages over alveolar macrophages as a cause of pulmonary disease in Simian immunodeficiency virus-infected rhesus macaques. Journal of Immunology (Baltimore, Md : 1950). 2015;**195**(10):4884-4891

[26] Cai Y, Sugimoto C, Liu DX, Midkiff CC, Alvarez X, Lackner AA, et al. Increased monocyte turnover is associated with interstitial macrophage accumulation and pulmonary tissue damage in SIV-infected rhesus macaques. Journal of Leukocyte Biology. 2015;**97**(6):1147-1153

[27] Shapouri-Moghaddam A, Mohammadian S, Vazini H, Taghadosi M, Esmaeili SA, Mardani F, et al. Macrophage plasticity, polarization, and function in health and disease. Journal of Cellular Physiology. 2018;**233**(9):6425-6440

[28] Röszer T. Understanding the biology of self-renewing macrophages. Cells. 2018;7(8):1-21

[29] Hashimoto D, Chow A, Noizat C, Teo P, Beasley MB, Leboeuf M, et al. Tissue-resident macrophages self-maintain locally throughout adult life with minimal contribution from circulating monocytes. Immunity. 2013;**38**(4):792-804

[30] Takahashi N, Ardeshir A, Holder GE, Cai Y, Sugimoto C, Mori K, et al. Comparison of predictors for terminal disease progression in SIV/

SHIV-infected rhesus macaques. AIDS (London, England). 2021;**35**:1021-1029

[31] Solius GM, Maltsev DI, Belousov VV, Podgorny OV. Recent advances in nucleotide analogue-based techniques for tracking dividing stem cells: An overview. Journal of Biological Chemistry. 2021;**297**(5):101345

[32] Petkov DI, Liu DX, Allers C, Didier PJ, Didier ES, Kuroda MJ. Characterization of heart macrophages in rhesus macaques as a model to study cardiovascular disease in humans. Journal of Leukocyte Biology. 2019;**106**(6):1241-1255

[33] Veazey R, Lackner A. The mucosal immune system and HIV-1 infection. AIDS R. 2003;**5**(4):245-252

[34] Pandrea I, Silvestri G, Apetrei C. AIDS in african nonhuman primate hosts of SIVs: A new paradigm of SIV infection. Current HIV Research. 2009;7(1):57-72

[35] Doitsh G, Greene WC. Dissecting how CD4^{+} T cells are lost during HIV infection. Cell Host & Microbe. 2016;**19**(3):280-291

[36] Kuroda MJ. Macrophages: Do they impact AIDS progression more than CD4^{+} T cells? Journal of Leukocyte Biology. 2010;**87**(4):569-573

[37] Kim WK, McGary CM, Holder GE, Filipowicz AR, Kim MM, Beydoun HA, et al. Increased expression of CD169 on blood monocytes and its regulation by virus and CD8 T cells in macaque models of HIV infection and AIDS. AIDS Research and Human Retroviruses. 2015;**31**(7):696-706

[38] Burdo TH, Soulas C, Orzechowski K, Button J, Krishnan A, Sugimoto C, et al. Increased monocyte turnover from bone marrow correlates with severity of SIV encephalitis and CD163 levels in plasma. PLoS Pathogens. 2010;**6**(4):e1000842

[39] Pahar B, Kuebler D, Rasmussen T, Wang X, Srivastav SK, Das A, et al. Quantification of viral RNA and DNA positive cells in tissues from Simian immunodeficiency virus/Simian human immunodeficiency virus infected controller and progressor rhesus macaques. Frontiers in Microbiology. 2019;**10**:2933

[40] Kim W-K, Corey S, Alvarez X, Williams K. Monocyte/macrophage traffic in HIV and SIV encephalitis. Journal of Leukocyte Biology. 2003;**74**(5):650-656

[41] Abreu C, Shirk EN, Queen SE, Beck SE, Mangus LM, Pate KAM, et al. Brain macrophages harbor latent, infectious simian immunodeficiency virus. AIDS (London, England). 2019;**33**(Suppl. 2):S181-S1s8

[42] Abreu CM, Veenhuis RT, Avalos CR, Graham S, Parrilla DR, Ferreira EA, et al. Myeloid and CD4^{+} T cells comprise the latent reservoir in antiretroviral therapy-suppressed SIVmac251-infected macaques. mBio. 2019;**10**(4):1-19

[43] Aggarwal A, McAllery S, Turville SG. Revising the role of myeloid cells in HIV pathogenesis. Current HIV/AIDS Reports. 2013;**10**(1):3-11

[44] Arainga M, Edagwa B, Mosley RL, Poluektova LY, Gorantla S, Gendelman HE. A mature macrophage is a principal HIV-1 cellular reservoir in humanized mice after treatment with long acting antiretroviral therapy. Retrovirology. 2017;**14**(1):17

[45] Damouche A, Lazure T, Avettand-Fenoel V, Huot N, Dejucq-Rainsford N, Satie AP, et al.

Adipose tissue is a neglected viral reservoir and an inflammatory site during chronic HIV and SIV infection. PLoS Pathogens. 2015;**11**(9):e1005153

[46] Freed EO, Martin MA. HIV-1 infection of non-dividing cells. Nature. 1994;**369**(6476):107-108

[47] Hassan J, Browne K, De Gascun C. HIV-1 in monocytes and macrophages: An overlooked reservoir? Viral Immunology. 2016;**29**(9):532-533

[48] Mitchell BI, Laws EI, Ndhlovu LC. Impact of myeloid reservoirs in HIV cure trials. Current HIV/AIDS Reports. 2019;**16**(2):129-140

[49] Pallikkuth S, Mohan M. Adipose tissue: Sanctuary for HIV/SIV persistence and replication. Trends in Microbiology. 2015;**23**(12):748-750

[50] Sharifi HJ, Furuya AM, de Noronha CM. The role of HIV-1 Vpr in promoting the infection of nondividing cells and in cell cycle arrest. Current Opinion in HIV and AIDS. 2012;**7**(2):187-194

[51] Busca A, Saxena M, Kryworuchko M, Kumar A. Anti-apoptotic genes in the survival of monocytic cells during infection. Current Genomics. 2009;**10**(5):306-317

[52] Honeycutt JB, Wahl A, Baker C, Spagnuolo RA, Foster J, Zakharova O, et al. Macrophages sustain HIV replication in vivo independently of T cells. The Journal of Clinical Investigation. 2016;**126**(4):1353-1366

[53] Malim MH, Bieniasz PD. HIV restriction factors and mechanisms of evasion. Cold Spring Harbor Perspectives in Medicine. 2012;**2**(5):a006940

[54] Cribbs SK, Lennox J, Caliendo AM, Brown LA, Guidot DM. Healthy HIV-1-infected individuals on highly active antiretroviral therapy harbor HIV-1 in their alveolar macrophages. AIDS Research Human Retroviruses. 2015;**31**(1):64-70

[55] Kim WK, Avarez X, Williams K. The role of monocytes and perivascular macrophages in HIV and SIV neuropathogenesis: Information from non-human primate models. Neurotoxicity Research. 2005;**8**(1-2):107-115

[56] Holder GE, McGary CM, Johnson EM, Zheng R, John VT, Sugimoto C, et al. Expression of the mannose receptor CD206 in HIV and SIV encephalitis: A phenotypic switch of brain perivascular macrophages with virus infection. Journal of Neuroimmune Pharmacology: The Official Journal of the Society on NeuroImmune Pharmacology. 2014;**9**(5):716-726

[57] Hurtrel B, Chakrabarti L, Hurtrel M, Montagnier L. Target cells during early SIV encephalopathy. Research Virology. 1993;**144**(1):41-46

[58] Smith MS, Niu Y, Li Z, Adany I, Pinson DM, Liu ZQ, et al. Systemic infection and limited replication of SHIV vaccine virus in brains of macaques inoculated intracerebrally with infectious viral DNA. Virology. 2002;**301**(1):130-135

[59] Fischer T, Wyatt CM, D'Agati VD, Croul S, McCourt L, Morgello S, et al. Mononuclear phagocyte accumulation in visceral tissue in HIV encephalitis: Evidence for increased monocyte/macrophage trafficking and altered differentiation. Current HIV Research. 2014;**12**(3):201-212

[60] Williams KC, Corey S, Westmoreland SV, Pauley D, Knight H, deBakker C, et al. Perivascular

macrophages are the primary cell type productively infected by simian immunodeficiency virus in the brains of macaques: Implications for the neuropathogenesis of AIDS. The Journal of Experimental Medicine. 2001;**193**(8):905-915

[61] Williams K, Burdo TH. Monocyte mobilization, activation markers, and unique macrophage populations in the brain: Observations from SIV infected monkeys are informative with regard to pathogenic mechanisms of HIV infection in humans. Journal of Neuroimmune Pharmacology : The Official Journal of the Society on NeuroImmune Pharmacology. 2012;**7**(2):363-371

[62] Lee SH, Starkey PM, Gordon S. Quantitative analysis of total macrophage content in adult mouse tissues. Immunochemical studies with monoclonal antibody F4/80. The Journal of Experimental Medicine. 1985;**161**(3):475-489

[63] Allers K, Fehr M, Conrad K, Epple HJ, Schurmann D, Geelhaar-Karsch A, et al. Macrophages accumulate in the gut mucosa of untreated HIV-infected patients. The Journal of Infectious Diseases. 2014;**209**(5):739-748

[64] Swan ZD, Bouwer AL, Wonderlich ER, Barratt-Boyes SM. Persistent accumulation of gut macrophages with impaired phagocytic function correlates with SIV disease progression in macaques. European Journal of Immunology. 2017;**47**(11):1925-1935

[65] Yearley JH, Pearson C, Shannon RP, Mansfield KG. Phenotypic variation in myocardial macrophage populations suggests a role for macrophage activation in SIV-associated cardiac disease. AIDS Research Human Retroviruses. 2007;**23**(4):515-524

[66] Walker JA, Sulciner ML, Nowicki KD, Miller AD, Burdo TH, Williams KC. Elevated numbers of CD163$^+$ macrophages in hearts of simian immunodeficiency virus-infected monkeys correlate with cardiac pathology and fibrosis. AIDS Research Human Retroviruses. 2014;**30**(7):685-694

[67] Walker JA, Beck GA, Campbell JH, Miller AD, Burdo TH, Williams KC. Anti-α4 integrin antibody blocks monocyte/macrophage traffic to the heart and decreases cardiac pathology in a SIV infection model of AIDS. Journal of the American Heart Association. 2015;**4**(7):1-11

[68] Deeks SG. HIV infection, inflammation, immunosenescence, and aging. Annual Review Medicine. 2011;**62**:141-155

[69] Deeks SG, Verdin E, McCune JM. Immunosenescence and HIV. Current Opinion in Immunology. 2012;**24**(4):501-506

[70] High KP, Brennan-Ing M, Clifford DB, Cohen MH, Currier J, Deeks SG, et al. HIV and aging: State of knowledge and areas of critical need for research. A report to the NIH Office of AIDS Research by the HIV and Aging Working Group. Journal of Acquired Immune Deficiency Syndrome. 2012;**60**(Suppl. 1):S1-S18

[71] Pathai S, Lawn SD, Gilbert CE, McGuinness D, McGlynn L, Weiss HA, et al. Accelerated biological ageing in HIV-infected individuals in South Africa: A case-control study. AIDS (London, England). 2013;**27**(15):2375-2384

[72] Herskowitz A, Willoughby S, Wu TC, Beschorner WE, Neumann DA, Rose NR, et al. Immunopathogenesis of HIV-1-associated cardiomyopathy. Clinical Immunology and Immunopathology. 1993;**68**(2):234-241

[73] Ho JE, Hsue PY. Cardiovascular manifestations of HIV infection. Heart (British Cardiac Society). 2009;**95**(14):1193-1202

[74] Sani MU. Myocardial disease in human immunodeficiency virus (HIV) infection: A review. Wiener Klinische Wochenschrift. 2008;**120**(3-4):77-87

[75] Zareba KM, Lipshultz SE. Cardiovascular complications in patients with HIV infection. Current Infectious Disease Reports. 2003;**5**(6):513-520

[76] Nishimura S, Manabe I, Nagasaki M, Eto K, Yamashita H, Ohsugi M, et al. $CD8^+$ effector T cells contribute to macrophage recruitment and adipose tissue inflammation in obesity. Nature Medicine. 2009;**15**(8):914-920

[77] Onodera T, Fukuhara A, Shin J, Hayakawa T, Otsuki M, Shimomura I. Eicosapentaenoic acid and 5-HEPE enhance macrophage-mediated Treg induction in mice. Scientific Reports. 2017;**7**(1):4560

[78] Wang L, Liu J, Zhang A, Cheng P, Zhang X, Lv S, et al. BVT.2733, a selective 11beta-hydroxysteroid dehydrogenase type 1 inhibitor, attenuates obesity and inflammation in diet-induced obese mice. PloS One. 2012;**7**(7):e40056

[79] Fahlberg M. The impact of Simian immunodeficiency virus on subcutaneous adipose tissue of rhesus macaues. Tulane University Theses and Dissertation Archive. 2018. https://digitallibrary.tulane.edu/islandora/object/tulane%3A110475

[80] Martinez-Pomares L, Platt N, McKnight AJ, da Silva RP, Gordon S. Macrophage membrane molecules: Markers of tissue differentiation and heterogeneity. Immunobiology. 1996;**195**(4-5):407-416

[81] Fabriek BO, Dijkstra CD, van den Berg TK. The macrophage scavenger receptor CD163. Immunobiology. 2005;**210**(2-4):153-160

[82] Stein M, Keshav S, Harris N, Gordon S. Interleukin 4 potently enhances murine macrophage mannose receptor activity: A marker of alternative immunologic macrophage activation. The Journal of Experimental Medicine. 1992;**176**(1):287-292

[83] Pallikkuth S, Mohan M. Adipose tissue: Sanctuary for HIV/SIV persistence and replication. Trends in Microbiology. 2015;**23**(12):748-750

[84] Kuźnik A, Październiok-Holewa A, Jewula P, Kuźnik N. Bisphosphonates-much more than only drugs for bone diseases. European Journal of Pharmacology. 2020;**866**:172773

[85] Burwitz BJ, Reed JS, Hammond KB, Ohme MA, Planer SL, Legasse AW, et al. Technical advance: Liposomal alendronate depletes monocytes and macrophages in the nonhuman primate model of human disease. Journal of Leukocyte Biology. 2014;**96**(3):491-501

Section 6

Macrophages in Neurological Diseases

Chapter 17

The Role of M1- and M2-Type Macrophages in Neurological and Infectious Diseases

Mary Dover, Michael Kishek, Miranda Eddins, Naneeta Desar and Milan Fiala

Abstract

Macrophages have a critical role in the outcome of neurological diseases, including neurodegenerative, autoimmune, vascular and microbial diseases. Macrophage role ranges from beneficial to pathogenic depending upon genetics, other components of innate and adaptive immunity, lifestyle and macrophage targets: aggregated molecules or bacterial and viral pathogens. Macrophages are attracted by chemokines to migrate into the brain and remove or inactivate pathogenic molecules. In the patients with neurodegenerative diseases, macrophages target aggregated molecules, amyloid-β_{1-42} (Aβ) and P-tau in Alzheimer's disease (AD), and superoxide dismutase-1 (SOD-1) in amyotrophic lateral sclerosis (ALS), but also have autoimmune targets. In AD and ALS patients, macrophages in the pro-resolution M1M2 state are adapted to brain clearance and homeostasis, whereas in the proinflammatory M1 state are modulate to an antiviral and antibacterial role, which may be associated with collateral damage to tissues. In HIV-1 and CoV2 viral infections, macrophages in M1 state are anti-viral but also pathogenic through inflammatory damage to the heart and the brain. In neurodegenerative diseases, the natural substances polyunsaturated fatty acids (PUFA), vitamins B and D, energy molecules, and flavonoids have beneficial effects on macrophage transcriptome and functions for brain clearance, but the effects are complex and depend on many variables.

Keywords: Alzheimer's disease, amyotrophic lateral sclerosis, inflammatory response, cytokines, macrophage, transcriptome, glycome

1. Introduction

Macrophages and dendritic cells are key players in activation of the innate and adaptive immune systems. In viral infections, such as HIV-1 and COVID-19, macrophages assume either a more protective or a pathogenic role depending on their classification.

Macrophages are polarized by cytokine signaling from CD4 T cells into the M1 or the M2 type. M1 macrophages are classically activated by interferon-γ (INF-γ), whereas M2 macrophages are activated by interleukin-4 (IL-4) and IL-13 [1].

M1 macrophages have a role in combating infection, whereas M2 macrophages in supporting homeostasis. This inflammatory response, while beneficial against microbes and aggregated molecules, when hyper-activated can lead to tissue damage in the lungs, heart, and brain.

Under conditions of high microbial activity, M1 promote inflammation, synthesize nitric oxide, and induce cytokine production IL-6, IL-12 and tumor necrosis factor (TNF). Type M2 macrophages secrete arginase-I, IL-10 and TGF-β and other anti-inflammatory cytokines promoting wound healing but also contributing to tumor growth. M1 macrophages phagocytize microbes and initiate an adaptive immune response by T cells while M2 macrophages induce collagen repair to maintain tissue repair [1].

The roles of M1 macrophages in opposing the disease and the M2 macrophages in promoting homeostasis, while evident in infectious diseases, is less evident in neurodegenerative diseases. Macrophages of AD patients were classified according to the ratio of cluster of differentiation (CD) surface markers: CD54+ CD80/CD163+ CD206 [2] as follows: the inflammatory M1 macrophage type has the ratio > 4, the anti-inflammatory M2 type has a ratio < 1. Both M1 and M2 are associated with progression of dementia. In AD patients, however, the intermediate M1M2 phenotype with a ratio between 1 and 4 is a pro-resolution type promoting homeostasis and protection against dementia. Infection or other stress can cause an imbalance in the expression of these two macrophage types, as seen by others [3].

Macrophages were first appreciated in tuberculosis, where the dual role of macrophages in containing vs. replicating *Mycobacterium tuberculosis* (Mtb) has been known for a century. A successful response to mycobacterial infection is a granuloma consisting of lymphocytes, macrophages, Langhans giant cells (fused macrophages around mycobacteria) and fibroblasts [4].

In recent years, the role of macrophages in neurodegenerative diseases, Alzheimer's disease (AD) and amyotrophic lateral sclerosis (ALS), has been appreciated as a result of immunochemical demonstration of central nervous system (CNS) invasion by peripheral blood monocyte/macrophages (MM) in AD patients [5]. Macrophage targets in AD are amyloid-beta (Aβ) and P-tau, while in ALS macrophage targets are aggregated superoxide dismutase (SOD-1) and microbial nucleic acids. Autologous DNA released into the cytoplasm could be a target in the cGAS-STING pathway [6].

This chapter will discuss the integral role and modulation of macrophage role in the therapy of neurodegenerative and infectious diseases. The natural substances polyunsaturated fatty acids (PUFA), circuminoids, vitamin D, and polyphenols improve macrophage transcriptome and functions for brain clearance in neurological diseases, but their mechanisms depend on many variables that are under study. The effects of natural substances on macrophage transcriptome and clearance of Aβ and P-tau could potentiate therapeutic outcome of monocl0nal antibodies, which increase phagocytosis but not degradation or export of Aβ and P-tau.

2. Macrophages of Alzheimer's disease patients fail in clearance of the AD brain

In AD patients, microglia are the first responders to accumulation of Aβ in the brain, which attract monocyte/macrophages (MM) from the blood into the CNS by chemokines, in particular CCL5 (RANTES) [7]. In non-demented individuals, post-mortem immunochemistry and results from a blood-brain barrier (BBB) model suggest that MM migrate across BBB in both directions, clear Aβ in plaques, degrade or export Aβ from the brain without disruption of BBB or accumulation of macrophages around vessels [5, 8], and deposit Aβ into cervical nodes or further downstream [9]. MM of healthy subjects with the pro-resolution M1M2 phenotype effectively upload Aβ into endosomes, fuse endosomes with lysosomes, and degrade Aβ by lysosomal enzymes. MM of AD patients are defective in internalization and degradation of Aβ in endosomes [8].

In the AD brain, MM immigrate into CNS through disrupted tight junctions between endothelial cells. In addition, opening of tight junctions in the blood-brain barrier (BBB) permits brain entry of fibrin and components of the complement. In the brain parenchyma, AD macrophages invade the plaques but upload Aβ only on its cell surface, do not transport Aβ into endosomes and fail to degrade Aβ. Clearance of individual Aβ plaques by macrophages is functionally stochastic, thus some plaques are not fully cleared [5]. After uploading Aβ, MM migrate to vessels but fail to emigrate across BBB, suffer apoptosis and release Aβ into vessels, which develop cerebrovascular angiopathy (CAA) (**Figure 1**) [10].

2.1 Natural substances have mixed results in prevention of Alzheimer's disease

Natural substances, prominently PUFA, have a long history in prevention of AD in the patients with mild cognitive impairment (MCI). PUFA supplementation had positive cognitive effects in MCI patients, but only in those with very mild MCI [11]. A large controlled clinical trial of PUFA supplementation, however, did not slow the rate of cognitive and functional decline in patients with mild to moderate Alzheimer disease [12].

Nevertheless, proven effects of PUFA on macrophage transcriptome and functions designate PUFA for immunotherapeutic studies controlled for baseline immune phenotype, APO E genotype, stage of disease, diet and lifestyle using a high-quality omega-fatty acid preparation protected against oxidation [2]. In an uncontrolled study of mild cognitive impairment (MCI) patients supplemented by the omega-3

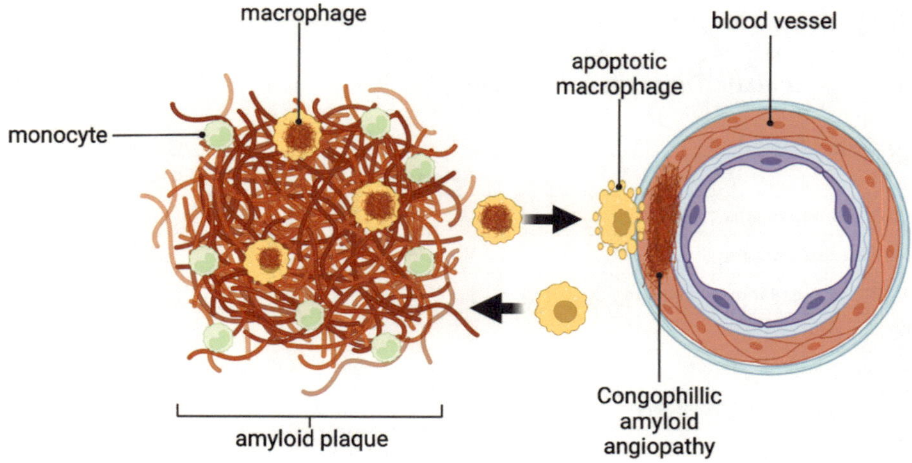

Figure 1.
Macrophage pathway in the AD brain. Created with BioRender.com.

fatty acid drink Smartfish, macrophage phenotype changed from either a highly inflammatory M1 or a very low non-inflammatory M2 to the desired pro-resolution M1/M2 (**Table 1**) [2]. Importantly, in this study, PUFA supplementation improved the cognitive status of MCI/AD patients for 4–17 months and protected against dementia for 4.5 years in certain patients [13]. In vivo supplementation and in vitro stimulation by the Smartfish drink stimulated the pro-resolution M1/M2 macrophage type with increased phagocytosis and energy [14].

A clinical study of supplementation with a high dose of vitamin B complex, including vitamins B6 (pyridoxine), B9 (folic acid), and B12 (cobalamin), showed a reduction in the rate of brain atrophy in MCI patients with elevated total homocysteine [15].

2.2 Alzheimer's disease patients' macrophages have transcriptomic defects that underlie their defective function

AD brain cells and macrophages lack energy due to oxidative damage and nitrosylation by reactive oxygen species (ROS) of the glycolytic enzyme transcripts GAPDH, *PKM1*, and *PDH*, and the citric acid cycle enzymes *ACO2* and *OGDH* [16]. The defects in macrophage transcriptome in protein-coding and regulatory sequences for energy, glycosylation, unfolded protein response, glymphatic system, Toll-like receptors, and other genes lead to macrophage malfunction and apoptosis [14]. Macrophages exhibit a faulty unfolded protein response (UPR) to endoplasmic reticulum (ER) stress from Aβ phagocytosis. These defects lead to macrophage apoptosis and inflammation [14].

2.3 Natural substances have positive effects on macrophage biochemistry

The anti-inflammatory molecule bisdemethoxycurcumin up regulated *MGAT3* transcripts and increased macrophage phagocytosis of Aβ. 1,25 dihydroxy vitamin D3 potentiated the 4,4-diisothiocyanostilbene-2,2-disulfonic acid-sensitive chloride channel ClC-3 currents essential for Aβ phagocytosis [17]. A clinical study of supplementation with a high dose of vitamin B complex, including vitamins B6 (pyridoxine), B9 (folic acid), and B12 (cobalamin), showed a reduction in the rate of brain atrophy in MCI patients with elevated total homocysteine [15].

RNA-seq analysis of single blood cell types in PUFA-supplemented MCI patients showed up-regulation of the transcripts for glycolysis, tricarboxylic acid cycle,

	AD patients	PUFA-supplemented AD patients
M1-type macrophages	↑	↓
M2-type macrophages	Variable	↑
M1/M2 pro-resolution-type macrophages	↓	↑↑
MGAT3 transcription	↓	↑↑
Inflammation	↑↑	↓
Aβ phagocytosis by macrophages	↓	↑

Table 1.
The effects of PUFA-supplementation on Alzheimer's disease (AD) patients.

OX-PHOS, nicotinamide dinucleotide (NAD^+) synthesis in monocytes, neutrophils, regulatory T cells, memory CD4 and CD8 T cells, and NK cells, but the most consistent effects across the whole spectrum were in monocytes/macrophages (MM). Importantly, the supplementation showed that PUFA provide energy for immune clearance of the brain throughout the diurnal cycle and even in hypo- or hyper-glycemia [13]. Both hypo- and hyper-glycemic glucose concentrations in the medium of macrophages *in vitro* inhibit Aβ phagocytosis, but phagocytosis is restored in presence of PUFA in the medium. Diabetic patients have an increased risk of AD and may benefit from PUFA supplementation to provide missing energy in hypoglycemia and to enhance correct glycation and protect against glucose adducts in hyperglycemia of mild cognitive impairment (MCI) patients.

2.4 Monoclonal antibodies and PUFA in therapy of AD

The approval of aducanumab in 2021 increased enthusiasm for immune therapy by monoclonal antibodies. Aducanumab cleared both soluble oligomers and aggregated Aβ in a dose- and time-dependent fashion according to amyloid positron emission tomography (PET) imaging and slowed disease progression [18]. Both aducanumab and another monoclonal antibody ponezumab, however, have been associated with cerebro-vascular amyloid angiopathy (CAA) in models and with amyloid-related imaging abnormalities (ARIA) in patients [19]. Although the exact mechanisms of CAA related to aducanumab are not known due to the lack of pathological and biochemical studies, this complication appears to be due to macrophage shuttling Aβ from plaques to vessels, failure of macrophages in Aβ degradation and macrophage apoptosis with a release of Aβ into CAA vessels [10]. As PUFA up regulate the transcription of Aβ degradation enzymes, PUFA supplementation could be synergistic with the monoclonal antibody therapy.

3. Macrophages in amyotrophic lateral sclerosis

In amyotrophic lateral sclerosis (ALS), macrophages target aggregated superoxide dismutase (SOD-1) [20] and may be targeting free autologous DNA in the cytoplasm.

Immunopathological studies of sporadic amyotrophic lateral sclerosis (sALS) patients demonstrated an inflammatory attack by macrophages, cytotoxic T cells, NK and mast cells on motor neurons in the spinal cord [21, 22]. The attack includes gray matter and white matter of the spinal cord as well as peripheral nerves. The invading macrophages are inflammatory expressing cyclooxygenase-2 (COX-2), inducible nitric oxide synthase (iNOS), IL-6 and TNF-α, and they attack both caspase-positive and caspase-negative neurons. In addition, cytotoxic CD8 T cells and NK cells participate in the autoimmune attack expressing the cytotoxic enzymes granzymes.

Aggregated superoxide dismutase-1 (SOD-1) stimulates peripheral blood mononuclear cells (PBMC) of sALS patients inducing IL-1, IL6, and IL23. These cytokines enhance production of the auto-immune pro-inflammatory cytokine IL-17A, which is increased in the serum and spinal cord of ALS patients [23]. The induction of inflammatory pathology in sALS by SOD-1 in aggregated form is an example that in neurodegenerative diseases the aggregated state of the putative culprits SOD-1 in ALS and amyloid-β and P-tau in Alzheimer's disease is sufficient for induction of inflammatory neuropathology.

4. Macrophages in HIV-1 infection

Trojan transport is the main path for virus penetration the blood-brain barrier in HIV-1 encephalitis. In addition, HIV-1 penetrates across coronary endothelia by transcytosis or by a paracellular route through disrupted tight junction protein ZO-1 [24].

Infiltration of target organs by inflammatory macrophages has a critical role in the progression of HIV-1 encephalitis and HIV-1 myocarditis. Other target organs in AIDS, the liver and the kidneys, are also infiltrated by macr0phages. In patients with HIV-1 encephalitis, cognitive impairment is proportionate to the number of macrophages infiltrating the brain [25]. In a study of postmortem heart tissues from 15 AIDS patients, the failing hearts showed significantly higher infiltration in the left ventricular myocardium by COX-2-positive and iNOS-positive macrophages compared to the functioning hearts. In the hearts with HIV-1 myocarditis, productive infection was exclusively in infiltrating macrophages and T cells, not in cardiomyocytes [26]. Significant infiltration of the failing heart by COX-2-positive macrophages (demonstrated using an antigen-retrieval technique) and production of inflammatory cytokines and mediators, such as NO, quinolinic acid, free radicals, is considered as the main mechanism of heart failure in HIV-1 myocarditis [26].

5. Macrophages in patients with COVID-19 infections

The recent epidemic of SARS-CoV-2 viral infection is associated with severe complications in subjects with risk factors, including older age, obesity, diabetes, renal failure; cancer; chronic obstructive pulmonary disease from smoking; and immunosuppressive conditions. In contrast, SARS-CoV-2 infected subjects without risk factors may suffer only mild pulmonary damage [27].

SARS-CoV-2 and previous coronaviruses responsible for severe acute respiratory syndrome (SARS) and the Middle East respiratory syndrome (MERS) induce inflammatory activation of monocytes/macrophages (MM). Patients with a low expression of interferon–$\alpha/\beta/\gamma$ in macrophages may suffer severe pulmonary damage by lung infiltration with inflammatory MM in a cytokine release syndrome (CRS), a.k.a. cytokine storm. MM are attracted into the lungs by chemokines produced by lung epithelia and fibroblasts. MM are activated by GM-CSF and IL-6, therefore, a blockade with IL-6 receptor antibody (tocilizumab, Actemra^{R}) is used in presence of a high inflammation [27]. CRS is related to the release of IL-1, IL-6 and nitric oxide (NO) from monocyte/macrophages, as shown in vitro and in an animal model by depletion of macrophages. CRS is similar to macrophage activation syndrome (MAS), a complication of several autoimmune diseases, in which well-differentiated macrophages show uncontrolled proliferation. CRS is also a complication of chimeric antigen receptor (CAR) therapy of B cell malignancies, in which macrophages produce IL-6, IL-1 and NO and where IL-1 blockade is therapeutic. COVID 19 pneumonia may be complicated by disseminated intravascular coagulation (DIC), therefore anticoagulation with enoxaparin (Lovenox^{R}) is routinely used in severe CoV2 infections.

In COVID-19 pneumonia, macrophages have a dual role with a beneficial antiviral role and a detrimental role through excessive release of inflammatory cytokines [28]. The lung has two types of macrophages, interstitial and alveolar macrophages. The alveolar macrophages with M1 type are pivotal in defense against pathogens by phagocytosis of microbes, enhancement of development of cytotoxic T cells and type I interferon production. The M2 type alveolar macrophages dampen the inflammation and repair the damage in association with other immune tissue cells. Macrophages infected by CoV2, however, accumulate lipid droplets in association with virus replication [29].

Angiotensin-converting enzyme 2 (ACE2) is a cell receptor for SARS and CoV-2 on lung epithelial cells. SARS-CoV-2 can infect monocytes and macrophages through ACE2-dependent and ACE2-independent pathways [27]. A second study with similar findings detected ACE2-expressing CD68+ and CD169+ macrophages containing SARS-CoV-2 nucleoprotein antigens in the sinuses of the lymph nodes of COVID-19 patients. These infected macrophages up regulated the pro-inflammatory cytokines IL-6 [30] and IL-1B [31]. The increased production of these cytokines by infected monocytes and macrophages induces hyper-inflammation and the onset of cytokine storm, leading to excess tissue damage and the potential harm of other vital organs in addition to the lungs (**Figure 2**) [27]. In addition, a subset of macrophages isolated from Covid-19 patients have been found to express genes that promote fibrosis generation and tissue repair. Therefore, the infection of infiltrating macrophages might not only be detrimental because of the promotion of acute inflammation, but also because of fibrotic complications that may arise and that have been observed in patients under mechanical ventilation. Long-term increases in the pro-inflammatory M1 type macrophages are associated with elevated reactive oxygen species (ROS) [32], which can produce harmful long-term side effects.

6. Macrophages in tuberculosis

Similar to in COVID-19 infections, macrophages play a dual role in tuberculosis. Macrophages permissive for *M. tuberculosis (*Mtb) replication, they may control and eliminate the infection in the presence of appropriate innate and acquired responses [4].

M1 and M2 macrophages are distinguished by their activation type. M1 cells are activated by the T helper type 1 (Th1) cells. These cells pertain to cell mediated immune responses and emit interleukin-2 (IL-2), IFN-γ, and lymphotoxins [33].

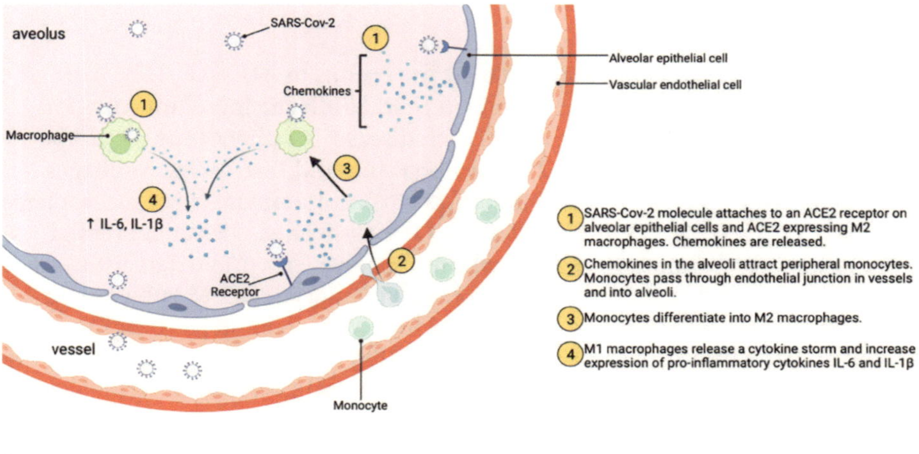

Figure 2.
Monocyte infiltration of the lungs with differentiation and activation of macrophages with production of cytokines and chemokines. Created with BioRender.com.

	Type 1 macrophages	Type 2 macrophages
Marker expression	CD80, CD54	CD163, CD206
Activation	Th1, INF-γ, GM-CSF	Th2, IL-4
Pro-inflammatory cytokines	High	Low
Antigen presentation	Yes	No
Production of ROS/NO	High	Low
Purpose	Destruction of microbes	Construct extracellular matrix

Table 2.
Type 1 and type 2 macrophage distinction.

Th1 cells lead to an increased M1 activation due to the production of IFN-y. Nitric oxide production is stimulated by the Th1 activation, rather than T helper type 2 (Th2) cells [34]. Th2 cells cause the activation of M2 macrophages. These cells are responsible for the stimulation of humoral immunity and secrete interleukin-4 (IL-4), interleukin-5 (IL-5), and interleukin-10 (IL-10). Th2 responses are a result of the production of ornithine which activates the M2 response allowing for tissue repair [1]. In tuberculosis, the intersection of Th1 and Th2 activation of M1 and M2 respectively leads to the immunity against pathogens. Along with the production of IFN-y, immunoglobulin A (Ig-A) is necessary for defense against tuberculosis (**Table 2**) [35].

Alveolar macrophages (AM) and dendritic cells phagocytize Mtb in the alveolar space in the lungs. Mtb is transmitted by macrophages to other organs via lymph nodes and blood vessels [36]. Alveolar macrophages present Mtb antigens to the adaptive immune cells to initiate an immune response. Subsequently, granulomas are formed because of the early inflammatory response caused by the AM [37]. Granulomas contain a variety of immune cells in order to contain the antigen. Some of the immune cells present in granulomas include foamy macrophages, epithelioid cells, neutrophils, and dendritic cells.

7. Conclusion

The phenotype of macrophages infiltrating the lesions in AD, ALS, HIV-1 myocarditis and encephalitis should be determined first, as it is the initial information necessary for analyzing macrophage role in each disease. M1 phenotype should be confirmed by staining of NOS, COX-2, TNF alpha, IL1, and IL-6 on macrophages.

Preliminary data suggest the following: (a) the pro-inflammatory M1 macrophage phenotype = CD54 + CD80/CD163 + CD206 > 4.0 is associated with an increased macrophage effector function in viral infections, but also with organ damage best known in HIV-1 myocarditis; b) the pro-resolution phenotype M1/M2 phenotype CD54 + CD80/CD163 + CD206 = in AD is associated with a beneficial role of macrophages in AD. The natural substances polyunsaturated fatty acids, vitamins B and D, energy molecules (carnitine), and flavonoids (resveratrol) may have individual health effects by improving macrophage transcriptome and macrophage pro-resolution type for brain clearance in AD, but the effects are complex and depend on many variables. In ALS patients, the M1/M2 phenotype promoted by fatty acids could be beneficial, but the data in human patients are not yet available.

Conflict of interest

The authors declare no conflict of interest.

Author details

Mary Dover, Michael Kishek, Miranda Eddins, Naneeta Desar and Milan Fiala*
Department of Integrative Physiology and Biology, UCLA School of Life Sciences, Los Angeles, California, USA

*Address all correspondence to: mfiala@ucla.edu

References

[1] Orecchioni M, Ghosheh Y, Pramod AB, Ley K. Macrophage polarization: Different gene signatures in M1(LPS+) vs. classically and M2(LPS–) vs. alternatively activated macrophages. Frontiers in Immunology. 2019;**10**(1084)

[2] Famenini S, Rigali EA, Olivera-Perez HM, Dang J, Chang MT, Halder R, et al. Increased intermediate M1-M2 macrophage polarization and improved cognition in mild cognitive impairment patients on omega-3 supplementation. The FASEB Journal. 2017;**31**(1):148-160

[3] Wang N, Liang H, Zen K. Molecular mechanisms that influence the macrophage M1-M2 polarization balance. Frontiers in Immunology. 2014;**5**:614

[4] Guirado E, Schlesinger LS, Kaplan G. Macrophages in tuberculosis: Friend or foe. Seminars in Immunopathology. 2013;**35**(5):563-583

[5] Fiala M, Liu QN, Sayre J, Pop V, Brahmandam V, Graves MC, et al. Cyclooxygenase-2-positive macrophages infiltrate the Alzheimer's disease brain and damage the blood-brain barrier. European Journal of Clinical Investigation. 2002;**32**(5):360-371

[6] Chen Q, Sun L, Chen ZJ. Regulation and function of the cGAS-STING pathway of cytosolic DNA sensing. Nature Immunology. 2016;**17**(10):1142-1149

[7] Persidsky Y, Ghorpade A, Rasmussen J, Limoges J, Liu XJ, Stins M, et al. Microglial and astrocyte chemokines regulate monocyte migration through the blood-brain barrier in human immunodeficiency virus-1 encephalitis. The American Journal of Pathology. 1999;**155**(5):1599-1611

[8] Fiala M, Cribbs DH, Rosenthal M, Bernard G. Phagocytosis of amyloid-beta and inflammation: Two faces of innate immunity in Alzheimer's disease. Journal of Alzheimer's Disease. 2007;**11**(4):457-463

[9] Nauen DW, Troncoso JC. Amyloid-beta is present in human lymph nodes and greatly enriched in those of the cervical region. Alzheimer's & Dementia. 2021

[10] Zaghi J, Goldenson B, Inayathullah M, Lossinsky AS, Masoumi A, Avagyan H, et al. Alzheimer disease macrophages shuttle amyloid-beta from neurons to vessels, contributing to amyloid angiopathy. Acta Neuropathologica. 2009;**117**(2):111-124

[11] Freund-Levi Y, Eriksdotter-Jönhagen M, Cederholm T, Basun H, Faxén-Irving G, Garlind A, et al. Omega-3 fatty acid treatment in 174 patients with mild to moderate Alzheimer disease: OmegAD study: A randomized double-blind trial. Archives of Neurology. 2006;**63**(10):1402-1408

[12] Quinn JF, Raman R, Thomas RG, Yurko-Mauro K, Nelson EB, Van Dyck C, et al. Docosahexaenoic acid supplementation and cognitive decline in Alzheimer disease: A randomized trial. Journal of the American Medical Association. 2010;**304**(17):1903-1911

[13] Lau YCC, Ding JA, Simental A, Mirzoyan H, Lee W, Diamante G, et al. Omega-3 fatty acids increase OXPHOS energy for immune therapy of Alzheimer disease patients. The FASEB Journal. 2020;**34**(8):9982-9994

[14] Olivera-Perez HM, Lam L, Dang J, Jiang W, Rodriguez F, Rigali E,

et al. Omega-3 fatty acids increase the unfolded protein response and improve amyloid-beta phagocytosis by macrophages of patients with mild cognitive impairment. The FASEB Journal. 2017;**31**(10):4359-4369

[15] Smith AD, Refsum H. Homocysteine, B vitamins, and cognitive impairment. Annual Review of Nutrition. 2016; **36**:211-239

[16] Butterfield DA, Halliwell B. Oxidative stress, dysfunctional glucose metabolism and Alzheimer disease. Nature Reviews. Neuroscience. 2019; **20**(3):148-160

[17] Fiala M, Liu PT, Espinosa-Jeffrey A, Rosenthal MJ, Bernard G, Ringman JM, et al. Innate immunity and transcription of MGAT-III and toll-like receptors in Alzheimer's disease patients are improved by bisdemethoxycurcumin. Proceedings of the National Academy of Sciences of the United States of America. 2007;**104**(31):12849-12854

[18] Crehan H, Lemere CA. Chapter 7 - Anti-amyloid-β immunotherapy for Alzheimer's Disease. In: Wolfe MS, editor. Developing Therapeutics for Alzheimer's Disease. Boston: Academic Press; 2016. pp. 193-226

[19] Sevigny J, Chiao P, Bussiere T, Weinreb PH, Williams L, Maier M, et al. The antibody aducanumab reduces Abeta plaques in Alzheimer's disease. Nature. 2016;**537**(7618):50-56

[20] Liu G, Fiala M, Mizwicki MT, Sayre J, Magpantay L, Siani A, et al. Neuronal phagocytosis by inflammatory macrophages in ALS spinal cord: Inhibition of inflammation by resolvin D1. American Journal of Neurodegenerative Disease. 2012;**1**(1):60-74

[21] Graves M, Fiala M, Dinglasan L, Nq L, Sayre J, Chiappelli F, et al. Inflammation in amyotrophic lateral sclerosis spinal cord and brain is mediated by activated macrophages, mast cells and T cells. Amyotrophic Lateral Sclerosis. 2004;**5**:1-7

[22] Chiot A, Zaïdi S, Iltis C, Ribon M, Berriat F, Schiaffino L, et al. Modifying macrophages at the periphery has the capacity to change microglial reactivity and to extend ALS survival. Nature Neuroscience. 2020;**23**(11):1339-1351

[23] Fiala M, Chattopadhay M, La Cava A, Tse E, Liu G, Lourenco E, et al. IL-17A is increased in the serum and in spinal cord CD8 and mast cells of ALS patients. Journal of Neuroinflammation. 2010;**7**(1):76-90

[24] Fiala M, Looney DJ, Stins M, Way DD, Zhang L, Gan X, et al. TNF-alpha opens a paracellular route for HIV-1 invasion across the blood-brain barrier. Molecular Medicine. 1997;**3**(8):553-564

[25] Lipton JD, Schafermeyer RW. Central nervous system infections. The usual and the unusual. Emergency Medicine Clinics of North America. 1995;**13**(2):417-443

[26] Liu QN, Reddy S, Sayre JW, Pop V, Graves MC, Fiala M. Essential role of HIV type 1-infected and cyclooxygenase 2-activated macrophages and T cells in HIV type 1 myocarditis. AIDS Research and Human Retroviruses. 2001;**17**(15):1423-1433

[27] Meidaninikjeh S, Sabouni N, Marzouni HZ, Bengar S, Khalili A, Jafari R. Monocytes and macrophages in COVID-19: Friends and foes. Life Sciences. 2021;**269**:119010

[28] Merad M, Martin JC. Pathological inflammation in patients with COVID-19: A key role for monocytes and macrophages. Nature Reviews. Immunology. 2020;**20**(6):355-362

[29] Park MD. Fatty monocytes in COVID-19. Nature Reviews. Immunology. 2020;**20**(11):649

[30] Park MD. Macrophages: A Trojan horse in COVID-19? Nature Reviews. Immunology. 2020;**20**(6):351

[31] Theobald SJ, Simonis A, Georgomanolis T, Kreer C, Zehner M, Eisfeld HS, et al. Long-lived macrophage reprogramming drives spike protein-mediated inflammasome activation in COVID-19. EMBO Molecular Medicine. 2021;**13**(8):e14150

[32] Deng Z, Shi F, Zhou Z, Sun F, Sun MH, Sun Q, et al. M1 macrophage mediated increased reactive oxygen species (ROS) influence wound healing via the MAPK signaling in vitro and in vivo. Toxicology and Applied Pharmacology. 2019;**366**:83-95

[33] Dlugovitzky D, Torres-Morales A, Rateni L, Farroni MA, Largacha C, Molteni O, et al. Circulating profile of Th1 and Th2 cytokines in tuberculosis patients with different degrees of pulmonary involvement. FEMS Immunology & Medical Microbiology. 1997;**18**(3):203-207

[34] Mills CD, Kincaid K, Alt JM, Heilman MJ, Hill AM. M-1/M-2 macrophages and the Th1/Th2 paradigm. Journal of Immunology. 2000;**164**(12):6166-6173

[35] Abebe F. Synergy between Th1 and Th2 responses during mycobacterium tuberculosis infection: A review of current understanding. International Reviews of Immunology. 2019;**38**(4):172-179

[36] Garcia-Romo GS, Pedroza-Gonzalez A, Lambrecht BN, Aguilar-Leon D, Estrada-Garcia I, Hernandez-Pando R, et al. Mycobacterium tuberculosis manipulates pulmonary APCs subverting early immune responses. Immunobiology. 2013; **218**(3):393-401

[37] Khan A, Singh VK, Hunter RL, Jagannath C. Macrophage heterogeneity and plasticity in tuberculosis. Journal of Leukocyte Biology. 2019;**106**(2):275-282

Section 7

Macrophages in Breast Cancer

Chapter 18

Targeted Regulation and Cellular Imaging of Tumor-Associated Macrophages in Triple-Negative Breast Cancer: From New Mechanistic Insights to Candidate Translational Applications

Anupama Hooda-Nehra, Tracey L. Smith, Alejandra I. Ferrer, Fernanda I. Staquicini, Wadih Arap, Renata Pasqualini and Pranela Rameshwar

Abstract

The complex interplay between immune cells and tumor cells within the tumor microenvironment (TME) can lead to disease progression. Specifically, signals generated in the TME can cause immunosuppression, promoting angiogenesis and immune evasion, which leads to tumor development. The interplay of M1 and M2 macrophage populations that coincide with these tumor markers is particularly important in the TME. Triple-negative breast cancer (TNBC) often presents as advanced disease, and these tumors are also often bereft of recognized molecular targets that can be found in other subtypes, limiting their therapeutic options. However, tumor-associated macrophages (TAMs) infiltration in TNBC is frequently observed. Moreover, a high density of TAMs, particularly M2 macrophages, is associated with poorer outcomes in various cancers, including TNBC. This provides a strong basis for exploiting TAMs as potential therapeutic targets. Specifically, efforts to increase M2 to M1 repolarization are promising therapeutic approaches in TNBC, and four recent studies wherein divergent approaches to target the M2-rich macrophage population and reverse immune subversion are described. These and similar efforts may yield promising diagnostic or therapeutic options for TNBC, a great clinical need.

Keywords: cancer, dormancy, bone marrow, microvesicle, macrophage, cytokine

IntechOpen

1. Introduction

The cellular microenvironment of metastatic solid tumors is composed of heterogeneous malignant cells and other supporting nonmalignant cells such as cancer-associated fibroblasts, angiogenic endothelial cells, mesenchymal stem cells, and pericytes, along with lymphoid and myeloid immune cells. The latter includes B- and T-cells, dendritic cells, and tumor-associated macrophages (TAMs).

TAMs form a major component of the tumor microenvironment (TME) and likely are the most abundant cell [1–3]. Macrophages, which are differentiated from monocytes, are heterogeneous and belong to the inherent myeloid cells present in TME. The roles and phenotypes of macrophages depend on their homeostatic and pathological microenvironment. Macrophages can aid in enhancing immunity by clearing cellular debris and tumor cells, as well as boosting adaptive immunity [4, 5]. In contrast, continued or prolonged activation of macrophages can result in a dysregulated host immune defense, ultimately resulting in pathogenetic outcomes [4].

Macrophages can release soluble factors such as cytokines and stimulate the complement system, contributing to inflammation [6]. In the case of a large tumor volume, the microenvironment can have low oxygen tension and acidic pH to create conditions that are identical to tissue damage seen in inflammatory conditions [7, 8]. In turn, the macrophages within an inflammatory microenvironment can initiate mechanisms to repair the "damaged tissue." These include triggers to initiate neoangiogenesis, tissue remodeling, and removal of dead and damaged cells as well as promoting immunosuppression [8–11]. In this regard, tumor growth can behave as an aberrant but complex interaction between tumor cells, immune system, and stromal cells in which proliferating and dying cells coexist similar to a wound [8, 9, 12].

The prognostic value of TAM infiltration in several different kinds of cancer, such as breast [13], lung [14], prostate [15], and gastric [16], has been demonstrated in various studies. Other studies reported on a correlation between TAM density and poor prognosis [17, 18]. Zhao et al. have also demonstrated that increased penetration of TAMs correlated with poor prognosis and reduced patient survival in breast cancer [19]. Further subset analysis has shown differential prognostic association between M1 and M2 macrophage phenotypes. A high M1 phenotype density has been shown to correlate with better prognosis due to the pro-inflammatory role of this subtype. In contrast, predominance of M2 phenotype correlated with a poorer overall survival as found in gastric cancer, partly due to their anti-inflammatory property, including increased regulatory T-cells [20].

Malignant transformation is associated with an "angiogenic switch," marked by an increase in the number of new blood vessels [21, 22]. Macrophages also appear to be important players in angiogenesis. TAMs may stimulate the tumor neovascularization by producing angiogenic factors. Leek et al. have shown a positive relationship between high vascular grade and increased macrophage infiltration in breast carcinoma, which leads to reduced disease-free survival and overall survival [23]. TAMs residing in hypoxic tumor areas have increased expression of vascular endothelial growth factor A (VEGFA) [24]. This correlates with TAM-mediated induction of metalloproteinases (MMPs), contributing to increased tumor angiogenesis, which is consistent with findings of TAMs as major source of MMP9 in a mouse model of human ovarian cancer [25]. Chen et al. have shown that a hypoxic TME can be crucial for preferential polarization of recruited macrophages into M2 subtype [26]. These recruited M2 macrophages significantly enhance tumor neovascularization while protecting the cancer cells of the immune system.

1.1 TAM polarization

Macrophages that express high levels of tumor necrosis factor (TNF), inducible nitric oxide synthase (iNOS), or major histocompatibility complex (MHC) class II molecules have been considered antitumorigenic. Expression of high levels of arginase-1 (ARG1), interleukin (IL)-10, CD163, CD204, or CD206 by macrophages has been associated with pro-tumorgenic behavior [27]. Macrophage polarization is an area of intense immunological research [28–30]. In a conventional dualistic approach, M1 macrophages refer to macrophages activated through lipopolysaccharide (LPS) or the polarizing cytokine interferon gamma (INFγ) [31, 32]. These are identified by the expression of "M1 marker genes" such as *NOS2*, *IL12*, and *MHC class II transactivator (CIITA)* [28]. M2 macrophages are IL-4 stimulated and typically express "M2 marker genes" such as *ARG1*, among other signal transducer and activator of transcription 6 (STAT6)-induced markers [8, 28–30, 32].

However, macrophages can express both ARG1 and NOS2 simultaneously, suggesting the inadequacy of the strict dichotomous model to address layers of complexity. This dualistic model has been replaced by a spectrum model, wherein M1 and M2 are thought to represent ends of a continuum. Heterogeneity in the microenvironment along with other development factors must be considered for TAM phenotyping. Metabolic changes within the TME have significant potential to change polarization of macrophages. It has been shown that oxidative pathways result in M2 polarized macrophages, whereas M1 macrophages depend more on glycolysis [6, 32].

2. Triple-negative breast cancer: an unmet need in contemporary cancer medicine

Breast cancer ranks as the second most common cancer type worldwide with higher incidence being seen in African Americans and Hispanics. Lifetime risk of breast cancer remains at one in every eight women equating to about 13% of American women developing breast cancer in their lifetime. It is estimated that in 2022, approximately 288,000 new cases of invasive breast cancer will be diagnosed in women within the United States and over 43,000 will die from their breast cancer (SEER database; http://cancer.gov).

Triple-negative breast cancer (TNBC) refers to tumors lacking expression of estrogen receptor (ER), progesterone receptor (PR), and receptor tyrosine-protein kinase erbB-2 (HER2), all of which are molecular targets of therapeutic agents, ensuring TNBC remains difficult to treat. Chemotherapy remains the mainstay for standard of care treatment of TNBC, with preferential use of platinum compounds in BRCA1/2 mutated breast cancer that are triple-negative. About 10–20% of all diagnosed breast cancers are triple-negative. TNBCs will often present with higher grade tumors that clinically correlate with a poorer outcome as compared to other breast cancer subtypes. In particular, patients with TNBC tend to present with clinically more advanced disease in the form of larger tumors and a higher burden of nodal involvement. This is reflective of their inherently aggressive nature [33]. Despite responses to treatment, these cancers can present with earlier relapses involving the visceral sites [34–39]. Despite multi-agent systemic treatment, fewer that 30% of patients with metastatic breast cancer survive longer than 5 years and virtually no patient with metastatic TNBC will be alive after that [40, 41]. Despite a higher risk of recurrence for TNBC, better clinical and pathological initial response to chemotherapy has been seen in TNBC compared to other breast tumors, an interesting but paradoxical contrast [41, 42]. In a large majority of residual TNBCs that persist after initial chemotherapy, there may be targetable pathway alterations that could serve as therapeutic targets [41, 43]. Use of poly ADP ribose polymerase (PARP) inhibitors, phosphoinositide 3-kinase (PI3K) inhibitors, mitogen-activated protein (MAP) kinase (MEK) inhibitors, heat-shock protein 90 (HSP90) inhibitors, histone deacetylase inhibitors, etc., are notable examples [41]. Some of these interventions have been approved by the US Food and Drug Administration (FDA) and others remain investigational. The standard of care for TNBC remains multiagent chemotherapy; however, use of PARP inhibitors (such as olaparib) and immune checkpoint inhibitors (such as pembrolizumab) have recently been incorporated as part of adjuvant or neoadjuvant potentially curative options approved in certain settings [39, 44–47]. Unfortunately, TNBC patients display remarkable clinical diversity, making treatment decisions challenging, as seen with the recent voluntary withdrawal of the expedited approval of atezolizumab in combination with chemotherapy against metastatic TNBC, despite initial approval for use in this setting. In summary, TNBC remains a major unmet need in contemporary cancer medicine.

2.1 PDL-1 and triple-negative breast cancer

Immunotherapy has been of interest and a focus for the development of therapeutics for many years. Clinical trials have yielded mixed results. Vaccine trials have exploited the idea of increasing immune system engagement by increasing tumor recognition by the immune system but without consistent results. Active engagement of the immune system using immunotherapies continues to be both of clinical and investigational interest [41].

TNBCs are known to have genomic instability and have been shown to have higher degree of tumor-infiltrating lymphocytes [48] along with increased expression of programmed cell death ligand 1 (PD-L1) in comparison with other breast tumor types [49, 50]. Immune tolerance regulation has been linked to PD-L1 and its receptor programmed cell death protein 1 (PD-1). PD-1 is a receptor expressed on the surface of cells, like T-cells in the adaptive immune environment. These cells can then bind to either PD-L1 or PD-L2 which can be found on both tumor cells and tumor-infiltrating cells. This can in turn induce inhibition and depletion of T-cells which limits the tumor cell clearance and allows the tumor cells to evade innate and adaptive immune mechanisms [51–53]. Therefore, inhibition of immune checkpoints can reverse the immunosuppressive environment to promote an effective local immune response [54, 55].

TNBC has been shown to harbor mutations and tumor-infiltrating lymphocytes, along with a higher expression of PD-L1, making immunotherapy an attractive therapeutic approach [56–58]. In KEYNOTE-012, a phase 1b study, the PD-1 inhibitor pembrolizumab was evaluated as monotherapy for TNBC patients whose tumors expressed PD-L1. An overall response rate of 19% was seen in the study with one complete response. There were four partial responses seen, and 29% of patients had stable disease on treatment [59]. KEYNOTE-086 further explored the use of pembrolizumab in patients with metastatic TNBC. This study characterized patients by treatment history for their metastatic disease as well as PD-L1 expression on tumor cells [53, 60]. Progression-free survival (PFS) was similar with an overall response of 4.7% in both PD-L1 positive and negative previously treated patients of Cohort A in this study. Cohort B consisted of untreated patients with positive PD-L1 expression and showed a higher overall response rate of 23.1% [53]. KEYNOTE-119 evaluated advanced TNBC patients with 1:1 randomization to single-agent pembrolizumab vs. physician choice of chemotherapy and failed to meet its primary endpoint [61]. KEYNOTE-522, a prospective randomized trial evaluating neoadjuvant and adjuvant pembrolizumab for patients with TNBC assigned to pembrolizumab plus chemotherapy and placebo plus chemotherapy in a 2:1 ratio, showed a pathological complete response of 64.8% vs. 51.2% between the two groups. Patients with early TNBC who had received pembrolizumab with neoadjuvant chemotherapy had a significantly higher complete pathological response compared to the group that received placebo with neoadjuvant chemotherapy [62, 63]. Atezolizumab, a monoclonal antibody targeting PD-L1, was the first immune checkpoint inhibitor to be approved in combination with Nab-paclitaxel for unresectable locally advanced and metastatic TNBC expressing PD-L1 [64]. Approval was withdrawn when results of IMpassion131 showed failure to meet the primary endpoint of PFS superiority compared to the frontline treatment. Additionally, there was no survival advantage seen in the PD-L1 positive population nor in the intention to treat population. In fact, the study investigators observed a negative trend for overall survival [65], highlighting the urgent need for new treatment options.

3. Targeted preclinical imaging and therapy of tumor-associated macrophages in models of triple-negative breast cancer

As immunotherapies targeting co-stimulatory blockade move to the forefront of cancer therapeutics, it becomes increasingly important to understand the contribution of inflammatory cells to tumor progression and their potential use for targeted therapy. As discussed earlier, TAMs are critical components of the TME in many solid tumors, including breast cancers, and play key roles in facilitating tumor progression and metastases [30]. This pro-tumor effect of TAM appears to be mediated by increased proliferation of tumor cells, angiogenesis, matrix remodeling, and the sustained release of growth factors and cytokines within the TME. Although both phenotypic and functional heterogeneity are well documented for the macrophage lineage, and the activation state can be clearly defined as a spectrum (see Section 1.2.), here we will utilize two distinct states of polarized activation to demonstrate macrophage targeting in translational experiments. Specifically, the classically activated (M1) macrophage acts in response to IFNγ and/or LPS, and the release of IL-12, IL-23, and tumor necrosis factor (TNF), resulting in efficient antigen presentation and antitumor activity. The alternatively activated (M2) macrophage was originally discovered to respond to IL-4 [66] and can be characterized by low IL-12 and high IL-10 expression, dampened inflammation, increased parasite clearance, tissue remodeling, and promotion of tumor progression [30].

Macrophage dysregulation is central to the pathogenesis of human TNBC. Given that TAMs are influenced by their TME, it becomes important to explore how disease-specific changes in TNBC, specifically the large TAM population within the TME, can be selectively exploited for clinical applications. Thus, a main goal of this book chapter is to provide a few recent selected examples of basic and applied research programs that study TAM biology in the setting of TNBC, toward bringing discoveries and new mechanistic insights into translational applications.

Here, we have highlighted four specific examples of reversal of immune subversion in TNBC and targeted cellular imaging in vivo of TAMs in preclinical models of disease, namely:

- Attenuating TNBC with a lysosome-targeted DNA nanodevice [67] (**Figure 1A**).
- Ligand-directed targeting a vitamin D receptor in the cell surface of TAMs in a TNBC model for tumor ablation and immune subversion reversal [39] (**Figure 1B**).
- Magnetic resonance imaging (MRI) of superparamagnetic iron oxide nanoparticle (SPION)-loaded TAMs in vivo in an isogenic mouse model of TNBC (**Figure 1C**) [68].
- Controlling TNBC dormancy through differentially activated TAM-derived exosomes and their cargo (**Figure 1D**) [69].

3.1 Attenuating TNBC with a lysosome-targeted DNA nanodevice

Cui et al. recently reported a novel approach to exploit the known lysosomal trapping phenomenon of DNA-based agents [67]. Nucleic acid therapies seem to be preferentially trafficked to the lysosome via the endo-lysosomal pathway [70, 71]. Rather than reinvent the wheel—re-engineer the nucleic acid—for alternative organelle targeting, the authors identified lysosomal functions that could be co-opted for an antitumor effect, specifically that an increase in cysteine protease activity in lysosomes diminishes antigen presentation on M2 macrophages, avoiding T-cell activation and tumor immunity [67].

Cui and team [67] completed a proteomic analysis of M1 and M2 macrophages to identify distinct markers of tumorigenesis associated with M2 polarization. In addition to validating known mitochondrial and adhesion proteins, the M2 macrophage-specific profile included a panel of elevated lysosomal proteins, findings confirmed in TAM samples from TNBC patients. Specific deletion of transcription factor EB (TFEB), a regulator of the concerted network of lysosomal enzymes responsible for degrading proteins [72] and transcriptional regulation of autophagosome-lysosome fusion and function [73], resulted in delayed tumor growth and decreased lysosomal activity, likely caused by increased antigen presentation by TAMs and the recruitment of $CD8^+$ T-cells [67].

The cysteine proteinase inhibitor E64 [74] was then selected to develop a therapeutic agent with the same effect as TFEB depletion [67]. Increased lysosomal cysteine protease activity is known to improve antigen cross-presentation [75], so E64, a specific inhibitor of cysteine proteases [76], was conjugated to a 38 base pair DNA sequence that could be picked up by scavenger receptors on TAMs for autophagolysosome processing [67]. The benefits of this approach would be twofold: 1) direct antitumor activity from immunomodulation [77] and 2) to sensitize cells to cancer drugs [78].

Trafficking of the E64-DNA compound to lysosomes was confirmed with a fluorescent reporter [67]. E64-DNA inhibited cysteine protease activity specifically, which increased antigen presentation and $CD8^+$ T-cell recruitment [77]. When tested in the E0771 TNBC tumor model, E64-DNA was able to selectively target TAMs, internalize via scavenger receptors, and localize to lysosomes. Further analyses revealed M2 macrophages were preferentially targeted. After E64-DNA administration, tumor growth was hampered, and the number of $CD8^+$ T effector cells increased, as did markers of both T-cell proliferation and activation. Further investigation confirmed that E64-DNA acts on the M2 macrophage population to reduce cysteine protease activity, which facilitates antigen presentation on the TAM cells, leading to activation of CD8+ T-cells and slowed tumor growth [67].

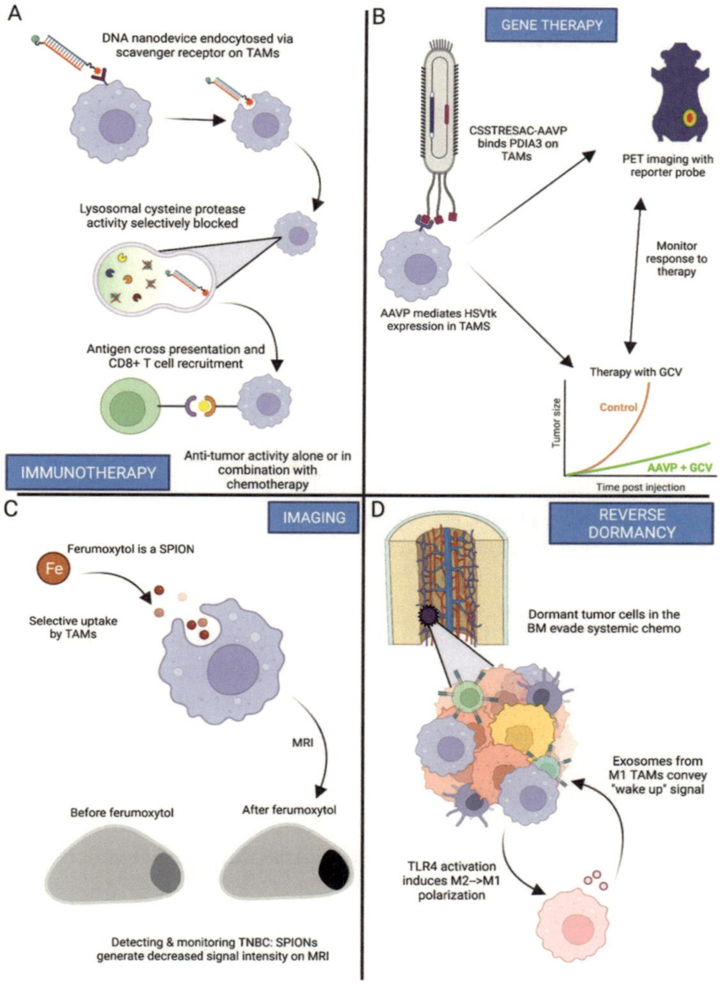

Figure 1.
Selected examples of targeting TAMs in TNBC for therapeutic or imaging applications in pre-clinical models of disease. (A) Administration of E64, an inhibitor or cysteine proteases, conjugated to DNA, leads to selective autophagocytosis and lysosomal uptake, where cysteine protease activity is blocked selectively, enabling TAMs to display tumor antigens and activate CD8+ T cells for anti-tumor activity [67]. (B) PDIA3 is a novel biomarker of TNBC, and it can be selectively targeted with the CSSTRESAC peptide ligand. CSSTRESAC displayed on a hybrid AAV/phage engineered to deliver HSVtk specifically homes to TAMs in EF43.fgf4-derived mammary tumors. Administration of appropriate HSVtk substrates for imaging (radiolabeled reporters) or suicide gene therapy (GCV) enables tumor monitoring and treatment [39]. (C) Ferumoxytol-contrasted MRI enables TNBC imaging and quantification and localization of the iron-containing TAM population in the TME of a mouse model of TNBC [68]. (D) Breast cancer metastasized to the bone marrow (BM) can become dormant, rendering the site invulnerable to circulating chemotherapy. Activating TLR4, for example by LPS administration, can repolarize M2 macrophages to M1. These M1 TAMs can secrete exosomes that interact with cancer stem cells to reverse their quiescent state, enabling effective anti-tumor therapy [69]. Created with BioRender.Com.

Finally, in addition to this nascent antitumor immunomodulatory activity, E64-DNA enhanced chemosensitivity, and combination therapy with E64-DNA and cyclophosphamide led to longer-term efficacy and tumor regression. The increase in tumor cell death provides a ready supply of antigens TAM presentation leading to antitumor immunity [67]. This report exemplifies the potential of exploiting what some might originally write off as a negative (lysosomal trapping of nucleic acids) to counterintuitively engineer an organelle-specific DNA conjugate for affecting lysosomal functions toward immunotherapeutic applications.

3.2 Ligand-directed targeting a vitamin D receptor in the cell surface of TAMs in a TNBC model for tumor ablation and immune subversion reversal

3.2.1 Viruses as therapeutic agents

The use of oncolytic viruses to selectively target cancer cells is fairly widespread. Multiple viruses have been selected or engineered for specific purposes, often tumor cell destruction with minimal impact to nonmalignant tissues. Some of the most common—and clinically advanced—are adenoviruses [79, 80] and adeno-associated viruses [81]. AAVP is a unique hybrid AAV and bacteriophage (phage) vector first described in 2006 [82]. AAVP contains cis-elements from AAV within the single-stranded phage genome that facilitates tumor-targeted delivery of a transgene cassette for noninvasive tumor imaging and/or therapy [82]. Unlike mammalian viruses that are conventionally used for gene therapy, AAVP has been extensively characterized and has several safety features built into the vector design, such as: (i) targeting peptides to ensure receptor-mediated transduction and tumor-specific gene expression, (ii) well-characterized fate of the genome (concatemerization and integration of intact genomes) [82], and (iii) the ability to avoid neutralization, as proven in repeat dose studies using pet dogs with spontaneous tumors [83] and several mouse models, including transgenic tumor models with intact immune systems [82, 84]. Receptor-mediated AAVP internalization is required for transduction, eliminating off-target effects, even during phage particle clearance through the reticuloendothelial system (RES), sparing healthy tissues while a strong promoter drives the transgene expression of the within tumors. In the following section, we report one translational approach utilizing AAVP to selectively target the TAM population for theranostic gene delivery.

3.2.2 Novel molecular markers of TAMs in TNBC

A recently reported study describing the identification and validation of the CSSTRESAC (single letter amino acid code) peptide and its receptor, a novel TAM biomarker, is summarized here. Staquicini et al. devised a combinatorial peptide library-based screening that allowed the identification of peptides selectively targeting the TAM-rich TME of mammary tumors [39]. Assuming that peptides binding to mammary tumors in vivo, but not to the corresponding breast cancer cells (BCCs) in vitro, would selectively target the TME, an in vivo combinatorial selection was performed by injecting a naive CX_7C (C, cysteine; X, any residue) phage peptide library into EF43.*fgf4* tumor bearing mice. These cells produce a rapidly growing, aggressive syngeneic model of TNBC that is highly infiltrated with F4/80$^+$ TAMs. After 24 hours, tumor homing peptides were recovered by bacterial infection, amplified, and re-injected for two additional rounds of screening. To facilitate the selection of microenvironment-specific binders, peptides enriched in the tumor were selected based on negative binding to the cancer cells. The peptide CSSTRESAC targeted tumors in vivo but did not bind EF43.*fgf4* breast cancer cells in vitro [85], suggesting specific targeting of the TME. Binding assays to cellular components of the TME showed that CSSTRESAC bound exclusively to F4/80$^+$ TAMs [39].

Peptide affinity chromatography and mass spectrometry identified protein disulfide-isomerase A3 (PDIA3) and vitamin D-binding protein (DBP) as targets of CSSTRESAC on the surface of TAMs. Because the CSSTRESAC phage bound specifically to the $CD11b^+$ $F4/80^+$ TAM population, and because PDIA3 was validated as its receptor, PDIA3 expression on the surface of TAMs was investigated. TAMs were isolated from EF43.*fgf4* tumors based on CD11b, IL-10, IL-12, and PDIA3 expression. Expression of PDIA3 on the surface of $CD11b^+$ $IL\text{-}10^{high}$ $IL\text{-}12^{low}$ macrophages was confirmed by flow cytometry, suggesting PDIA3 is a novel surface marker of M2-polarized macrophage [39]. With a novel ligand/receptor interaction confirmed in TAMs in the TNBC model, the diagnostic and therapeutic utility of this finding was then investigated.

Homing of CSSTRESAC phage to the tumors in two aggressive breast cancer models [86, 87] was robust and specific, and, when displayed on AAVP to deliver the Herpes simplex virus *thymidine kinase* (*HSVtk*) gene, markedly slowed tumor growth, at least partially due to ganciclovir (GCV)-mediated cell death via *HSVtk* suicide gene therapy (**Figure 1B**) [39]. HSVtk expression levels over time, as well as the response to GCV therapy, can be monitored with positron emission tomography (PET) using an HSVtk reporter probe such as $[^{18}F]$-FEAU [82, 88, 89] or $[^{124}I]$-FIAU [90].

Importantly, upon binding, the CSSTRESAC peptide—alone or displayed on phage—induced the expression of pro-inflammatory cytokines IL-6, TNF, and IL-1β in $CD11b^+$ $F4/80^+$ TAMs, reverting from an M2-rich macrophage population toward an inflammatory TME reminiscent of classical M1 macrophages and further inhibiting tumor growth (**Figure 2A**) [39]. Collectively, these data confirm the binding specificity of the CSSTRESAC peptide to the TME, specifically the M2 macrophage population expressing PDIA3 on the cell surface, and the potential for an immunoregulatory response that shifts the cytokine profile toward an inflammatory M1 population and further induces antitumor activity.

Extrapolating from publicly available datasets, high *PDIA3* transcript expression levels in TNBC patients were associated with markers of immune suppression and M2 polarity as well as angiogenic markers associated with poor prognosis, confirming the potential clinical utility of CSSTRESAC-based therapeutic agents [39]. With these promising data confirming the ability to target the TAM population of the TME specifically, the potential effects of CSSTRESAC-targeted agents in TNBC warrant further investigation, for both immunoregulatory and theranostic applications.

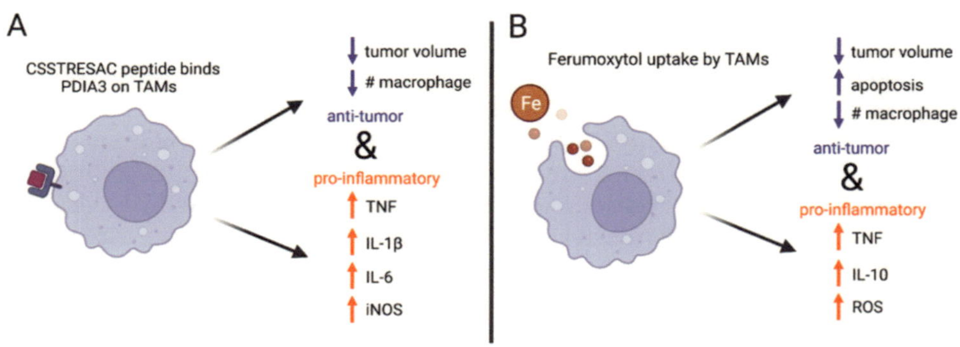

Figure 2.
Immunomodulation roles of CSSTRESAC and ferumoxytol remain untapped. (A) The CSSTRESAC peptide alone or displayed on phage/AAVP functions in an immunoregulatory role in TAMs in an EF43.fgf4-derived mouse model of TNBC. After treatment with CSSTRESAC, the tumors decrease in volume, and the macrophages revert from an M2-rich population to an M1-polarized population with the expression of several pro-inflammatory cytokines [39]. (B) Similarly, iron agents like ferumoxytol can trigger re-polarization from M2 to M1 TAMs after phagocytosis; IL-10 levels drop while levels TNF and other inflammatory cytokines increase [91–93]. Created with BioRender.com.

3.3 MRI of superparamagnetic iron oxide nanoparticle (SPION)-loaded TAMs in vivo in an isogenic mouse model of TNBC

Breast cancer patients undergo a series of imaging studies in order to diagnose disease, monitor disease progression, and evaluate responses to therapy. The presence of TAMs in the microenvironment of TNBC, in particular, promotes tumor growth and metastasis formation. Accordingly, a method of imaging this cell population specifically would be of clinical interest, particularly relating to response to immunotherapies utilized in these patients. Sillerud et al. recently reported one such approach, wherein an iron (Fe) nanoparticle is selectively phagocytosed by TAMs in mouse models of breast cancer for visualization by MRI [68]. A decrease in signal is detectable with T2-weighted MRI, and the spatial and temporal dynamics of particle uptake can be quantified and monitored [68].

Ferumoxytol is a superparamagnetic iron oxide nanoparticle (SPION) that has been approved by the FDA for patients with iron-deficient anemia. Its off-label use as a contrast agent for MRI has been studied for almost two decades in parallel with its role as an iron replacement therapy [91, 92, 94–96]. Importantly, a multicenter study found ferumoxytol was generally well tolerated and safe for administration [93].

More importantly, both M1 and M2 macrophages—but not tumor cells—can internalize ferumoxytol [97]. When combined with work done to validate ferumoxytol uptake and detection in lymphomas and sarcomas, known to have $CD68^+$ and $CD163^+$ TAM populations, ferumoxytol can function as an "imaging biomarker for TAM" [98]. When in a macrophage-rich TME, ferumoxytol might also induce some cytotoxicity and M1 macrophage polarization, making the tumor more susceptible to immunotherapeutic agents [99–101] (**Figure 2B**). Yet another application of clinical importance would be to use MRI to image ferumoxytol-containing TAMs as a surrogate for tumor localization. Specifically, on T2-weighted MRI, ferumoxytol produces a decrease in signal, darkening dramatically from a hyperintense image at baseline [68].

The EF43.*fgf4* mouse model of TNBC [87] introduced earlier was utilized for this work as well [68]. Initially, tumor and nonmalignant tissues were imaged at baseline, and then tumor and off-site ferumoxytol accumulation after administration was assessed. By 24 hours, dramatic contrast changes were evident in the MR signal from the tumor, while no significant change was evident in the control tissues (**Figure 1C**) [68]. This decrease was most evident in T2-weighted images, with about a 10-fold difference from baseline starting 1 day after ferumoxytol administration and remaining evident up to 4 days later, before returning to baseline by 7 days. The level of iron within the tumors can be quantified, revealing the distribution of TAMs in the tumor [68]. Higher levels of macrophages, and M2 macrophages in particular, are associated with metastatic potential, resistance to treatment, and an overall worse prognosis [102], information that would be relevant for clinicians and patients. Further elucidation of the role of ferumoxytol in M2 to M1 polarization [99] could broaden treatment options or otherwise combine Fe-based imaging with immunotherapies, chemotherapies, etc., for theranostic applications [103, 104].

3.4 Controlling TNBC dormancy through differentially activated TAM-derived exosomes and their cargo

3.4.1 Breast cancer dormancy in bone marrow

Breast cancer cells (BCCs) preferentially disseminate to the bone marrow (BM) [105]. The BM niche contributes to the survival of BCCs by allowing their transition into dormancy [106]. Dormant BCCs can remain undetected for extended periods by acquiring a cancer stem cell (CSC) phenotype [107]. Cancer stem cells (CSCs) share properties with nonmalignant stem cells such as self-renewal, cell cycle quiescence, and drug resistance [108]. Reactivation of dormant BCCs/CSCs in BM is associated with poor patient prognosis and results in cancer resurgence [109, 110]. Targeting dormant BCCs/CSCs is challenging because current treatments mostly target the active cycling cells [111]. Additionally, dormant BCCs home to the endosteal niche of the BM close to endogenous hematopoietic stem cells (HSCs) and utilize strategies similar to those of the endogenous HSCs to survive and remain dormant [105, 112]. More importantly, the method of survival includes the marrow microenvironment with macrophages comprising a major component of the supporting cells. Thus, any treatment aimed to eliminate the BCCs can also target the survival and/or function of the HSCs found within the same niche. This could result in disruption of hematopoietic activity, which will affect the individual's immune system and other organ functions that require immune competence. Hence, it is imperative to elucidate the precise mechanisms of communication between cells in the BM microenvironment and BCCs to understand how dormancy is achieved and how the same microenvironment can reverse the dormant phase. Such understanding will lead to effective methods to selectively eliminate malignant stem cells without harm to the endogenous HSCs.

The BM is a complex organ composed of various niches that aid in hematopoietic activity and maintain dormancy [112–114]. The cellular component of the BM niche includes mesenchymal stem cells, fibroblasts, and macrophages, all contributing to the survival of BCC dormancy [69, 115, 116]. Intercellular communication between BM niche cells and BCCs is fundamental for BC dormancy [105]. The interaction between components of the BM niche and BCCs can be direct through intercellular communication such as gap junctions and/or contact-independent, which involves soluble and insoluble factors such as cytokines and microvesicles (i.e. exosomes). Both forms of the aforementioned interactions facilitate and maintain BC dormancy [116, 117]. Disrupting these interactions can reverse the dormant phenotype of BCCs resulting in cancer recurrence [115, 118, 119]. The next section addresses the role of macrophages in BC dormancy and provides evidence supporting that intercellular communication between the niche and BCCs is essential for dormancy.

3.4.2 Role of macrophages in breast cancer dormancy

BCCs recruit macrophages to the TME by upregulating chemokines such as C-C motif chemokine ligand 2 (CCL2) [120]. Recruited macrophages have been shown to modulate BC dormancy or reversal. For instance, Ma et al. demonstrated that a macrophage subset expressing high levels of CD204 and IL-4 receptor facilitated BC metastasis to the bone [121]. Depletion of this macrophage subset halted BCC proliferation [121]. Depletion of $CD11b^{+}$ $VEGFR^{high}$ $CCR2^{high}$ macrophages prevented extravasation and growth of BCCs within the lungs [122]. This macrophage subset is significantly present in lungs with BC metastasis compared to healthy lungs [122]. Although these findings are related to BC metastasis to the lung, it is plausible that a similar mechanism is occurring upon BC metastasis to the BM or bone.

Endogenous BM-derived macrophages have a crucial role in BC dormancy and can be polarized into M1 or M2 phenotype depending on microenvironmental cues [69]. Classically activated macrophages (M1) exert antitumor response in BC, whereas alternatively activated (M2) macrophages employ a pro-tumorigenic effect [123]. However, with respect to dormancy, M2 macrophages maintain cycling quiescence

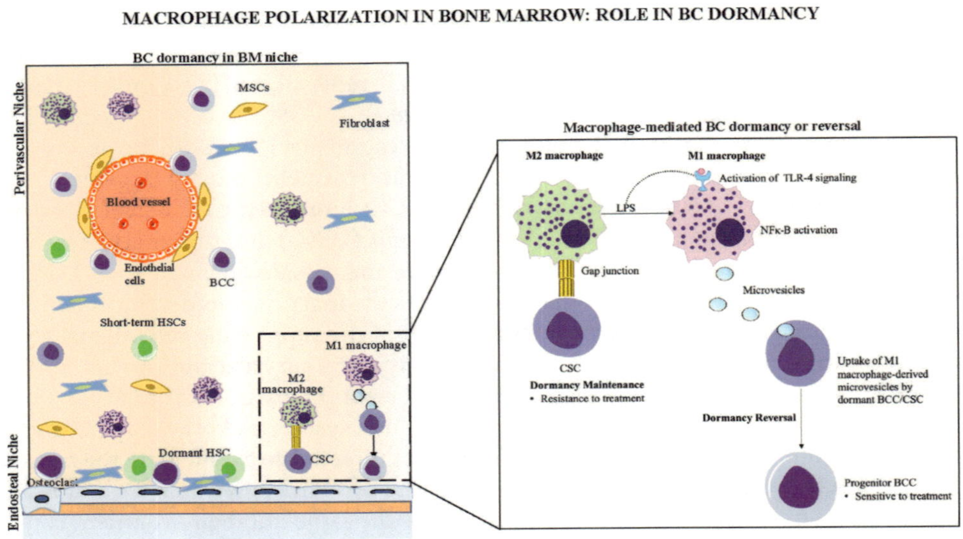

Figure 3.
Left panel shows the bone marrow cavity and the predominant region for dormant breast cancer cells within the endosteal niche. The established dormant phenotype is highlighted in boxed region, which is enlarged. The latter shows M2 macrophage sustaining gap junctional-mediated dormancy. Activation of M2 macrophages to M1 type release microvesicles to reverse dormancy.

whereas M1 macrophages can reverse dormancy [69]. Such polarization has been demonstrated when the toll-like receptor was activated, suggesting that infectious agents that activate these receptors could be a method to reverse dormancy.

M1 macrophages facilitate reversed dormancy by releasing microvesicles that promote NF-κB signaling in quiescent BCCs to mediate cell cycle activation (**Figure 3**) [69]. As a result, M1-derived microvesicles sensitized BCCs to chemotherapy by reducing BCC stemness. Conversely, M2 macrophages form gap junctions with CSCs to support dormancy and chemoresistance of BC in BM [69]. Mechanistically, the polarization of M2 macrophages into an M1 phenotype was shown to be mediated by LPS, which activated toll-like receptor 4 signaling. This study showed the role of contact-dependent and contact-independent interactions between BCCs and macrophages in BC dormancy.

In TNBC cells, macrophage polarization toward an M2 phenotype is facilitated by the oncogene multiple copies in T-cell malignancy-1 (MCT-1) [124]. Silencing of MCT-1 in TNBC reduced overall tumor volume and the total number of M2 macrophages within the TME [124]. Interestingly, MCT-1 enhances mammosphere formation in TNBC cells through IL-6 signaling. Blockade of IL-6 signaling with the IL-6 receptor (IL-6R) monoclonal antibody tocilizumab reduced mammosphere formation and downregulated MCT-1 expression [124]. Another strategy to target MCT-1 expression was shown by miRNA-34a reducing stemness in TNBC cells and prevented M2 polarization. Macrophage polarization in the TME can also be mediated by oncometabolites such as lactate which enhance BCC proliferation through the ERK/STAT3 signaling pathway [125]. Pharmacological inhibition of ERK/STAT3 with selumetinib and stattic, respectively, abrogated lactate levels within the TME and prevented macrophage polarization to M2 phenotype [125]. Collectively, these studies provided evidence of the importance of macrophage polarization in BC dormancy and reversal.

As stated earlier, the chemokine CCL2 is crucial in macrophage recruitment to the TME. Thus, efforts to prevent macrophage recruitment and polarization in the TME aimed to target the chemoattractant CCL2. However, although preclinical studies showed promising results and effectively abrogated macrophage recruitment to the TME, anti-CCL2 antibodies failed in clinical studies [126]. Therefore, studies need to be conducted to develop strategies to target macrophage recruitment or polarization into M2 phenotype to inhibit tumor progression.

4. Conclusion

Macrophages are key to the behavior of tumors and metastatic dissemination. TNBC, while missing specific targetable markers amenable to treatment, is rife with a potentially vulnerable population of macrophages, M2 polarized macrophages in particular. This population in primary tumor sites can be specifically and selectively targeted to (1) induce antitumor immunity and drug sensitivity, (2) produce a theranostic gene for imaging and treatment of the TAM population, and (3) image TAMs in TNBC for diagnosis or assessing response to therapy. Furthermore, M2 macrophages interact with non-hematopoietic cells in BM to maintain cellular quiescence/dormancy, which can be selectively repolarized to an M1 type population to reverse tumor cell quiescence/dormancy and enable systemic therapy.

Acknowledgements

This work was supported by grant awards from METAvivor Foundation and New Jersey Commission on Cancer Research.

Conflict of interest

FIS, RP, and WA are inventors on a pending patent application related to the CSSTRESAC peptide and associated technology. They are entitled to royalty payments from licensing or commercialization. RP and WA are founders and equity stockholders of PhageNova Bio, which has licensed this IP. RP is the Chief Scientific Officer and a paid consultant for PhageNova Bio. These conflicts are managed by Rutgers, The State University of New Jersey. The remaining authors declare no conflicts of interest.

Author details

Anupama Hooda-Nehra[1,2], Tracey L. Smith[1,3], Alejandra I. Ferrer[2,4], Fernanda I. Staquicini[1,3], Wadih Arap[1,2*], Renata Pasqualini[1,3] and Pranela Rameshwar[1,2*]

1 Rutgers Cancer Institute of New Jersey, Newark, NJ, USA

2 Division of Hematology/Oncology, Department of Medicine, Rutgers New Jersey Medical School, Newark, NJ, USA

3 Division of Cancer Biology, Department of Radiation Oncology, Rutgers New Jersey Medical School, Newark, NJ, USA

4 Rutgers School of Graduate Studies, New Jersey Medical School, Newark, NJ, USA

*Address all correspondence to: wadih.arap@rutgers.edu and rameshwa@njms.rutgers.edu

References

[1] Cassetta L, Pollard JW. Targeting macrophages: Therapeutic approaches in cancer. Nature Reviews. Drug Discovery. 2018;**17**(12):887-904. DOI: 10.1038/nrd.2018.169

[2] Mantovani A, Marchesi F, Malesci A, Laghi L, Allavena P. Tumour-associated macrophages as treatment targets in oncology. Nature Reviews. Clinical Oncology. 2017;**14**(7):399-416. DOI: 10.1038/nrclinonc.2016.217

[3] Wang M, Zhao J, Zhang L, et al. Role of tumor microenvironment in tumorigenesis. Journal of Cancer. 2017;**8**(5):761-773. DOI: 10.7150/jca.17648

[4] Cendrowicz E, Sas Z, Bremer E, Rygiel TP. The role of macrophages in cancer development and therapy. Cancers (Basel). 2021;**13**(8):1946. DOI: 10.3390/cancers13081946

[5] Lewis CE, Pollard JW. Distinct role of macrophages in different tumor microenvironments. Cancer Research. 2006;**66**(2):605-612. DOI: 10.1158/0008-5472.CAN-05-4005

[6] Baradaran A, Asadzadeh Z, Hemmat N, et al. The cross-talk between tumor-associated macrophages and tumor endothelium: Recent advances in macrophage-based cancer immunotherapy. Biomedicine & Pharmacotherapy. 2022;**146**:112588. DOI: 10.1016/j.biopha.2021.112588

[7] Zitvogel L, Kepp O, Kroemer G. Immune parameters affecting the efficacy of chemotherapeutic regimens. Nature Reviews. Clinical Oncology. 2011;**8**(3):151-160. DOI: 10.1038/nrclinonc.2010.223

[8] Ostuni R, Kratochvill F, Murray PJ, Natoli G. Macrophages and cancer: From mechanisms to therapeutic implications. Trends in Immunology. 2015;**36**(4):229-239. DOI: 10.1016/j.it.2015.02.004

[9] Noy R, Pollard JW. Tumor-associated macrophages: From mechanisms to therapy. Immunity. 2014;**41**(1):49-61. DOI: 10.1016/j.immuni.2014.06.010

[10] Dvorak HF. Tumors: Wounds that do not heal. Similarities between tumor stroma generation and wound healing. The New England Journal of Medicine. 1986;**315**(26):1650-1659. DOI: 10.1056/NEJM198612253152606

[11] Murray PJ, Wynn TA. Protective and pathogenic functions of macrophage subsets. Nature Reviews. Immunology. 2011;**11**(11):723-737. DOI: 10.1038/nri3073

[12] McAllister SS, Weinberg RA. The tumour-induced systemic environment as a critical regulator of cancer progression and metastasis. Nature Cell Biology. 2014;**16**(8):717-727. DOI: 10.1038/ncb3015

[13] Mahmoud SM, Lee AH, Paish EC, et al. Tumour-infiltrating macrophages and clinical outcome in breast cancer. Journal of Clinical Pathology. 2012;**65**(2):159-163. DOI: 10.1136/jclinpath-2011-200355

[14] Zhang BC, Gao J, Wang J, et al. Tumor-associated macrophages infiltration is associated with peritumoral lymphangiogenesis and poor prognosis in lung adenocarcinoma. Medical Oncology. 2011;**28**(4):1447-1452. DOI: 10.1007/s12032-010-9638-5

[15] Nonomura N, Takayama H, Nakayama M, et al. Infiltration of tumour-associated macrophages in

prostate biopsy specimens is predictive of disease progression after hormonal therapy for prostate cancer. BJU International. 2011;**107**(12):1918-1922. DOI: 10.1111/j.1464-410X.2010.09804.x

[16] Zhang J, Yan Y, Yang Y, et al. High infiltration of tumor-associated macrophages influences poor prognosis in human gastric cancer patients, associates with the phenomenon of EMT. Medicine (Baltimore). 2016;**95**(6):e2636. DOI: 10.1097/MD.0000000000002636

[17] Pantano F, Berti P, Guida FM, et al. The role of macrophages polarization in predicting prognosis of radically resected gastric cancer patients. Journal of Cellular and Molecular Medicine. 2013;**17**(11):1415-1421. DOI: 10.1111/jcmm.12109

[18] Zhang H, Wang X, Shen Z, et al. Infiltration of diametrically polarized macrophages predicts overall survival of patients with gastric cancer after surgical resection. Gastric Cancer. 2015;**18**(4):740-750. DOI: 10.1007/s10120-014-0422-7

[19] Zhao X, Qu J, Sun Y, et al. Prognostic significance of tumor-associated macrophages in breast cancer: A meta-analysis of the literature. Oncotarget. 2017;**8**(18):30576-30586. DOI: 10.18632/oncotarget.15736

[20] Yin S, Huang J, Li Z, et al. The prognostic and Clinicopathological significance of tumor-associated macrophages in patients with gastric cancer: A meta-analysis. PLoS One. 2017;**12**(1):e0170042. DOI: 10.1371/journal.pone.0170042

[21] Hanahan D. Hallmarks of cancer: New dimensions. Cancer Discovery. 2022;**12**(1):31-46. DOI: 10.1158/2159-8290.CD-21-1059

[22] Hanahan D, Folkman J. Patterns and emerging mechanisms of the angiogenic switch during tumorigenesis. Cell. 1996;**86**(3):353-364. DOI: 10.1016/s0092-8674(00)80108-7

[23] Leek RD, Lewis CE, Whitehouse R, et al. Association of macrophage infiltration with angiogenesis and prognosis in invasive breast carcinoma. Cancer Research. 1996;**56**(20):4625-4629

[24] Laoui D, Van Overmeire E, Di Conza G, et al. Tumor hypoxia does not drive differentiation of tumor-associated macrophages but rather fine-tunes the M2-like macrophage population. Cancer Research. 2014;**74**(1):24-30. DOI: 10.1158/0008-5472.CAN-13-1196

[25] Huang S, Van Arsdall M, Tedjarati S, et al. Contributions of stromal metalloproteinase-9 to angiogenesis and growth of human ovarian carcinoma in mice. Journal of the National Cancer Institute. 2002;**94**(15):1134-1142. DOI: 10.1093/jnci/94.15.1134

[26] Chen XJ, Wu S, Yan RM, et al. The role of the hypoxia-Nrp-1 axis in the activation of M2-like tumor-associated macrophages in the tumor microenvironment of cervical cancer. Molecular Carcinogenesis. 2019;**58**(3):388-397. DOI: 10.1002/mc.22936

[27] Mantovani A, Sozzani S, Locati M, Allavena P, Sica A. Macrophage polarization: Tumor-associated macrophages as a paradigm for polarized M2 mononuclear phagocytes. Trends in Immunology. 2002;**23**(11):549-555. DOI: 10.1016/s1471-4906(02)02302-5

[28] Lawrence T, Natoli G. Transcriptional regulation of macrophage polarization: Enabling diversity with identity. Nature Reviews. Immunology.

2011;**11**(11):750-761. DOI: 10.1038/nri3088

[29] Martinez FO, Helming L, Gordon S. Alternative activation of macrophages: An immunologic functional perspective. Annual Review of Immunology. 2009;**27**:451-483. DOI: 10.1146/annurev.immunol.021908.132532

[30] Biswas SK, Mantovani A. Macrophage plasticity and interaction with lymphocyte subsets: Cancer as a paradigm. Nature Immunology. 2010;**11**(10):889-896. DOI: 10.1038/ni.1937

[31] Orecchioni M, Ghosheh Y, Pramod AB, Ley K. Macrophage polarization: Different gene signatures in M1(LPS+) vs. classically and M2(LPS-) vs. Alternatively Activated Macrophages. Frontiers in Immunology. 2019;**10**:1084. DOI: 10.3389/fimmu.2019.01084

[32] Viola A, Munari F, Sanchez-Rodriguez R, Scolaro T, Castegna A. The metabolic signature of macrophage responses. Frontiers in Immunology. 2019;**10**:1462. DOI: 10.3389/fimmu.2019.01462

[33] Malorni L, Shetty PB, De Angelis C, et al. Clinical and biologic features of triple-negative breast cancers in a large cohort of patients with long-term follow-up. Breast Cancer Research and Treatment. 2012;**136**(3):795-804. DOI: 10.1007/s10549-012-2315-y

[34] Coughlin SS. Epidemiology of breast cancer in women. Advances in Experimental Medicine and Biology. 2019;**1152**:9-29. DOI: 10.1007/978-3-030-20301-6_2

[35] Dent R, Trudeau M, Pritchard KI, et al. Triple-negative breast cancer: Clinical features and patterns of recurrence. Clinical Cancer Research. 2007;**13**(15 Pt 1):4429-4434. DOI: 10.1158/1078-0432.CCR-06-3045

[36] Dietze EC, Sistrunk C, Miranda-Carboni G, O'Regan R, Seewaldt VL. Triple-negative breast cancer in African-American women: Disparities versus biology. Nature Reviews. Cancer. 2015;**15**(4):248-254. DOI: 10.1038/nrc3896

[37] Newman LA, Kaljee LM. Health disparities and triple-negative breast cancer in African American women: A review. JAMA Surgery. 2017;**152**(5):485-493. DOI: 10.1001/jamasurg.2017.0005

[38] Schettini F, Giuliano M, De Placido S, Arpino G. Nab-paclitaxel for the treatment of triple-negative breast cancer: Rationale, clinical data and future perspectives. Cancer Treatment Reviews. 2016;**50**:129-141. DOI: 10.1016/j.ctrv.2016.09.004

[39] Staquicini FI, Hajitou A, Driessen WH, et al. Targeting a cell surface vitamin D receptor on tumor-associated macrophages in triple-negative breast cancer. eLife. 2021;**10**:e65145. DOI: 10.7554/eLife.65145

[40] Bonotto M, Gerratana L, Poletto E, et al. Measures of outcome in metastatic breast cancer: Insights from a real-world scenario. The Oncologist. 2014;**19**(6):608-615. DOI: 10.1634/theoncologist.2014-0002

[41] Bianchini G, Balko JM, Mayer IA, Sanders ME, Gianni L. Triple-negative breast cancer: Challenges and opportunities of a heterogeneous disease. Nature Reviews. Clinical Oncology. 2016;**13**(11):674-690. DOI: 10.1038/nrclinonc.2016.66

[42] Carey LA, Dees EC, Sawyer L, et al. The triple negative paradox: Primary tumor chemosensitivity of breast

cancer subtypes. Clinical Cancer Research. 2007;**13**(8):2329-2334. DOI: 10.1158/1078-0432.CCR-06-1109

[43] Balko JM, Giltnane JM, Wang K, et al. Molecular profiling of the residual disease of triple-negative breast cancers after neoadjuvant chemotherapy identifies actionable therapeutic targets. Cancer Discovery. 2014;**4**(2):232-245. DOI: 10.1158/2159-8290.CD-13-0286

[44] Garrido-Castro AC, Lin NU, Polyak K. Insights into molecular classifications of triple-negative breast cancer: Improving patient selection for treatment. Cancer Discovery. 2019;**9**(2):176-198. DOI: 10.1158/2159-8290.CD-18-1177

[45] Khan MA, Jain VK, Rizwanullah M, Ahmad J, Jain K. PI3K/AKT/mTOR pathway inhibitors in triple-negative breast cancer: A review on drug discovery and future challenges. Drug Discovery Today. 2019;**24**(11):2181-2191. DOI: 10.1016/j.drudis.2019.09.001

[46] Lyons TG, Traina TA. Emerging novel therapeutics in triple-negative breast cancer. Advances in Experimental Medicine and Biology. 2019;**1152**:377-399. DOI: 10.1007/978-3-030-20301-6_20

[47] Marra A, Viale G, Curigliano G. Recent advances in triple negative breast cancer: The immunotherapy era. BMC Medicine. 2019;**17**(1):90. DOI: 10.1186/s12916-019-1326-5

[48] Loi S, Sirtaine N, Piette F, et al. Prognostic and predictive value of tumor-infiltrating lymphocytes in a phase III randomized adjuvant breast cancer trial in node-positive breast cancer comparing the addition of docetaxel to doxorubicin with doxorubicin-based chemotherapy: BIG 02-98. Journal of Clinical Oncology. 2013;**31**(7):860-867. DOI: 10.1200/JCO.2011.41.0902

[49] Wimberly H, Brown JR, Schalper K, et al. PD-L1 expression correlates with tumor-infiltrating lymphocytes and response to neoadjuvant chemotherapy in breast cancer. Cancer Immunology Research. 2015;**3**(4):326-332. DOI: 10.1158/2326-6066.CIR-14-0133

[50] Ali HR, Glont SE, Blows FM, et al. PD-L1 protein expression in breast cancer is rare, enriched in basal-like tumours and associated with infiltrating lymphocytes. Annals of Oncology. 2015;**26**(7):1488-1493. DOI: 10.1093/annonc/mdv192

[51] Karn T, Jiang T, Hatzis C, et al. Association between genomic metrics and immune infiltration in triple-negative breast cancer. JAMA Oncology. 2017;**3**(12):1707-1711. DOI: 10.1001/jamaoncol.2017.2140

[52] Safonov A, Jiang T, Bianchini G, et al. Immune gene expression is associated with genomic aberrations in breast cancer. Cancer Research. 2017;**77**(12):3317-3324. DOI: 10.1158/0008-5472.CAN-16-3478

[53] Shen M, Pan H, Chen Y, et al. A review of current progress in triple-negative breast cancer therapy. Open Medicine (Wars). 2020;**15**(1):1143-1149. DOI: 10.1515/med-2020-0138

[54] Hanahan D, Weinberg RA. Hallmarks of cancer: The next generation. Cell. 2011;**144**(5):646-674. DOI: 10.1016/j.cell.2011.02.013

[55] Nicolini A, Ferrari P, Rossi G, Carpi A. Tumour growth and immune evasion as targets for a new strategy in advanced cancer. Endocrine-Related Cancer. 2018;**25**(11):R577-R604. DOI: 10.1530/ERC-18-0142

[56] Mittendorf EA, Philips AV, Meric-Bernstam F, et al. PD-L1 expression in triple-negative breast cancer. Cancer Immunology Research. 2014;**2**(4):361-370. DOI: 10.1158/2326-6066.CIR-13-0127

[57] Denkert C, von Minckwitz G, Darb-Esfahani S, et al. Tumour-infiltrating lymphocytes and prognosis in different subtypes of breast cancer: A pooled analysis of 3771 patients treated with neoadjuvant therapy. The Lancet Oncology. 2018;**19**(1):40-50. DOI: 10.1016/S1470-2045(17)30904-X

[58] Luen S, Virassamy B, Savas P, Salgado R, Loi S. The genomic landscape of breast cancer and its interaction with host immunity. Breast. 2016;**29**:241-250. DOI: 10.1016/j.breast.2016.07.015

[59] Nanda R, Chow LQ, Dees EC, et al. Pembrolizumab in patients with advanced triple-negative breast cancer: Phase Ib KEYNOTE-012 study. Journal of Clinical Oncology. 2016;**34**(21):2460-2467. DOI: 10.1200/JCO.2015.64.8931

[60] Adams S, Schmid P, Rugo HS, et al. Pembrolizumab monotherapy for previously treated metastatic triple-negative breast cancer: Cohort a of the phase II KEYNOTE-086 study. Annals of Oncology. 2019;**30**(3):397-404. DOI: 10.1093/annonc/mdy517

[61] Winer EP, Lipatov O, Im SA, et al. Pembrolizumab versus investigator-choice chemotherapy for metastatic triple-negative breast cancer (KEYNOTE-119): A randomised, open-label, phase 3 trial. The Lancet Oncology. 2021;**22**(4):499-511. DOI: 10.1016/S1470-2045(20)30754-3

[62] Schmid P, Cortes J, Dent R, et al. Event-free survival with Pembrolizumab in early triple-negative breast cancer. The New England Journal of Medicine. 2022;**386**(6):556-567. DOI: 10.1056/NEJMoa2112651

[63] Schmid P, Cortes J, Pusztai L, et al. Pembrolizumab for early triple-negative breast cancer. The New England Journal of Medicine. 2020;**382**(9):810-821. DOI: 10.1056/NEJMoa1910549

[64] Schmid P, Adams S, Rugo HS, et al. Atezolizumab and nab-paclitaxel in advanced triple-negative breast cancer. The New England Journal of Medicine. 2018;**379**(22):2108-2121. DOI: 10.1056/NEJMoa1809615

[65] Miles D, Gligorov J, Andre F, et al. Primary results from IMpassion131, a double-blind, placebo-controlled, randomised phase III trial of first-line paclitaxel with or without atezolizumab for unresectable locally advanced/metastatic triple-negative breast cancer. Annals of Oncology. 2021;**32**(8):994-1004. DOI: 10.1016/j.annonc.2021.05.801

[66] Stein M, Keshav S, Harris N, Gordon S. Interleukin 4 potently enhances murine macrophage mannose receptor activity: A marker of alternative immunologic macrophage activation. The Journal of Experimental Medicine. 1992;**176**(1):287-292. DOI: 10.1084/jem.176.1.287

[67] Cui C, Chakraborty K, Tang XA, et al. A lysosome-targeted DNA nanodevice selectively targets macrophages to attenuate tumours. Nature Nanotechnology. 2021;**16**(12):1394-1402. DOI: 10.1038/s41565-021-00988-z

[68] Sillerud LO, Neuwelt AJ, Staquicini FI, Arap W, Pasqualini R. Repurposing Ferumoxytol as a breast cancer-associated macrophage tracer with five-dimensional quantitative [Fe]MRI of SPION dynamics. Cancers (Basel). 2021;**13**(15):3802. DOI: 10.3390/cancers13153802

[69] Walker ND, Elias M, Guiro K, et al. Exosomes from differentially activated macrophages influence dormancy or resurgence of breast cancer cells within bone marrow stroma. Cell Death & Disease. 2019;**10**(2):59. DOI: 10.1038/s41419-019-1304-z

[70] Bonam SR, Wang F, Muller S. Lysosomes as a therapeutic target. Nature Reviews. Drug Discovery. 2019;**18**(12):923-948. DOI: 10.1038/s41573-019-0036-1

[71] Li J, Fan C. A DNA nanodevice boosts tumour immunity. Nature Nanotechnology. 2021;**16**(12):1306-1307. DOI: 10.1038/s41565-021-01002-2

[72] Song W, Wang F, Savini M, et al. TFEB regulates lysosomal proteostasis. Human Molecular Genetics. 2013;**22**(10):1994-2009. DOI: 10.1093/hmg/ddt052

[73] Settembre C, Di Malta C, Polito VA, et al. TFEB links autophagy to lysosomal biogenesis. Science. 2011;**332**(6036):1429-1433. DOI: 10.1126/science.1204592

[74] Barrett AJ, Kembhavi AA, Brown MA, et al. L-trans-Epoxysuccinyl-leucylamido(4-guanidino)butane (E-64) and its analogues as inhibitors of cysteine proteinases including cathepsins B, H and L. Biochemical Journal. 1982;**201**(1):189-198. DOI: 10.1042/bj2010189

[75] Honey K, Rudensky AY. Lysosomal cysteine proteases regulate antigen presentation. Nature Reviews. Immunology. 2003;**3**(6):472-482. DOI: 10.1038/nri1110

[76] Matsumoto K, Mizoue K, Kitamura K, et al. Structural basis of inhibition of cysteine proteases by E-64 and its derivatives. Biopolymers. 1999;**51**(1):99-107. DOI: 10.1002/(SICI)1097-0282(1999)51:1<99::AID-BIP11>3.0.CO;2-R

[77] Medd PG, Chain BM. Protein degradation in MHC class II antigen presentation: Opportunities for immunomodulation. Seminars in Cell & Developmental Biology. 2000;**11**(3):203-210. DOI: 10.1006/scdb.2000.0162

[78] Piao S, Amaravadi RK. Targeting the lysosome in cancer. Annals of the New York Academy of Sciences. 2016;**1371**(1):45-54. DOI: 10.1111/nyas.12953

[79] Cao GD, He XB, Sun Q, et al. The oncolytic virus in cancer diagnosis and treatment. Frontiers in Oncology. 2020;**10**:1786. DOI: 10.3389/fonc.2020.01786

[80] Jin S, Wang Q, Wu H, Pang D, Xu S. Oncolytic viruses for triple negative breast cancer and beyond. Biomarker Research. 2021;**9**(1):71. DOI: 10.1186/s40364-021-00318-4

[81] Hacker UT, Bentler M, Kaniowska D, Morgan M, Buning H. Towards clinical implementation of adeno-associated virus (AAV) vectors for cancer gene therapy: Current status and future perspectives. Cancers (Basel). 2020;**12**(7):1889. DOI: 10.3390/cancers12071889

[82] Hajitou A, Trepel M, Lilley CE, et al. A hybrid vector for ligand-directed tumor targeting and molecular imaging. Cell. 2006;**125**(2):385-398. DOI: 10.1016/j.cell.2006.02.042

[83] Paoloni MC, Tandle A, Mazcko C, et al. Launching a novel preclinical infrastructure: Comparative oncology trials consortium directed therapeutic targeting of TNFalpha to cancer vasculature. PLoS One. 2009;**4**(3):e4972. DOI: 10.1371/journal.pone.0004972

[84] Smith TL, Yuan Z, Cardo-Vila M, et al. AAVP displaying octreotide for ligand-directed therapeutic transgene delivery in neuroendocrine tumors of the pancreas. Proceedings of the National Academy of Sciences of the United States of America. 2016;**113**(9):2466-2471. DOI: 10.1073/pnas.1525709113

[85] Giordano RJ, Cardo-Vila M, Lahdenranta J, Pasqualini R, Arap W. Biopanning and rapid analysis of selective interactive ligands. Nature Medicine. 2001;**7**(11):1249-1253. DOI: 10.1038/nm1101-1249

[86] Guy CT, Cardiff RD, Muller WJ. Induction of mammary tumors by expression of polyomavirus middle T oncogene: A transgenic mouse model for metastatic disease. Molecular and Cellular Biology. 1992;**12**(3):954-961. DOI: 10.1128/mcb.12.3.954-961.1992

[87] Hajitou A, Baramova EN, Bajou K, et al. FGF-3 and FGF-4 elicit distinct oncogenic properties in mouse mammary myoepithelial cells. Oncogene. 1998;**17**(16):2059-2071. DOI: 10.1038/sj.onc.1202126

[88] Soghomonyan S, Hajitou A, Rangel R, et al. Molecular PET imaging of HSV1-tk reporter gene expression using [18F]FEAU. Nature Protocols. 2007;**2**(2):416-423. DOI: 10.1038/nprot.2007.49

[89] Ferrara F, Staquicini DI, Driessen WHP, et al. Targeted molecular-genetic imaging and ligand-directed therapy in aggressive variant prostate cancer. Proceedings of the National Academy of Sciences of the United States of America. 2016;**113**(45):12786-12791. DOI: 10.1073/pnas.1615400113

[90] Dobroff AS, D'Angelo S, Eckhardt BL, et al. Towards a transcriptome-based theranostic platform for unfavorable breast cancer phenotypes. Proceedings of the National Academy of Sciences of the United States of America. 2016;**113**(45):12780-12785. DOI: 10.1073/pnas.1615288113

[91] Langsjoen J, Neuwelt A, Eberhardt S, et al. A comparison of ferumoxytol with gadolinium as contrast agents for the diagnostic magnetic resonance imaging of osteomyelitis. Magnetic Resonance Imaging. 2020;**71**:45-54. DOI: 10.1016/j.mri.2020.04.012

[92] Ramanathan RK, Korn RL, Raghunand N, et al. Correlation between Ferumoxytol uptake in tumor lesions by MRI and response to Nanoliposomal irinotecan in patients with advanced solid tumors: A pilot study. Clinical Cancer Research. 2017;**23**(14):3638-3648. DOI: 10.1158/1078-0432.CCR-16-1990

[93] Nguyen KL, Yoshida T, Kathuria-Prakash N, et al. Multicenter safety and practice for off-label diagnostic use of Ferumoxytol in MRI. Radiology. 2019;**293**(3):554-564. DOI: 10.1148/radiol.2019190477

[94] Li W, Tutton S, Vu AT, et al. First-pass contrast-enhanced magnetic resonance angiography in humans using ferumoxytol, a novel ultrasmall superparamagnetic iron oxide (USPIO)-based blood pool agent. Journal of Magnetic Resonance Imaging. 2005;**21**(1):46-52. DOI: 10.1002/jmri.20235

[95] Bashir MR, Bhatti L, Marin D, Nelson RC. Emerging applications for ferumoxytol as a contrast agent in MRI. Journal of Magnetic Resonance Imaging. 2015;**41**(4):884-898. DOI: 10.1002/jmri.24691

[96] Finn JP, Nguyen KL, Hu P, Ferumoxytol vs. Gadolinium agents for contrast-enhanced MRI: Thoughts on

evolving indications, risks, and benefits. Journal of Magnetic Resonance Imaging. 2017;**46**(3):919-923. DOI: 10.1002/jmri.25580

[97] Cao Q, Yan X, Chen K, et al. Macrophages as a potential tumor-microenvironment target for noninvasive imaging of early response to anticancer therapy. Biomaterials. 2018;**152**:63-76. DOI: 10.1016/j.biomaterials.2017.10.036

[98] Aghighi M, Theruvath AJ, Pareek A, et al. Magnetic resonance imaging of tumor-associated macrophages: Clinical translation. Clinical Cancer Research. 2018;**24**(17):4110-4118. DOI: 10.1158/1078-0432.CCR-18-0673

[99] Zanganeh S, Hutter G, Spitler R, et al. Iron oxide nanoparticles inhibit tumour growth by inducing pro-inflammatory macrophage polarization in tumour tissues. Nature Nanotechnology. 2016;**11**(11):986-994. DOI: 10.1038/nnano.2016.168

[100] Kroner A, Greenhalgh AD, Zarruk JG, et al. TNF and increased intracellular iron alter macrophage polarization to a detrimental M1 phenotype in the injured spinal cord. Neuron. 2014;**83**(5):1098-1116. DOI: 10.1016/j.neuron.2014.07.027

[101] Zhou Y, Que KT, Zhang Z, et al. Iron overloaded polarizes macrophage to proinflammation phenotype through ROS/acetyl-p53 pathway. Cancer Medicine. 2018;**7**(8):4012-4022. DOI: 10.1002/cam4.1670

[102] Santoni M, Romagnoli E, Saladino T, et al. Triple negative breast cancer: Key role of tumor-associated macrophages in regulating the activity of anti-PD-1/PD-L1 agents. Biochimica Et Biophysica Acta. Reviews on Cancer. 2018;**1869**(1):78-84. DOI: 10.1016/j.bbcan.2017.10.007

[103] Huang Y, Hsu JC, Koo H, Cormode DP. Repurposing ferumoxytol: Diagnostic and therapeutic applications of an FDA-approved nanoparticle. Theranostics. 2022;**12**(2):796-816. DOI: 10.7150/thno.67375

[104] Mohanty S, Yerneni K, Theruvath JL, et al. Nanoparticle enhanced MRI can monitor macrophage response to CD47 mAb immunotherapy in osteosarcoma. Cell Death & Disease. 2019;**10**(2):36. DOI: 10.1038/s41419-018-1285-3

[105] Walker ND, Patel J, Munoz JL, et al. The bone marrow niche in support of breast cancer dormancy. Cancer Letters. 2016;**380**(1):263-271. DOI: 10.1016/j.canlet.2015.10.033

[106] Ghajar CM, Peinado H, Mori H, et al. The perivascular niche regulates breast tumour dormancy. Nature Cell Biology. 2013;**15**(7):807-817. DOI: 10.1038/ncb2767

[107] Sosa MS, Bragado P, Aguirre-Ghiso JA. Mechanisms of disseminated cancer cell dormancy: An awakening field. Nature Reviews. Cancer. 2014;**14**(9):611-622. DOI: 10.1038/nrc3793

[108] Reya T, Morrison SJ, Clarke MF, Weissman IL. Stem cells, cancer, and cancer stem cells. Nature. 2001;**414**(6859):105-111. DOI: 10.1038/35102167

[109] Risson E, Nobre AR, Maguer-Satta V, Aguirre-Ghiso JA. The current paradigm and challenges ahead for the dormancy of disseminated tumor cells. Nature Cancer. 2020;**1**(7):672-680. DOI: 10.1038/s43018-020-0088-5

[110] Redig AJ, McAllister SS. Breast cancer as a systemic disease: A view of metastasis. Journal of Internal Medicine. 2013;**274**(2):113-126. DOI: 10.1111/joim.12084

[111] Blagosklonny MV. Target for cancer therapy: Proliferating cells or stem cells. Leukemia. 2006;**20**(3):385-391. DOI: 10.1038/sj.leu.2404075

[112] Bushnell GG, Deshmukh AP, den Hollander P, et al. Breast cancer dormancy: Need for clinically relevant models to address current gaps in knowledge. NPJ Breast Cancer. 2021;**7**(1):66. DOI: 10.1038/s41523-021-00269-x

[113] Jagannathan-Bogdan M, Zon LI. Hematopoiesis. Development. 2013;**140**(12):2463-2467. DOI: 10.1242/dev.083147

[114] Morrison SJ, Scadden DT. The bone marrow niche for haematopoietic stem cells. Nature. 2014;**505**(7483):327-334. DOI: 10.1038/nature12984

[115] Bliss SA, Sinha G, Sandiford OA, et al. Mesenchymal stem cell-derived exosomes stimulate cycling quiescence and early breast cancer dormancy in bone marrow. Cancer Research. 2016;**76**(19):5832-5844. DOI: 10.1158/0008-5472.CAN-16-1092

[116] Sandiford OA, Donnelly RJ, El-Far MH, et al. Mesenchymal stem cell-secreted extracellular vesicles instruct stepwise dedifferentiation of breast cancer cells into dormancy at the bone marrow perivascular region. Cancer Research. 2021;**81**(6):1567-1582. DOI: 10.1158/0008-5472.CAN-20-2434

[117] Sinha G, Ferrer AI, Moore CA, Naaldijk Y, Rameshwar P. Gap junctions and breast cancer dormancy. Trends in Cancer. 2020;**6**(4):348-357. DOI: 10.1016/j.trecan.2020.01.013

[118] Lim PK, Bliss SA, Patel SA, et al. Gap junction-mediated import of microRNA from bone marrow stromal cells can elicit cell cycle quiescence in breast cancer cells. Cancer Research. 2011;**71**(5):1550-1560. DOI: 10.1158/0008-5472.CAN-10-2372

[119] Sinha G, Ferrer AI, Ayer S, et al. Specific N-cadherin-dependent pathways drive human breast cancer dormancy in bone marrow. Life Science Alliance. 2021;**4**(7):e202000969. DOI: 10.26508/lsa.202000969

[120] Linde N, Casanova-Acebes M, Sosa MS, et al. Macrophages orchestrate breast cancer early dissemination and metastasis. Nature Communications. 2018;**9**(1):21. DOI: 10.1038/s41467-017-02481-5

[121] Ma RY, Zhang H, Li XF, et al. Monocyte-derived macrophages promote breast cancer bone metastasis outgrowth. The Journal of Experimental Medicine. 2020;**217**(11):e20191920. DOI: 10.1084/jem.20191820

[122] Qian B, Deng Y, Im JH, et al. A distinct macrophage population mediates metastatic breast cancer cell extravasation, establishment and growth. PLoS One. 2009;**4**(8):e6562. DOI: 10.1371/journal.pone.0006562

[123] Boutilier AJ, Elsawa SF. Macrophage polarization states in the tumor microenvironment. International Journal of Molecular Sciences. 2021;**22**(13):6995. DOI: 10.3390/ijms22136995

[124] Weng YS, Tseng HY, Chen YA, et al. MCT-1/miR-34a/IL-6/IL-6R signaling axis promotes EMT progression, cancer stemness and M2 macrophage polarization in triple-negative breast cancer. Molecular Cancer. 2019;**18**(1):42. DOI: 10.1186/s12943-019-0988-0

[125] Mu X, Shi W, Xu Y, et al. Tumor-derived lactate induces M2 macrophage polarization via the activation of the

ERK/STAT3 signaling pathway in breast cancer. Cell Cycle. 2018;**17**(4):428-438. DOI: 10.1080/15384101.2018.1444305

[126] Lim SY, Yuzhalin AE, Gordon-Weeks AN, Muschel RJ. Targeting the CCL2-CCR2 signaling axis in cancer metastasis. Oncotarget. 2016;**7**(19):28697-28710. DOI: 10.18632/oncotarget.7376

Section 8

Stem Cells-Derived Macrophages

Chapter 19

Pluripotent Stem Cell Derived Macrophages: Current Applications and Future Perspectives

Shyam Sushama Jose and Lesley M. Forrester

Abstract

The ability to derive macrophages from human-induced pluripotent stem cells (iPSCs) provides an unlimited source of genotype-specific cells with the potential to play a role in advancing our understanding of macrophage biology in both homeostasis and disease. While sharing many of the functional characteristics of monocyte-derived macrophages, iPSC-derived macrophages have also been shown to have phenotypical and functional features associated with tissue resident macrophages. These features present new opportunities to develop models of human disease and to understand the role of developmental or tissue context in innate immune cell function. iPSCs-derived macrophages have also been identified as a highly attractive source for cell and gene therapy in the treatment of diverse degenerative diseases based on their anti-inflammatory activity, their ability to clear scarred cells by phagocytosis, and providing extracellular matrices. We review and present a concise discussion on macrophage differentiation from stem cells highlighting their advantages over classical monocyte-derived macrophages in modelling organ specific macrophages. We summarize the various disease models utilizing iPSCs-derived macrophages including hereditary syndromes and host-pathogen interactions in tissue repair and the strategies used to mimic pathological phenotypes. Finally, we describe the pre-clinical studies that have addressed the application of iPSCs-derived macrophages as a therapeutic intervention.

Keywords: iPSCs, macrophages, polarization, inflammation, regeneration, cell therapy

1. Introduction

Macrophages were historically considered as specialized immune cells that are resident in every tissue. They are professional phagocytic cells and are considered to be one of the most evolutionary conserved components of the innate immune system [1]. However, studies of the past two decades identified several additional functions of macrophages particularly those involved in maintaining tissue homeostasis such as wound healing and regeneration [2]. Macrophage populations within the tissue were originally assumed to be continuously replaced by the differentiation of monocytes derived from peripheral blood [3, 4]. However recent studies using methods such as lineage tracing and single cell transcriptomics have established that several macrophage populations resident in organs including brain, lung, intestine and liver, originate from yolk-sac (YS) myeloid precursor cells that were seeded within the tissues during early embryonic hematopoiesis [5]. These myeloid precursors differentiate into macrophages (microglia in case of brain) within their resident tissue site, and are self-maintained throughout the life course of the organism [5]. Tissue resident macrophages (TRMs) are functionally distinct from macrophages derived from the more accessible circulating blood monocytes but their yolk sac origin makes them difficult to study [5]. In order to successfully study these cells *in vitro*, researchers have develop methods that permit functional TRMs to be isolated [5]. *In vitro* strategies to replicate the tissue resident differentiation of macrophages in a way that mimics their tissue specific developmental and differentiation pathways have been developed using a variety of growth factors and cytokines [6]. However, cells produced using these methods do not completely recapitulate the properties of TRMs and it would be challenging to scale up and produce large numbers of cells.

The ground-breaking discovery that human somatic cells could be reprogramed into induced pluripotent stem cells (iPSCs) that are capable of differentiating into any cell type has revolutionized many areas of medical research including macrophage biology [7]. Several studies have shown that human iPSCs can be differentiated into macrophage populations that are phenotypically and functionally comparable to human macrophages. The major advantage of the iPSCs-derived macrophages is that they share some phenotypic and functional profiles with both tissue resident macrophages and monocyte derived macrophages (MDMs) [8]. Here, we review the potential of iPSCs derived macrophages in both classical immune function as well as their tissue repair and regeneration properties. We summarize the various protocols that have been used for macrophage production from iPSCs, discuss their disease modeling potential including hereditary and pathogen associated diseases and describe some of the pre-clinical trials lay the foundations for their use in cell therapies.

2. Human induced pluripotent stem cells for macrophage production *in vitro*

The generation of iPSCs from adult somatic cells by the introduction of four genes encoding the "Yamanaka" transcription factors, octamer-binding transcription factor 3/4 (OCT3/4), sex determining region Y-box 2 (SOX2), Kruppel-like factor 4 (KLF4), and myelocytomatosis viral oncogene homolog (MYC), was first reported in 2006 [9]. Resultant iPSCs were shown to be comparable to embryonic stem cells (ESCs), thus providing an ethical strategy for creating clonal PSC lines that did not involve the destruction of human embryos [10]. Initially reprogramming of somatic cells to iPSCs was successfully performed using genome integrating retroviral or lentiviral vectors such as retroviruses and lentiviruses [7]. Though viral integration was efficient, it was associated with risks of random mutational insertions into the genome. Alternate non-viral integration methods such as plasmids, synthetic mRNA, minicircle DNA molecules and small chemical molecules to generate iPSCs reduced random mutations but the efficiency of generating iPSCs was low [7, 8]. Sendai virus is now commonly used for iPSC generation as its replication is limited within the cytoplasm and it does not integrate into the genome. Initially skin fibroblasts were used for reprogramming iPSCs, but other easily accessible cells such as peripheral blood monocytes and renal epithelial cells from urine have been successfully used as the starting cells [11, 12]. iPSCs are able to be differentiated into the three embryonic germ layers namely ectoderm, endoderm and mesoderm and can differentiate into somatic cells associated with all cell lineages [13].

Following the generation of stable iPSCs, their pluripotent properties are maintained using specific growth factors [9]. Removal of these maintenance factors results in spontaneous differentiation and, under appropriate conditions the formation of 3-dimensional (3D) embryoid bodies (EBs) that are considered to mimic early embryogenesis [14]. Differentiation factors such as cytokines and small molecules have been used to stimulate specific differentiation pathways resulting in the production of cells displaying phenotypes and gene expression patterns of almost any cell type including cells of the blood and immune system [15].

Doetschman and colleagues were the first to report that hematopoietic cell types could be produced from mouse embryonic stem cells (ESCs) by demonstrating structures resembling blood islands in cystic embryoid bodies (EBs) that were comparable to the primitive wave of hematopoiesis in the yolk sac [16]. Differentiation protocols were subsequently developed and refined to include the use of feeder cells, extracellular matrices and specific growth factors [17–20]. Many of these protocols failed to generate the long-term reconstituting hematopoietic stem cells (HSCs) associated with the definitive wave of hematopoietic development and a significant amount of research has gone into addressing this problem in both the mouse and human systems [21–24]. The production of macrophages was reported even in the first, rather crude differentiation protocols with the ability to harvest on regular basis for several weeks represented a significant advance in the field [18, 25]. The fact that these differentiation protocols most likely mimic the primitive wave of hematopoiesis it is not surprising that resultant cells have some features that are comparable to TRMs.

The production of macrophages from human iPSCs is now well established and they are considered to have features associated with both YS-derived TRMs as well as MDMs [5]. As iPSCs can been maintained indefinitely in culture and can be readily genetically manipulated, they can therefore provide an inexhaustible source of macrophages carrying any desired genetic alteration. The first protocols that were developed involved the co-culture of iPSCs with OP9 mouse stromal cell monolayers to induce hematopoietic differentiation, followed by expansion of myeloid progenitors and selective differentiation into macrophages by using growth factors to differentiate dendritic cells and macrophages [26, 27]. These protocols were further modified to establish embryoid body (EB)-based protocols for IPSC-derived macrophage differentiation. We have used a modified serum-free protocol in which EB-based hematopoiesis is used to generate monocyte-like cells in suspension that can then be differentiated into mature macrophages [28]. Briefly, differentiation from human iPSCs is initiated by the removal of pluripotency factors and the addition of stem cell factor (SCF), bone morphogenetic protein (BMP)-4 and vascular endothelial growth factor (VEGF) to induce EB formation. The addition of interleukin (IL)-3 and macrophage colony stimulating factor (M-CSF) to EBs that are then plated down onto the culture plates results in the production of monocyte precursors that are released into suspension. Monocyte-like cells are then plated down and differentiated into mature macrophages by the addition of M-CSF [29]. iPSCs derived macrophages express macrophage-specific markers including cluster of differentiation (CD)11b, CD163, and CD169 [30]. Macrophages generated from iPSCs that carried the Zeiss Green reporter gene integrated into the adeno-associated virus integration site 1 (*AAVS1*) locus showed that neither expression of the reporter nor the targeting of the *AAVS1* locus affected of macrophage phenotype confirming the idea that genetically manipulated macrophages can be generated using this strategy [30].

2.1 iPSCs-derived macrophages share features of MDM

Yeung and colleagues demonstrated that the iPSCs-derived macrophages exhibited gene expression profiles and responsiveness to external stimuli that were comparable to MDMs. Their data demonstrated that untreated iPSCs-derived macrophages and MDMs expressed 12,599 human genes overlapping and a further 93% of these genes were expressed to a similar level [31]. This pattern of gene expression iPSCs-derived macrophages and MDMs remained consistent even after stimulation, as upon *Chlamydia trachomatis* infection, the two cell types had more than 2000 differentially expressed genes in common [31].

iPSCs-derived macrophages secrete comparable levels of cytokines as MDMs upon stimulation with pattern recognition receptors such as toll-like receptor (TLR) agonist [32]. They are able to phagocytose live *Salmonella typhi* or fungal particles like zymosan [30, 33]. Most importantly, iPSCs-derived macrophages retain plasticity which is one of the key characteristic of macrophages [34]. Naive macrophages express an M0-like steady state phenotype, which can be switch to either an inflammatory (M1) or immunosuppressive (M2) function based on their microenvironment. It is proposed that due to the genetic and functional similarities between iPSCs-derived macrophages and primary macrophages, the former could be used as a tool to model macrophage polarization in inflammatory diseases and genetic diseases such as autosomal recessive disorders. A study from Matsuo et al modeling a disease *fibro dysplasia ossificans progressiva* using iPSCs derived macrophages showed the potential of 2D and 3D based differentiation of macrophages having a differential role in their polarization potential [35]. While the 2D iPSCs-derived macrophages could be polarized to either M1 or M2, the 3D differentiated macrophages showed a mixed M1 and M2 like functional features, highlighting the complexity of macrophage plasticity.

2.2 iPSCs derived macrophages model tissue resident macrophages

Although iPSCs-derived macrophages have demonstrated similar phenotypic, functional, and transcriptomic characteristics to MDMs as discussed above, they are also reported to have comparable characteristics to tissue resident macrophages (TRMs). This TRM like phenotype gives iPSCs-derived macrophages an advantage over other models such as MDMs or monocytic cell lines such as THP-1. It has been recognized that the standard hematopoietic differentiation protocols of iPSCs resemble the primitive rather than definitive wave of hematopoiesis *in vivo* [36]. To confirm this theory, Vanhee and colleagues used a reporter PSC line with myeloblastosis proto-oncogene with a green fluorescent protein (*MYB-eGFP*), a marker for definitive hematopoietic stem cell (HSC)-dependent hematopoiesis, and as expected the *in vitro* generation of EB-based iPSCs derived macrophages lacked *MYB*+ HSCs [37]. The results were further validated by demonstrating that clustered regularly interspaced short palindromic repeats and its associated protein 9 (CRISPR/Cas9) knockout of *MYB* in human iPSCs, did not impact macrophage differentiation [38]. The theory was further verified in experiments where two important transcription regulators of YS hematopoiesis transcription factor PU.1 encoding gene *SPI1* and Runt-related transcription factor 1 gene *RUNX1* were knocked out in iPSCs, they were unable to produce mature macrophages [37, 38]. Several studies have indicated the TRM nature of iPSCs-derived macrophages is based on *in vitro* microglia modeling. Indeed, several cytokine mediated iPSCs to microglia-like cell differentiation protocols were published in recent years using coculture with iPSCs-derived neurons and astrocytes or using conditioned media from those cell types to recapitulate organ-specific microenvironment [39]. Takata and colleagues further demonstrated by macrophages derived from iPSCs using a protocol that specifically resembles primitive hematopoiesis and yolk sac macrophages that they are very similar to TRMs [5]. They did this by engrafting iPSCs derived macrophages into the mouse brain which then underwent functional and morphological changes to become microglia, while the iPSCs derived macrophages engrafted to the lung of the Pulmonary Alveolar Proteinosis (PAP) mouse model matured into alveolar macrophages. This study showed that the iPSC-derived macrophages developed to microglia-like cells *in vivo* and showed genomic profile similar to that of both human adult and foetal microglia, while in the lung of the PAP mouse model they eliminated the surfactant protein that had accumulated as a result of the disease. Our lab recently used iPSCs-derived macrophages to model the erythroblastic Island (EBI) niche *in vitro* by genetic programming with the transcription factor, KLF1 [29].

2.3 iPSCs derived macrophages in disease modeling

Another important feature of human iPSCs derived macrophages is that iPSCs are amenable to genetic engineering and thus can be manipulated to be model genetic disease. Disease modeling can be achieved either through the production of iPSCs from patients carrying disease-causing mutations and/or specific genome-wide associations or by targeted gene edited using the (CRISPR)/Cas9 system. iPSCs-derived macrophages are increasingly being used to study genetic disease, including validation of known causative genes or identifying novel mutations associated with single nucleotide polymorphisms (SNPs) [40]. iPSCs-derived macrophages helped overcome the limitations of the poor availability of disease-specific primary macrophages in studying these rare genetic diseases. The ability to derive macrophages from iPSCs provided new opportunities to develop models relevant to human genetics, resulting in a progressive accumulation of studies describing macrophage functions in both tissue homeostasis and disease. For example, patient iPSCs-derived macrophages have been utilized to investigate several genetically inherited diseases including Blau Syndrome, Tangier disease and Gaucher disease. In additions there are studies where a diseased condition such as Dyskeratosis Congenita has been generated in iPSCs using genetic engineering technology and macrophages or myeloid cells derived from these used to understand the disease mechanism [41–44]. **Table 1** lists some of the genetic studies performed using patient iPSCs-derived macrophages, that would not have been possible using primary cells.

As well as generating valuable disease models these studies also described the novel approach of immortalizing iPSCs-derived myeloid cells using transducing lentiviral vectors that encoded genes *MYC*, polycomb complex protein gene *BMI1* and mouse double minute 2 homolog gene *MDM2,* creating a strategy to generate monocytic cell lines, with the diseased phenotype [53]. These iPSC-derived immortalized myeloid cell lines have the advantage that they can be stored and differentiated into terminally differentiated progenies and expanded from one experimental batch with reduced financial and labour costs, overcoming many of the hurdles associated with iPSCs.

2.4 iPSCs-derived macrophages in host-pathogen interactions

iPSCs-derived macrophages have also been used widely in studies relating to their classical role in infection biology. iPSCs-derived macrophages can polarized

Studies utilizing iPSCs derived macrophages for disease modeling		
Disease	**Research findings**	**References**
Tangier Disease (TD)	iPSC-derived macrophages from TD patients recapitulate the clinical defect of failed cholesterol efflux resulting in reverse cholesterol transport.	[45]
	TD effect of reverse cholesterol transport in macrophages derived from CRISPR/Cas9 induced adenosine triphosphate binding cassette subfamily A member 1 gene (*ABCA1*) knockout iPSCs.	[43]
Gaucher disease (GD)	iPSCs-derived macrophages from GD patients exhibited delayed clearance of phagocytosed RBC which was reversed when treated with recombinant glucocerebrosidase enzyme.	[42]
	Reversal of GD phenotype in iPSCs-derived macrophages using small-molecule chaperone drug.	[46]
Chronic granulomatous disease	iPSCs-derived macrophages from dihydronicotinamide-adenine dinucleotide phosphate (NADPH) oxidase defective patient showed normal phagocytic properties unlike patient MDMs, however showed a lack in reactive oxygen species production, correlating with clinical diagnosis.	[47]
Blau syndrome	iPSCs-derived macrophages from nucleotide-binding oligomerization domain-containing protein 2 (*NOD2*) mutated patient showed ligand-independent pro-inflammatory cytokine production *in vitro* upon Interferon (IFN)-γ treatment. The cytokine production was terminated upon NOD2 mutation correction by CRISPR/Cas9.	[41]
Type 1 diabetes	iPSCs-derived macrophages from Diabetic patient showed potential for antigen presentation to proinsulin-specific T cell receptors from donor-matched islet-infiltrating T cells.	[48]
Familial Mediterranean fever	Patient iPSCs-derived macrophages exhibited the disease characteristics including enhanced IL-1β secretion and hyperactivation of the pyrin inflammasome.	[49]
Mendelian Susceptibility to Mycobacterial Disease (MSMD)	iPSCs-derived macrophages from MSMD patients with autosomal recessive complete- and partial IFN-γR2 deficiency, partial IFN-γR1 deficiency and complete STAT1 deficiency demonstrated varying phenotypes including cytokine secretion for the partial and complete deficiencies.	[50]
Idiopathic Parkinson's disease	Patient iPSCs-derived microglia to confirmed findings in patients brain tissue of having elevated *IL1B, IL10* and NLRP3 expression after *in vitro* LPS stimulation. iPSCs-derived microglia showed high phagocytic capacity under basal conditions that was exacerbated upon stimulation with LPS.	[51]
Chronic infantile neurologic cutaneous and articular syndrome	iPSCs-derived macrophages from NLRP3 mutated patient showed the disease relevant phenotype of abnormal IL-1β secretion which were inhibited by anti-inflammatory compounds.	[52]
	Immortalized iPSCs-derived myeloid cells from patient recapitulated the disease phenotypes *in vitro.*	[53]

Table 1.
Summary of studies that have used iPSCs-derived monocytes and macrophages for in vitro modeling of genetic diseases.

to a pro-inflammatory or anti-inflammatory phenotype by treating with lipopolysaccharide (LPS)/IFN-γ or IL-4/IL-10, respectively [30]. These features make them a powerful *in vitro* tool to study bacterial, viral, and parasitic infections and their resultant immune responses. Hale et al infected iPSC-derived macrophages with *Salmonella enterica serovar Typhimurium* (*S. Typhimurium*) and *S. Typhi* and reported comparable data to that observed using the commonly used human monocyte-like THP1 cell line thus opening the way for their application to other bacterial infections [33].

One such example was the study of the interaction between *Staphylococcus aureus* toxin leukocidins with macrophages, which are the initial targets during *S. aureus* lung infection [54]. iPSCs-derived macrophages were susceptible to the leukocidins and triggered NLPR3 inflammasome activation resulting in IL-1β secretion and eventual cell death. CRISPR/Cas9-mediated deletion of the leukocidin receptor, complement component 5a receptor 1 (C5aR1) also known as CD88 protected the macrophages from cytotoxicity [54]. Another bacterial study using the iPSCs-derived macrophages model was on *C. trachomatis,* which causes bacterial sexually transmitted infections and preventable blindness worldwide. Yeung and colleagues demonstrated that iPSC-derived macrophages supported the full infectious life cycle of *C. trachomatis in vitro* in a manner that resembled the infection of human blood *in vivo* [31]. Using transcriptomic and proteomic profiling of the macrophage they identified that the key players in response to chlamydial infection are type I interferon and interleukin 10. This was further confirmed by knocking-out IRF5 and IL-10RA in iPSCs, which resulted in limited chlamydial infection in genetically-deficient macrophages. Though the studies mentioned above showed that bacterial infection studies using iPSCs-derived macrophages are comparable with the data generated using MDMs, one recent study clearly highlights an additional advantage of using iPSCs-derived macrophages. Nenasheva et al reported that iPSCs-derived macrophages differed from MDMs by an low-activated/low- polarized naïve-like (HLA-DR^{low} CD14^{+}CD16^{int}) phenotype compared to the HLA-DR^{high} CD14^{+}CD16^{+} phenotype of mature macrophages shown by MDMs, where HLA-DR stands for human leukocyte antigen – DR isotype [8]. These naïve-like iPSCs-derived macrophages were transcriptionally similar to pulmonary macrophages and restricted *Mycobacterium tuberculosis* growth *in vitro* by >75% higher phagocytic potential than MDMs [8]. Similarly, a study from Hong et al also showed that iPSCs-derived macrophages perform the immunological functions in response to Bacillus Calmette-Guérin a vaccine against *M. tuberculosis*, similar to MDMs by undergoing apoptosis, increased production of nitric oxide and elevated expression of Tumor necrosis factor (TNF)-α, thus demonstrating their suitability as a potential drug target [55].

Viruses require a specific cellular host for replication and so the readily available supply of infectable cells is crucial in viral research. iPSCs are ideal for this purpose because they can be differentiated into the specific cell type associated with an infectious agent, including endothelial cells for cytomegalovirus, neurons for herpes simplex virus, hepatocytes for hepatitis viruses, CD4 T-cells for human immunodeficiency virus (HIV) [56]. The field of HIV research has used iPSCs-derived macrophages widely. Using various genetic editing techniques, Kambal *et al* and Ye *et al* introduced mutations into C-C chemokine receptor type 5 (CCR5), the major coreceptor required for macrophage trophic strains of HIV and demonstrated that monocytes and macrophages differentiated from CCR5-mutated iPSCs were resistant to HIV-1 challenge [57, 58]. Kang et al confirmed this study by demonstrating that CCR5-mutant iPSCs derived macrophages showed unique and enhanced resistance to CCR5-tropic HIV challenge but were susceptible to CCR4-tropic viruses [59]. One of the most elegant studies that utilized human PSCs-derived macrophages characterized the molecular and cellular basis involved in both Zika and Dengue viral infections [60]. Using macrophages derived from both human ESCs and iPSCs, Lang et al showed that though both these viruses are closely related, their mechanism of infection was different. Zika virus disrupts the nuclear factor κB (NF-κB)-migration inhibitory factor (MIF) positive feedback loop by inhibiting the NF-κB signaling pathway and thus the infected macrophages exhibit prolonged migration but expressed low levels of pro-inflammatory cytokines and chemokines. In contrast, Dengue virus strongly activates MIF secretion and results in decreased macrophage migration. In summary the characteristics of iPSCs-derived macrophages together with genetic editing tools such as CRISPR/Cas9 has significantly enhanced our ability to study host–pathogen interactions as well as the role of human genetic variations in influencing the susceptibility to specific pathogens and disease outcomes.

2.5 iPSCs-derived macrophages in cell and regenerative therapy

Several studies performed in the last decade identified macrophages to have a prominent role in tissue repair and regeneration by their injury response features including clearing cell debris by phagocytosis, activating and resolving inflammation and promoting fibrosis by providing growth factors [61, 62]. For example the transplantation of mouse bone marrow-derived macrophages into a CCL4 mediated advanced liver injury mice model resulted in the reduction of fibrosis by increased recruitment of host effector cells such as neutrophils and secretion of regenerative factors such as matrix metallopeptidase 9 (MMP9), insulin-like growth factor 1 (IGF-1), M-CSF, vascular endothelial growth factor (VEGF) and IL10 [63]. Similarly exogenous macrophage treatments were shown to promote injury resolution in a several murine models of inflammatory and degenerative diseases including pulmonary fibrosis and osteochondral defect [64, 65]. This successful demonstration of macrophage therapy in pre-clinical models led to the use of autologous macrophages in therapeutic interventions in clinical studies against chronic liver injury and neurodegenerative diseases [66, 67]. It is thought that these repair functions are performed by the anti-inflammatory or resolving M2-polarized macrophages and several studies identified iPSCs-derived macrophages to be able to be polarized into an M2-phenotype similar to MDMs [30]. The polarization potential together with their ability for unrestricted production makes the iPSCs-derived macrophages ideal candidates for future cell therapies. Some of the studies highlighting these *in vivo* studies using iPSCs-derived macrophages as exogenous interventions are summarized in **Table 2**.

Studies from our lab demonstrated that *in vitro* generated macrophages from mouse ESCs had the capacity for repair *in vivo* in a murine model of liver fibrosis [68]. Using a chemokine (C-C motif) ligands 4 (CCL4)-mediated liver injury model, the effect of injecting ESCs-derived macrophages or bone marrow derived macrophages (BMDMs) were assessed. ESCs-derived macrophages had a higher capacity to repopulate the Kupffer cell compartment of injured liver compared to BMDMs, supporting the theory that PSC-derived macrophages have a phenotype more akin to tissue resident macrophages. In addition, markers of liver damage were significantly lowered in mice that received ESCs-derived macrophages compared to controls indicating their reparative capacity. Another study assessed the effects of human iPSCs-derived macrophages polarized to an M1 or M2 phenotype on CCL4-induced fibrosis

Studies demonstrating iPSCs derived macrophages as therapeutic interventions		
Disease	**Research findings**	**References**
Liver Fibrosis	Mouse ESC-derived macrophages showed repair capacity in CCL4 murine model.	[68]
	M1 and M2 polarized human iPSCs-derived macrophages ameliorated fibrosis in an immunodeficient CCL4 murine model.	[69]
Pulmonary Alveolar Proteinosis (PAP)	Mouse iPSCs-derived macrophages gained an alveolar phenotype lung of PAP model and improved alveolar protein deposition.	[34]
	Human iPSCs–derived macrophages transplanted into the lung of humanized PAP mice showed *in situ* differentiation to an alveolar macrophage-like phenotype and disease remission.	[70]
	Human iPSCs-derived macrophages engrafted into the lung of the PAP mouse model differentiated into alveolar macrophages and eliminated disease associated surfactant proteins.	[5]
	Macrophages derived from gene corrected PAP patient-derived iPSCs showed restoration of normal phenotype.	[71]
Inflammatory Bowel Diseases (IBDs)	Very early onset of IBDs in patients leads to decreased bacterial killing ability in macrophages, which was reverted by the pharmacological inhibition of PGE2 synthesis and PGE2 receptor blockade.	[72]
	Genetic correction of patient iPSCs-derived macrophages *in vitro* led to reinitiating of the anti-inflammatory response and reduction of IBD associated traits.	[73]
Solid Tumors	Engineered iPSCs-derived CAR-macrophages with antigen-dependent anti-cancer functions demonstrated pro-inflammatory/ anti-tumor state, enhanced clearance of tumor cells by phagocytosis.	[74]
	Designer iPSCs-derived macrophage cell line to secrete IFN-β (opinion)	[75]

Table 2.
Summary of studies that have used iPSCs-derived macrophages as a source of therapeutic cells and/or to study mechanism of disease.

of immunodeficient recombination activating gene knock-out ($Rag2^{-/-}\ \gamma c^{-/-}$) mice [69]. These human iPSCs-M1 (in presence of IFN-γ and LPS) and M2 (in presence of IL-4 and IL-13) macrophage subtypes demonstrate distinct pro-inflammatory and anti-inflammatory phenotypes at both gene and protein level, which was confirmed by their RNA-seq analysis. Interestingly administration of both M1 and M2-polarized macrophages led to reduced liver fibrosis and inflammation. iPSCs-M2 as expected demonstrated a stronger downregulation of clinically relevant fibrotic markers. However, the profound antifibrogenic potential and resolution in the presence of iPSCs-M1 was unexpected based on currently thinking on the reparative phenotype of macrophages. The scenario of iPSCs-M1 showing a resolving phenotype could be corroborated by a previous study reporting the therapeutic potential of M1 polarized BM-derived macrophages to ameliorate fibrosis by the recruitment of endogenous macrophages as well as promote apoptosis through mediators of inflammation including MMPs, transforming growth factors (TGFs) and TNF related apoptosis inducing ligand (TRAIL) [73]. This could be the situation as the iPSCs-M1 macrophages in this study were shown to secrete MMP9 and TGF-β [69]. However more detailed study is required to understand the mechanisms underlying this resolving capacity of iPSCs-M1 macrophages. Nevertheless, the study clearly confirms the potential of iPSCs-derived M2 macrophages as a therapeutic option against liver fibrosis.

The therapeutic potential of iPSCs-derived macrophages has also been assessed in lung fibrosis particularly in the case of pulmonary alveolar proteinosis (PAP). Hereditary PAP is a disorder known to be originated by a defect in the *CSF2RA* gene coding for the granulocyte-macrophage colony-stimulating factor (GM-CSF) receptor alpha-chain (CD116). Happle et al demonstrated for the first time that transplantation of human iPSCs–derived macrophages into the lung of a humanized PAP mice model led to their pulmonary engraftment and their differentiation to an alveolar macrophage like phenotype in situ [70]. They also showed that this engraftment resulted in a reduction of alveolar proteinosis as measured by diminished protein content and surfactant protein D levels, decreased turbidity of the BAL fluid, and reduced surfactant deposition in the lungs of transplanted humanized PAP model mice. Similar results were observed using the aid of wild type murine iPSCs-derived macrophage *in vivo* transplantation to a CD116 (CSF2RA) deficient PAP mice model resulted in the former's integration into the diseased lung, gaining an alveolar macrophage phenotype and improving alveolar protein deposition [34]. Kuhn et al gene-corrected patient-derived PAP-specific iPSCs carrying a defective *CSF2RA* gene using targeted insertion of a codon-optimized CSF2RA-cDNA into the *AAVS1* locus [71]. This strategy resulted in robust expression of the *CSF2RA* gene in both undifferentiated iPSCs as well as in differentiated macrophages. The authors further demonstrated that these genetically-modified macrophages showed that the exogenous CSF2RA protein was functional by STAT5 phosphorylation and GM-CSF uptake studies, supporting the idea that these functionally restored iPSCs-derived macrophages could serve as a source for an autologous cell-based gene therapy for the treatment of PAP.

Inflammatory bowel disease (IBD) is another group of inflammatory syndromes where the potential role of iPSCs-derived macrophage mediated therapy has been evaluated. Studies have demonstrated that these macrophages can be used in disease modeling and to reduce the disease pathology *in vitro*. A recent study showed that macrophages derived from an infantile-onset IBD patient iPSCs were unable to phosphorylate signal transducer and activator of transcription 3 (STAT3), and failed to reduce LPS induced inflammatory cytokines even in the presence of exogenous IL-10 [72]. These macrophages exhibited a functional defect in their ability to kill *S. Typhimurium*, but were rescued by the introduction of a functional *IL10RB* gene. The study also showed that macrophages derived from patient iPSCs produced higher amounts of eicosanoid prostaglandin E2 (PGE2) after LPS stimulation and that pharmacological inhibition of PGE2 synthesis and PGE2 receptor blockade enhanced their bacterial killing ability. This study identified a regulatory interaction between IL-10 and PGE2 and that their dysregulation contributed to IBD pathogenesis. Gene correction in an independently-derived iPSC line from another IL10RB^{-}deficient IBD patient led to reconstitution of the anti-inflammatory response - reinitiating the IL-10RB expression, IL-10-inducible phosphorylation of STAT3, and subsequent SOCS3 expression [76]. This second study also showed that LPS-mediated TNF-α secretion could be modulated by IL-10 stimulation in gene-edited iPSCs-derived macrophages. Taken together, these established iPSC-derived macrophages based IBD models provide the opportunity to identify and validate new curative molecular and cellular therapies against IBD and other inflammatory syndromes.

The iPSCs-derived macrophage strategy has also been applied to the exciting field of cancer immunotherapy. Chimera antigen receptor (CAR)-T cells and NK cells re shown to have potent cytotoxicity against tumor cells with CAR-T cell therapy having gained great success in the clinic [77]. Recently CAR-macrophages have been developed by engineering an adenoviral vector to express a CAR targeted against human epidermal growth factor receptor 2, (a biomarker in many solid tumors) and imparted a sustained pro-inflammatory (M1) phenotype [78]. The model showed great success by demonstrating antigen-specific phagocytosis and tumor clearance *in vitro* as well as decreasing tumor burden and prolonged overall survival in two solid tumor xenograft models [78]. These successful pre-clinical data have led to an Phase-1 clinical trial using HER2 re-targeted CAR-macrophages for the treatment of solid tumors [77]. Other examples of iPSC-derived CAR-macrophages with antigen-dependent anti-cancer functions include those expressing either CD19 and mesothelin-specific fusion receptors [74]. CAR-macrophages demonstrated functions including expression and secretion of cytokines, polarization toward the pro-inflammatory/anti-tumor state, enhanced phagocytosis of tumor cells, and in anti-cancer cell activity *in vivo* when stimulated by tumor antigens. These data demonstrate the technology platform of iPSC-derived CAR-macrophage to eliminate cancer cells. These CAR engineered iPSCs-derived macrophages is a ground breaking technology in cancer immunotherapy and when combined with novel methods of bioreactor based bulk macrophage differentiation from iPSCs will provide an unlimited source of therapeutic cells [79].

3. Conclusion

In summary, the phenotypic, functional, and transcriptomic characteristics of iPSCs-derived macrophages share many similarities with both tissue resident macrophages and MDMs. The unlimited replication potential of iPSCs and the ease of genetic manipulation thus provides a valuable platform for disease modeling, drug screening, and studying the mechanisms of infection biology in various genetic backgrounds. Their autologous nature and polarization potential could also make them ideal tools for cell and regeneration therapy. iPSCs-derived macrophages have enormous potential in advancing our understanding of diseases that involve human macrophages and to date have demonstrated proof of principle utility in the development of disease models and in novel cell therapies. The use of iPSCs-derived macrophages does not eliminate the need for other models such as MDMs or BM-derived macrophages, but rather provides a complementary or alternative approach to further ensure validity and reproducibility. Together with genetic manipulations techniques such as CRISPR/Cas9 they can facilitate clinical and therapeutic translation for diseases such as liver fibrosis or inflammatory lung diseases where macrophages play an important clinical modulatory role. This is well highlighted by a research article under peer-review where M2 polarized iPSCs-derived macrophages are studied in context with COVID19 therapy [80]. The clinical potential of the macrophage cell therapy is highlighted by several clinical trials approved for autologous macrophages as intervention in various diseases including chronic liver injury, spinal cord injury, non-acute stroke, chronic anal fissure and as an anti-fibrotic treatment following COVID-19 infection [clinicaltrials.gov]. The future of iPSCs-derived macrophage therapy could be focused toward increasing their universality or increasing their better storage and differentiation as demonstrated by the studies of developing iPSCs-derived myeloid lines, continuous differentiation or cryopreservation [53, 81, 82]. An overview of the iPSCs-derived macrophages features and applications covered in this review is summarized as **Figure 1**.

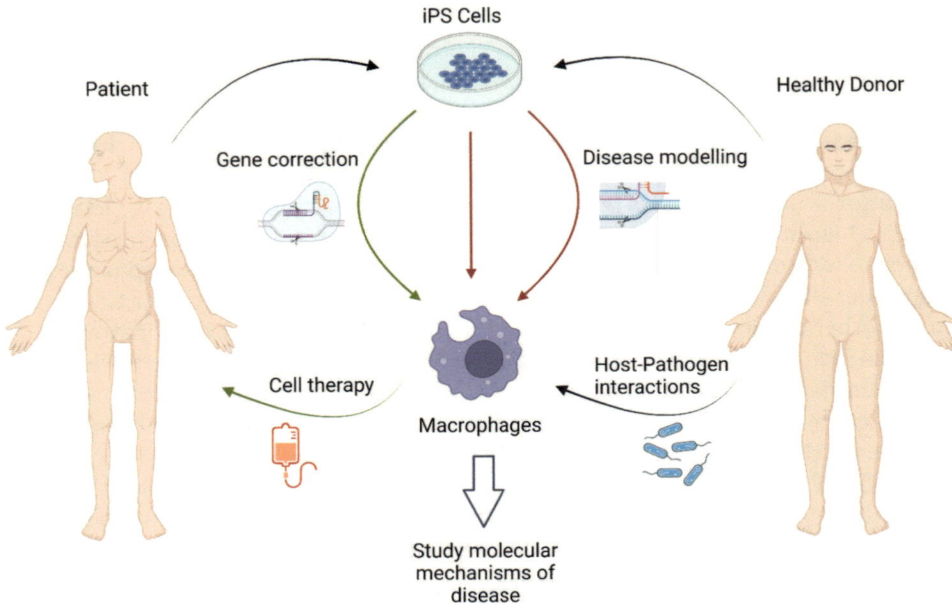

Figure 1.
Summary of iPSCs-derived macrophages attributes and applications.

Acknowledgements

This work was funded by the UK Medical Research Council (MR/T013923/1) and **Figure 1** was created using BioRender.com

Conflict of interest

The authors declare no conflict of interest.

Author details

Shyam Sushama Jose and Lesley M. Forrester*
Centre for Regenerative Medicine, Institute for Regeneration and Repair, University of Edinburgh, Edinburgh, Scotland

*Address all correspondence to: l.forrester@ed.ac.uk

References

[1] Murray PJ. Macrophage polarization. Annual Review of Physiology. 2017;**79**(1):541-566. DOI: 10.1146/annurev-physiol-022516-034339

[2] Wynn TA, Vannella KM. Macrophages in tissue repair, regeneration, and fibrosis. Immunity. 2016;**44**(3):450-462

[3] Gordon S, Taylor PR. Monocyte and macrophage heterogeneity. Nature reviews. Immunology. 2005;5(12):953-964. DOI: 10.1038/nri1733

[4] Frederic G, Steffen J, Miriam M, Klaus L. Development of monocytes, macrophages, and dendritic cells. Science. 2010;**327**(5966):656-661. DOI: 10.1126/science.1178331

[5] Takata K, Kozaki T, Lee CZW, Thion MS, Otsuka M, Lim S, et al. Induced-pluripotent-stem-cell-derived primitive macrophages provide a platform for modeling tissue-resident macrophage differentiation and function. Immunity. 2017;**47**(1):183-198.e6

[6] Rajab N, Rutar M, Laslett AL, Wells CA. Designer macrophages: Pitfalls and opportunities for modelling macrophage phenotypes from pluripotent stem cells. Differentiation. 2018;**104**:42-49

[7] Lewandowski J, Kurpisz M. Techniques of human embryonic stem cell and induced pluripotent stem cell derivation. Archivum Immunologiae et Therapiae Experimentalis (Warsz). 2016;**64**(5):349-370. DOI: 10.1007/s00005-016-0385-y

[8] Nenasheva T, Gerasimova T, Serdyuk Y, Grigoreva E, Kosmiadi G, Nikolaev A, et al. Macrophages derived from human induced pluripotent stem cells are low-activated "naïve-like" cells capable of restricting mycobacteria growth. Frontiers in Immunology. 2020;**11**:1016

[9] Takahashi K, Yamanaka S. Induction of pluripotent stem cells from mouse embryonic and adult fibroblast cultures by defined factors. Cell. 2006;**126**(4):663-676

[10] Chin MH, Pellegrini M, Plath K, Lowry WE. Molecular analyses of human induced pluripotent stem cells and embryonic stem cells. Cell Stem Cell. 2010;**7**(2):263-269

[11] Uhm K-O, Jo EH, Go GY, Kim S-J, Choi HY, Im YS, et al. Generation of human induced pluripotent stem cells from urinary cells of a healthy donor using a non-integration system. Stem Cell Research. 2017;**21**:44-46

[12] Isogai S, Yamamoto N, Hiramatsu N, Goto Y, Hayashi M, Kondo M, et al. Preparation of induced pluripotent stem cells using human peripheral blood monocytes. Cellular Reprogramming. 2018;**20**(6):347-355. DOI: 10.1089/cell.2018.0024

[13] Ackermann M, Liebhaber S, Klusmann J-H, Lachmann N. Lost in translation: Pluripotent stem cell-derived hematopoiesis. EMBO Molecular Medicine. 2015;**7**(11):1388-1402

[14] Guo N-N, Liu L-P, Zheng Y-W, Li Y-M. Inducing human induced pluripotent stem cell differentiation through embryoid bodies: A practical and stable approach. World Journal of Stem Cells. 2020;**12**(1):25-34

[15] Phetfong J, Supokawej A, Wattanapanitch M, Kheolamai P,

U-pratya Y, Issaragrisil S. Cell type of origin influences iPSC generation and differentiation to cells of the hematoendothelial lineage. Cell and Tissue Research. 2016;**365**(1):101-112. DOI: 10.1007/s00441-016-2369-y

[16] Doetschman TC, Eistetter H, Katz M, Schmidt W, Kemler R. The in vitro development of blastocyst-derived embryonic stem cell lines: Formation of visceral yolk sac, blood islands and myocardium. Development. 1985;**87**(1):27-45. DOI: 10.1242/dev.87.1.27

[17] Wiles MV, Keller G. Multiple hematopoietic lineages develop from embryonic stem (ES) cells in culture. Development. 1991;**111**(2):259-267. DOI: 10.1242/dev.111.2.259

[18] Schmitt RM, Bruyns E, Snodgrass HR. Hematopoietic development of embryonic stem cells in vitro: Cytokine and receptor gene expression. Genes & Development. 1991;**5**(5):728-740

[19] Johansson BM, Wiles MV. Evidence for involvement of activin A and bone morphogenetic protein 4 in mammalian mesoderm and hematopoietic development. Molecular and Cellular Biology. 1995;**15**(1):141-151. DOI: 10.1128/MCB.15.1.141

[20] Toru N, Hiroaki K, Tasuku H. Generation of lymphohematopoietic cells from embryonic stem cells in culture. Science. 1994;**265**(5175):1098-1101. DOI: 10.1126/science.8066449

[21] Choi K, Yu J, Smuga-otto K, Salvagiotto G, Rehrauer W, Vodyanik M, et al. Hematopoietic and endothelial differentiation of human induced pluripotent stem cells. Stem Cells. 2009;**27**(3):559-567

[22] Kennedy M, Firpo M, Choi K, Wall C, Robertson S, Kabrun N, et al. A common precursor for primitive erythropoiesis and definitive haematopoiesis. Nature. 1997;**386**(6624):488-493. DOI: 10.1038/386488a0

[23] Sturgeon CM, Ditadi A, Awong G, Kennedy M, Keller G. Wnt signaling controls the specification of definitive and primitive hematopoiesis from human pluripotent stem cells. Nature Biotechnology. 2014;**32**(6):554-561. DOI: 10.1038/nbt.2915

[24] Ng ES, Azzola L, Bruveris FF, Calvanese V, Phipson B, Vlahos K, et al. Differentiation of human embryonic stem cells to HOXA+ hemogenic vasculature that resembles the aorta-gonad-mesonephros. Nature Biotechnology. 2016;**34**(11):1168-1179. DOI: 10.1038/nbt.3702

[25] Wiles MVBT-M, in E. Embryonic stem cell differentiation in vitro. In: Guide to Techniques in Mouse Development. London, United Kingdom: Academic Press; 1993. pp. 900-918

[26] Choi K-D, Vodyanik M, Slukvin II. Hematopoietic differentiation and production of mature myeloid cells from human pluripotent stem cells. Nature Protocols. 2011;**6**(3):296-313. DOI: 10.1038/nprot.2010.184

[27] Senju S, Haruta M, Matsumura K, Matsunaga Y, Fukushima S, Ikeda T, et al. Generation of dendritic cells and macrophages from human induced pluripotent stem cells aiming at cell therapy. Gene Therapy. 2011;**18**(9):874-883. DOI: 10.1038/gt.2011.22

[28] Lopez-Yrigoyen M, May A, Ventura T, Taylor H, Fidanza A, Cassetta L, et al. Production and characterization of human macrophages from pluripotent stem cells. JoVE. 2020;**158**:e61038

[29] Lopez-Yrigoyen M, Yang C-T, Fidanza A, Cassetta L, Taylor AH, McCahill A, et al. Genetic programming of macrophages generates an in vitro model for the human erythroid Island niche. Nature Communications. 2019;**10**(1):881. DOI: 10.1038/s41467-019-08705-0

[30] Lopez-Yrigoyen M, Fidanza A, Cassetta L, Axton RA, Taylor AH, Meseguer-Ripolles J, et al. A human iPSC line capable of differentiating into functional macrophages expressing ZsGreen: a tool for the study and in vivo tracking of therapeutic cells. Philosophical Transactions of the Royal Society B Biological Sciences. 2018;**373**(1750):20170219. DOI: 10.1098/rstb.2017.0219 [Online]

[31] Yeung ATY, Hale C, Lee AH, Gill EE, Bushell W, Parry-Smith D, et al. Exploiting induced pluripotent stem cell-derived macrophages to unravel host factors influencing Chlamydia trachomatis pathogenesis. Nature Communications. 2017;**8**(1):15013. DOI: 10.1038/ncomms15013

[32] Zhang H, Xue C, Shah R, Bermingham K, Hinkle CC, Li W, et al. Functional analysis and transcriptomic profiling of iPSC-derived macrophages and their application in modeling mendelian disease. Circulation Research. 2015;**117**(1):17-28. DOI: 10.1161/CIRCRESAHA.117.305860

[33] Hale C, Yeung A, Goulding D, Pickard D, Alasoo K, Powrie F, et al. Induced pluripotent stem cell derived macrophages as a cellular system to study salmonella and other pathogens. PLoS One. 2015;**10**(5):e0124307. DOI: 10.1371/journal.pone.0124307

[34] Mucci A, Lopez-Rodriguez E, Hetzel M, Liu S, Suzuki T, Happle C, et al. iPSC-derived macrophages effectively treat pulmonary alveolar proteinosis in Csf2rb-deficient mice. Stem Cell Reports. 2018;**11**(3):696-710

[35] Matsuo K, Lepinski A, Chavez RD, Barruet E, Pereira A, Moody TA, et al. ACVR1R206H extends inflammatory responses in human induced pluripotent stem cell-derived macrophages. Bone. 2021;**153**:116129

[36] Lim WF, Inoue-Yokoo T, Tan KS, Lai MI, Sugiyama D. Hematopoietic cell differentiation from embryonic and induced pluripotent stem cells. Stem Cell Research & Therapy. 2013;**4**(3):71. DOI: 10.1186/scrt222

[37] Vanhee S, De Mulder K, Van Caeneghem Y, Verstichel G, Van Roy N, Menten B, et al. In vitro human embryonic stem cell hematopoiesis mimics MYB-independent yolk sac hematopoiesis. Haematologica. 2015;**100**(2 SE-Articles):157-166

[38] Buchrieser J, James W, Moore MD. Human induced pluripotent stem cell-derived macrophages share ontogeny with MYB-independent tissue-resident macrophages. Stem Cell Reports. 2017;**8**(2):334-345

[39] Zhang H, Reilly MP. Human induced pluripotent stem cell–derived macrophages for unraveling human macrophage biology. Arteriosclerosis, Thrombosis, and Vascular Biology. 2017;**37**(11):2000-2006. DOI: 10.1161/ATVBAHA.117.309195

[40] Bassett AR. Editing the genome of hiPSC with CRISPR/Cas9: Disease models. Mammalian Genome. 2017;**28**(7):348-364. DOI: 10.1007/s00335-017-9684-9

[41] Takada S, Kambe N, Kawasaki Y, Niwa A, Honda-Ozaki F, Kobayashi K, et al. Pluripotent stem cell models of Blau

syndrome reveal an IFN-γ–dependent inflammatory response in macrophages. The Journal of Allergy and Clinical Immunology. 2018;**141**(1):339-349.e11

[42] Panicker LM, Miller D, Park TS, Patel B, Azevedo JL, Awad O, et al. Induced pluripotent stem cell model recapitulates pathologic hallmarks of Gaucher disease. Proceedings of the National Academy of Sciences. 2012;**109**(44):18054 LP-18018059

[43] Gupta RM, Meissner TB, Cowan CA, Musunuru K. Genome-edited human pluripotent stem cell–derived macrophages as a model of reverse cholesterol transport—brief report. Arteriosclerosis, Thrombosis, and Vascular Biology. 2016;**36**(1):15-18. DOI: 10.1161/ATVBAHA.115.305956

[44] Jose SS, Tidu F, Burilova P, Kepak T, Bendickova K, Fric J. The telomerase complex directly controls hematopoietic stem cell differentiation and senescence in an induced pluripotent stem cell model of telomeropathy. Frontiers in Genetics. 2018;**9**:345

[45] Zhang H, Rodriguez S, Wang L, Wang S, Serezani H, Kapur R, et al. Sepsis induces hematopoietic stem cell exhaustion and myelosuppression through distinct contributions of TRIF and MYD88. Stem Cell Reports. 2016;**6**:1-17. DOI: 10.1016/j.stemcr.2016.05.002

[46] Elma A, Emerson M, Grisel L, Nima M, Ehud G, et al. Macrophage models of gaucher disease for evaluating disease pathogenesis and candidate drugs. Science Translational Medicine. 2014;**6**(240):240ra73-240ra73. DOI: 10.1126/scitranslmed.3008659

[47] Jiang Y, Cowley SA, Siler U, Melguizo D, Tilgner K, Browne C, et al. Derivation and functional analysis of patient-specific induced pluripotent stem cells as an in vitro model of chronic granulomatous disease. Stem Cells. 2012;**30**(4):599-611. DOI: 10.1002/stem.1053

[48] Joshi K, Elso C, Motazedian A, Labonne T, Schiesser JV, Cameron F, et al. Induced pluripotent stem cell macrophages present antigen to proinsulin-specific T cell receptors from donor-matched islet-infiltrating T cells in type 1 diabetes. Diabetologia. 2019;**62**(12):2245-2251. DOI: 10.1007/s00125-019-04988-6

[49] Shiba T, Tanaka T, Ida H, Watanabe M, Nakaseko H, Osawa M, et al. Functional evaluation of the pathological significance of MEFV variants using induced pluripotent stem cell–derived macrophages. The Journal of Allergy and Clinical Immunology. 2019;**144**(5):1438-1441.e12

[50] Haake K, Neehus A-L, Buchegger T, Kühnel MP, Blank P, Philipp F, et al. Patient iPSC-derived macrophages to study inborn errors of the IFN-γ responsive pathway. Cell. 2020;**9**:483

[51] Badanjak K, Mulica P, Smajic S, Delcambre S, Tranchevent L-C, Diederich N, et al. iPSC-derived microglia as a model to study inflammation in idiopathic parkinson's disease. Frontiers in Cell and Developmental Biology. 2021;**9**:740758

[52] Tanaka T, Takahashi K, Yamane M, Tomida S, Nakamura S, Oshima K, et al. Induced pluripotent stem cells from CINCA syndrome patients as a model for dissecting somatic mosaicism and drug discovery. Blood. 2012;**120**(6):1299-1308. DOI: 10.1182/blood-2012-03-417881

[53] Seki R, Ohta A, Niwa A, Sugimine Y, Naito H, Nakahata T, et al. Induced pluripotent stem cell-derived monocytic

cell lines from a NOMID patient serve as a screening platform for modulating NLRP3 inflammasome activity. PLoS One. 2020;**15**(8):e0237030. DOI: 10.1371/journal.pone.0237030

[54] Chow SH, Deo P, Yeung ATY, Kostoulias XP, Jeon Y, Gao M-L, et al. Targeting NLRP3 and Staphylococcal pore-forming toxin receptors in human-induced pluripotent stem cell-derived macrophages. Journal of Leukocyte Biology. 2020;**108**(3):967-981. DOI: 10.1002/JLB.4MA0420-497R

[55] Hong D, Ding J, Li O, He Q, Ke M, Zhu M, et al. Human-induced pluripotent stem cell-derived macrophages and their immunological function in response to tuberculosis infection. Stem Cell Research & Therapy. 2018;**9**(1):49. DOI: 10.1186/s13287-018-0800-x

[56] Baquir B, An AY, Lee AHY, REW H. Human-induced pluripotent stem cell–derived macrophages for studying infection biology and immunology. In: Birbrair ABT-CP in iPSC-derived CT. In: Advances in Stem Cell Biology. London, United Kingdom: Academic Press; 2021. pp. 1-22

[57] Ye L, Wang J, Beyer AI, Teque F, Cradick TJ, Qi Z, et al. Seamless modification of wild-type induced pluripotent stem cells to the natural CCR5Δ32 mutation confers resistance to HIV infection. Proceedings of the National Academy of Sciences. 2014;**111**(26):9591 LP-9599596

[58] Kambal A, Mitchell G, Cary W, Gruenloh W, Jung Y, Kalomoiris S, et al. Generation of HIV-1 resistant and functional macrophages from hematopoietic stem cell–derived induced pluripotent stem cells. Molecular Therapy. 2011;**19**(3):584-593

[59] Kang H, Minder P, Park MA, Mesquitta W-T, Torbett BE, Slukvin II. CCR5 disruption in induced pluripotent stem cells using CRISPR/Cas9 provides selective resistance of immune cells to CCR5-tropic HIV-1 virus. Molecular Therapy Nucleic Acids. 2015;**4**:e268

[60] Lang J, Cheng Y, Rolfe A, Hammack C, Vera D, Kyle K, et al. An hPSC-derived tissue-resident macrophage model reveals differential responses of macrophages to ZIKV and DENV infection. Stem Cell Reports. 2018;**11**(2):348-362

[61] Goodridge HS. Induced pluripotent stem cell derived myeloid phagocytes: Disease modeling and therapeutic applications. Drug Discovery Today. 2014;**19**(6):774-780

[62] Oishi Y, Manabe I. Macrophages in inflammation, repair and regeneration. International Immunology. 2018;**30**(11):511-528. DOI: 10.1093/intimm/dxy054

[63] Thomas JA, Pope C, Wojtacha D, Robson AJ, Gordon-Walker TT, Hartland S, et al. Macrophage therapy for murine liver fibrosis recruits host effector cells improving fibrosis, regeneration, and function. Hepatology. 2011;**53**(6):2003-2015. DOI: 10.1002/hep.24315

[64] Yang J, Zhang X, Chen J, Heng BC, Jiang Y, Hu X, et al. Macrophages promote cartilage regeneration in a time-and phenotype-dependent manner. Journal of Cellular Physiology. 2022. DOI: 10.1002/jcp.30694 [Online ahead of print]

[65] Pechkovsky DV, Prasse A, Kollert F, Engel KMY, Dentler J, Luttmann W, et al. Alternatively activated alveolar macrophages in pulmonary fibrosis—mediator production and intracellular signal transduction. Clinical Immunology. 2010;**137**(1):89-101

[66] Brennan PN, MacMillan M, Manship T, Moroni F, Glover A, Graham C, et al. Study protocol: A multicentre, open-label, parallel-group, phase 2, randomised controlled trial of autologous macrophage therapy for liver cirrhosis (MATCH). BMJ Open. 2021;**11**(11):e053190

[67] Chernykh ER, Shevela EY, Starostina NM, Morozov SA, Davydova MN, Menyaeva EV, et al. Safety and therapeutic potential of M2 macrophages in stroke treatment. Cell Transplantation. 2016;**25**(8):1461-1471. DOI: 10.3727/096368915X690279

[68] Haideri SS, McKinnon AC, Taylor AH, Kirkwood P, Starkey Lewis PJ, O'Duibhir E, et al. Injection of embryonic stem cell derived macrophages ameliorates fibrosis in a murine model of liver injury. npj. Regenerative Medicine. 2017;**2**(1):14. DOI: 10.1038/s41536-017-0017-0

[69] Pouyanfard S, Meshgin N, Cruz LS, Diggle K, Hashemi H, Pham TV, et al. Human induced pluripotent stem cell-derived macrophages ameliorate liver fibrosis. Stem Cells. 2021;**39**(12):1701-1717. DOI: 10.1002/stem.3449

[70] Happle C, Lachmann N, Ackermann M, Mirenska A, Göhring G, Thomay K, et al. Pulmonary transplantation of human induced pluripotent stem cell–derived macrophages ameliorates pulmonary alveolar proteinosis. American Journal of Respiratory and Critical Care Medicine. 2018;**198**(3):350-360. DOI: 10.1164/rccm.201708-1562OC

[71] Kuhn A, Ackermann M, Mussolino C, Cathomen T, Lachmann N, Moritz T. TALEN-mediated functional correction of human iPSC-derived macrophages in context of hereditary pulmonary alveolar proteinosis. Scientific Reports. 2017;**7**(1):15195. DOI: 10.1038/s41598-017-14566-8

[72] Mukhopadhyay S, Heinz E, Porreca I, Alasoo K, Yeung A, Yang H-T, et al. Loss of IL-10 signaling in macrophages limits bacterial killing driven by prostaglandin E2. The Journal of Experimental Medicine. 2019;**217**(2):e20180649. DOI: 10.1084/jem.20180649

[73] Ma P-F, Gao C-C, Yi J, Zhao J-L, Liang S-Q, Zhao Y, et al. Cytotherapy with M1-polarized macrophages ameliorates liver fibrosis by modulating immune microenvironment in mice. Journal of Hepatology. 2017;**67**(4):770-779

[74] Zhang L, Tian L, Dai X, Yu H, Wang J, Lei A, et al. Pluripotent stem cell-derived CAR-macrophage cells with antigen-dependent anti-cancer cell functions. Journal of Hematology & Oncology. 2020;**13**(1):153. DOI: 10.1186/s13045-020-00983-2

[75] Senju S, Koba C, Haruta M, Matsunaga Y, Matsumura K, Haga E, et al. Application of iPS cell-derived macrophages to cancer therapy. Oncoimmunology. 2014;**3**(3):e27927. DOI: 10.4161/onci.27927

[76] Hoffmann D, Sens J, Brennig S, Brand D, Philipp F, Vollmer Barbosa P, et al. Genetic correction of IL-10RB deficiency reconstitutes anti-inflammatory regulation in iPSC-derived macrophages. Journal of Personalized Medicine. 2021;**11**:221

[77] Mazza R, Maher J. Prospects for development of induced pluripotent stem cell-derived CAR-targeted immunotherapies. Archivum Immunologiae et Therapiae Experimentalis (Warsz). 2021;**70**(1):2. DOI: 10.1007/s00005-021-00640-7

[78] Klichinsky M, Ruella M, Shestova O, Lu XM, Best A, Zeeman M, et al. Human chimeric antigen receptor macrophages for cancer immunotherapy. Nature Biotechnology. 2020;**38**(8):947-953. DOI: 10.1038/s41587-020-0462-y

[79] Ackermann M, Kempf H, Hetzel M, Hesse C, Hashtchin AR, Brinkert K, et al. Bioreactor-based mass production of human iPSC-derived macrophages enables immunotherapies against bacterial airway infections. Nature Communications. 2018;**9**(1):5088. DOI: 10.1038/s41467-018-07570-7

[80] Duan F, Guo L, Yang L, Han Y, Thakur A, Nilsson-Payant BE, et al. Modeling COVID-19 with human pluripotent stem cell-derived cells reveals synergistic effects of anti-inflammatory macrophages with ACE2 inhibition against SARS-CoV-2. Res Sq. 2020:rs.3.rs-rs62758 [Preprint repository article ahead of peer-review]

[81] Ackermann M, Rafiei Hashtchin A, Manstein F, Carvalho Oliveira M, Kempf H, Zweigerdt R, et al. Continuous human iPSC-macrophage mass production by suspension culture in stirred tank bioreactors. Nature Protocols. 2022;**17**(2):513-539. DOI: 10.1038/s41596-021-00654-7

[82] Munn C, Burton S, Dickerson S, Bakshy K, Strouse A, Rajesh D. Generation of cryopreserved macrophages from normal and genetically engineered human pluripotent stem cells for disease modelling. PLoS One. 2021;**16**(4):e0250107. DOI: 10.1371/journal.pone.0250107